AF443406

MEDICAL APPLICATIONS OF LASERS

MEDICAL APPLICATIONS OF LASERS

edited by

D. R. Vij
and
K. Mahesh
Department of Physics
Kurukshetra University
136119 Kurukshetra
India

KLUWER ACADEMIC PUBLISHERS
Boston / Dordrecht / London

Distributors for North, Central and South America:
Kluwer Academic Publishers
101 Philip Drive
Assinippi Park
Norwell, Massachusetts 02061 USA
Telephone (781) 871-6600
Fax (781) 871-6528
E-Mail <kluwer@wkap.com>

Distributors for all other countries:
Kluwer Academic Publishers Group
Distribution Centre
Post Office Box 322
3300 AH Dordrecht, THE NETHERLANDS
Telephone 31 78 6392 392
Fax 31 78 6546 474
E-Mail <services@wkap.nl>

Electronic Services <http://www.wkap.nl>

Library of Congress Cataloging-in-Publication Data

Medical applications of lasers / edited by D. R. Vij and K. Mahesh.
   p. ; cm.
  Includes bibliographical references and index
  ISBN 0-7923-7662-5 (alk. Paper)
   1.   Lasers in medicine. 2. Lasers in surgery. I Vij, D. R. II Mahesh, K., 1940-
  {DNLM: 1. Lasers—therapeutic use. 2. Laser Surgery. WB 480 M488 2002}
  R857.L37 M435 2002
610'.28—dc21

                         2001050835

Table of Contents

Preface

A careful review of the literature covering various aspects of applications of lasers in science and technology reveals that lasers are being applied very widely throughout the entire gamut of physical medicine. After surveying the current developments taking place in the field of medical applications of lasers, it was considered appropriate to bring together these efforts of international research scientists and experts into one volume.

It is with this aim that the editors have prepared this volume which brings current research and recent developments to the attention of a wide spectrum of readership associated with hospitals, medical institutions and universities world wide, including also the medical instrument industry. Both teachers and students in the medical faculties will especially find this compendium quite useful.

This book is comprised of eleven chapters. All of the important medical applications of lasers are featured. The editors have made every effort that individual chapters are self-contained and written by experts. Emphasis has been placed on straight and simple presentation of the subject matter so that even the new entrants into the field will find the book of value.

The first chapter deals with the elements of laser emission process. In the second chapter on laser-tissue interaction, the authors emphasize Monte Carlo simulation of laser-tissue. Models of laser-tissue propagation are discussed along with the thermal and mechanical damage to tissues. The remaining chapters deal with the use of lasers in the various fields in medicine, such as ophthalmology, cardiology, tomography, urology, lithrotripsy, dermatology, dentistry and gynecology. The last chapter on laser safety in medicine describes the various hazards associated with the use of lasers, and the required safety methods and procedures.

This book represents a valuable contribution by outstanding researchers in their individual fields. It has an international flavor inasmuch as the contributors are drawn from the U.S.A., U.K., Germany, Canada, Japan, India, Russia Israel and Kuwait.

It is our pleasant duty to express our gratitude to the various authors who made this book possible by contributing respective chapters in the fields of their expertise. We are indebted to all those authors and publishers who freely granted permissions to reproduce their copyrighted works. The patient encouragement of the staff at Kluwer Academic Publishers is also thankfully acknowledged. Last but not least, we wish to express our deep appreciation to our wives (Dr. (Mrs.) Meenakshi Vij and Dr. (Mrs.) Brijesh Kumari Gupta respectively) for their indispensable support, encouragement, and patience during the completion of the task of writing and editing the book.

D. R. Vij

Kurukshetra, India K. Mahesh

Contributing Authors

Ken Barat, Lawrence Berkeley National Laboratory, Berkeley, California, U.S.A., E-mail: klbarat@lbl.gov

Steven F. Barrett, Department of Electrical Engineering, University of Wyoming, Laramie, Wyoming, U.S.A., E-mail : steveb@uwyo.edu

Geoffrey Dougherty, Department of Radiologic Sciences, Kuwait University, Sulaibikhat 90805, KUWAIT, E-mailgeoff@hsc.kuniv.edu.kw

Shmuel Einav, Department of Biomedical Engineering , Tel Aviv University, Tel Aviv 69978 , ISRAEL, E-mail: einav@eng.tau.ac.il

A.K. Hemal, Department of Urology, All India Institute of Medical Sciences, Ansari Nagar, New Delhi - 110 029, INDIA , E-mail: akhemal@hotmail.com

K. Mahesh, Department of Physics, Kurukshetra University, Kurukshetra - 136 119 , INDIA

Ronald B. Moore, Division of Urology, Department of Surgery, University of Alberta, Edmonton, Alberta, CANADA, Fax : (780) 432-8333
E-mail: ronald.moore@cancerboard.ab.ca

Markolf H. Niemz, Mannheim Biomedical Engineering Laboratories,University of Heidelberg, Theodor-Kutzer-Ufer, 68135, Mannheim,GERMANY
E-mail : Mark.Niemz@URZ.UNI-HEIDELBERG.DE

Masayoshi Okada, Former Director, Kobe University School of Medicine, 1-1-39-103, Sumiyoshihonmachi, Higashinada-ku, Kobe 658-0051, JAPAN, Fax : +81-78-856-0123

Terence Ryan, Oxford Brookes University, Oxford, U.K.

S. K. Sharma, Director, Postgraduate Institute of Medical Education and Research, Chandigarh , INDIA, E-mail: medist@pgi.chd.nic.in

Alka Sinha, Department of Obstetrics and Gynaecology, All India Institute of Medical Sciences, New Delhi, INDIA

D. Takkar, Department of Obstetrics and Gynaecology, All India Institute of Medical Sciences, New Delhi, INDIA, E-mail: dtakkar@vsnl.com

Valery V. Tuchin, Department of Optics, Saratov State University, Astrakhanskaya, 83, Saratov, Russian Federation, E-mail: tuchin@sgu.ssu.runnet.ru

D. R. Vij, Department of Physics, Kurukshetra University, Kurukshetra-136119, INDIA, E-mail: drv@vidya.kuk.ernet.in

Ashley J. Welch, Department of Electrical Engineering, The University of Texas at Austin, Austin, U.S.A., E-mail: welch@mail.utexas.edu

Tim A. Wollin, Division of Urology, Department of Surgery, University of Alberta, Edmonton, Alberta, CANADA, E-mail : twollin@ualberta.ca

Cameron H. G. Wright, Department of Electrical Engineering. U.S. Air Force Academy , Colorado, U.S.A., E mail: cameron.wright@usafa.af.mil

Dmitry A. Zimnyakov, Department of Optics, Saratov State University, Russian Federation, E-mail : zimnyakov@sgu.ssu.runnet.ru

Chapter 1

ELEMENTS OF LASER EMISSION PROCESS

K. Mahesh and D. R. Vij,
Department of Physics, Kurukshetra University, INDIA

1.1   INTRODUCTION

Lasers are now associated with the global technological Society in much the same way as perhaps the nuclear energy, x-rays and radioisotopes are. Traditionally, the medical sciences have been the domain of physicians and surgeons although, during the past four decades, deep and wide inroads have been made by physicists and technologists associated with research and development in health sciences. A whole lot of medical instrumentation and procedures, of great value and significance in health sciences, have developed that have direct origin in physics.

The present book covers in details several areas in health sciences that are being explored and serviced by lasers. The authors of the present chapter, being main stream physicists, consider as useful and pertinent to describe and explain various physical features of lasers. The description, it is hoped, will enable both teachers and students of medical faculty to appreciate better the role that lasers are being made to play in the domain of physical medicine . Medical students will indeed see this chapter as an essential reading.

Study and knowledge of optical properties of lasers and optical characteristics of the target bio-tissue is indeed central to the medical applications of lasers. In fact, the dependence of absorption of the laser light by the target bio-tissue on its wavelength constitutes the elements of technology of laser surgery. Two major consequences following laser absorption by the biological tissue are tissue-ablation and tissue-fusion. Careful combination of laser wave-length and its delivery system (which defines the delivery parameters such as pulse energy, pulse width, and inter-pulse interval) eminently achieves a given clinical task with reasonable precision . It is, therefore, important to construct a simple understanding of several physical concepts and parameters associated with laser beams and laser devices.

1.2   COMPONENTS OF A LASER SOURCE

Laser light, like ordinary light, is an electromagnetic wave, i.e., it consists of time varying electric and magnetic fields whose vector-directions are perpendicular to each other. The direction of propagation of light is perpendicular to both these field-vectors (**E** and **B**) as illustrated in Figure 1. The plane in which electric field **E** oscillates, is called the plane of polarization.

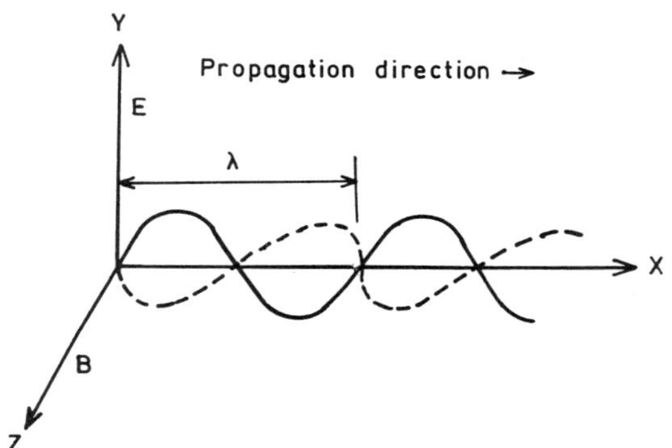

Figure 1. Oscillatory electric and magnetic fields in x-y and x-z planes respectively. x- denotes the wave propagation direction .

There is, however, a very important fundamental difference in the mechanism of light emission by the source of ordinary light and that of the laser light. While the emission from the ordinary light source is spontaneous and the light spreads isotropically (uniformally) in all directions in space; emission from the laser source is stimulated and the emitted light beam is highly directional with extremely low divergence in space (except for the semi-conductor laser). Figure 2 provides a schematic illustration of the two types of sources of light .

It is interesting to note that whereas **E** and **B** vectors both constitute an electromagnetic wave, the physical processes such as photochemical, photo-electronic and physiological effects are mainly caused by the electric field **E**.

Various laser devices have been invented which are capable of delivering laser beams ranging from ultraviolet (UV) to the far-infrared (IR) region including the visible range between 0.48 to 0.78 μm.

A typical laser source comprises of three primary components; (i) the active medium (or a lasing medium) which can be a solid, gas or a liquid medium; (ii) an excitation source , also known as the pump which causes higher population of atoms/molecules in the excited state as compared to the ground state (popularly known as *population inversion*); and (iii) the feedback mechanism of the emitted photons which is usually provided by and mirror reflection (see Figure 3).

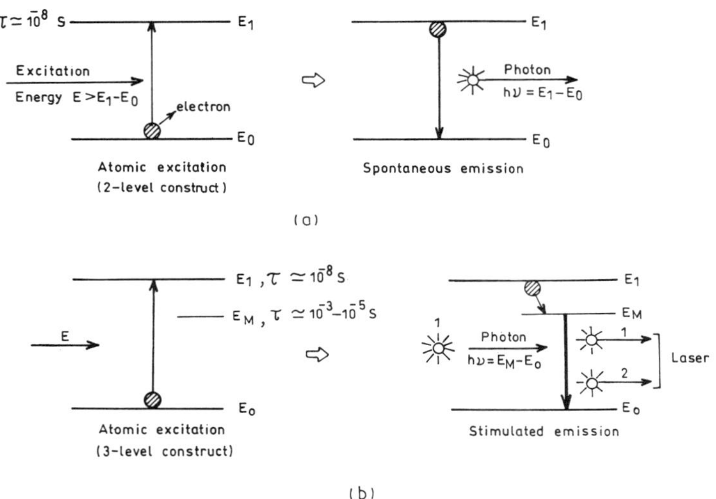

Figure 2. Spontaneous and stimulated emission processes of light. (a) Emission-process of ordinary light, τ is the electron life time in energy state E_1; (b) Stimulated emission process of light, (1) stimulating photon (one of the emitted photon will act as the stimulating photon which induces further emission), (2) induced photon; E_M – metastable state having considerably longer life time than the excited state. Presence of metastable state provides for the inversion of atomic population (number of atoms in the higher energy state being larger than in the ground state). The emitted photon takes the direction of the stimulating photon.

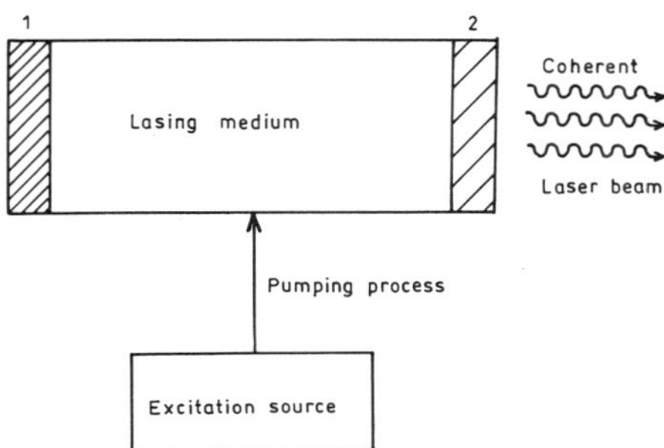

Figure 3. Primary components of a laser source. 1- total reflecting mirror, 2- partially reflecting mirror.

1.3   LASER AMPLIFICATION

Electromagnetic waves produced inside the lasing medium are all coherent having the same phase as they traverse in space (spatial coherence) and time (temporal coherence) and as such their amplitudes add up giving rise to a loss-less brightness of the laser beam. This brightness stays all along; spatially and temporally. If A is the amplitude for a wave then, say, for two coherent waves, the added amplitude is equal to $2A$. The resulting beam intensity is, therefore, proportional to $4A^2$. If N_1 and N_2 are the population of atoms/molecules (can be termed as lasing atoms/molecules) in the two lower and higher levels respectively (also, can be termed as the lasing levels) then $N_2 > N_1$ in the state of population inversion (see Figure 4) the amplification factor χ of the laser device can be expressed as:

$$\chi = \sigma (N_2 - N_1) \tag{1}$$

where σ is the probability of induced transition from higher to lower level. According to the Boltzmann distribution law, $N_1 = N \exp[-E_1/k_B T]$ and $N_2 = N \exp[-E_2/k_B T]$. Hence $(N_2/N_1) = \exp[-(E_2 - E_1)/k_B T]$, where $N_1 + N_2 + \ldots = N$.

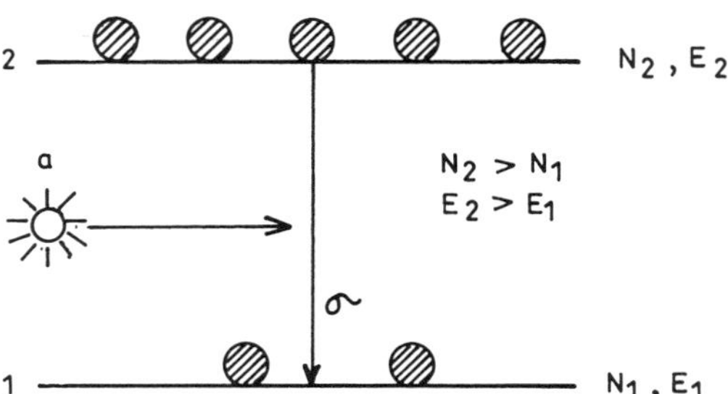

Figure 4. Lasing levels (1 and 2); a - photon inducing transition from 2 to 1 with transition probability σ.

1.4   BEAM DIVERGENCE

Anisotropy is inherent in the basic mechanism of laser process. The emitted photon takes the direction of some photon moving perpendicular to the reflecting mirror and inducing (i.e., stimulating) the emission. On account of coherence, a high degree of collimation (i.e., all waves travelling parallel to each other) is achieved. A laser beam, therefore, possesses a high degree of directionality.

If $\theta_{1/2}$ is the angle of divergence of the laser beam at a point where laser power density* is reduced to half of its value at the emerging point, then $\theta_{1/2}$ defines the directionality of the beam.

$$\theta_{1/2} = 1.22\lambda/D \tag{2}$$

where D is the diameter of the beam and λ is the laser wavelength (see Figure 5). For ruby laser, $\lambda = 0.69\ \mu m$ and taking $D = 1$ cm, $\theta = 8.5 \times 10^{-5}$ radians.

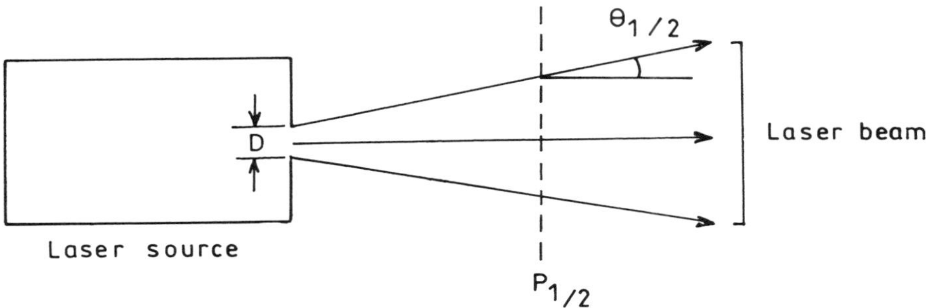

Figure 5.   Diagram depicting beam divergence. $P_{1/2}$ is a plane where laser power density is reduced to half.

1.5   MONOCHROMATICITY

Laser spectral lines (laser intensity versus wavelength profile is a laser spectral line) are very narrow because the laser light exhibits a high degree of monochromaticity as compared to the ordinary light. In simple terms, the color of a given laser light is highly pure to the exclusion of any other color in the light. The degree of monochromaticity μ is defined as:

$$\mu = \lambda_o/\Delta\lambda = \Delta v/v_o \tag{3}$$

where $\Delta\lambda$ (or Δv) is the line width as shown in Figure 6. Since $\Delta\lambda$ for a laser line is very small, the value of μ for the laser light is very large.

---

*The power output of a laser source as also the power delivered by a laser beam at the target location is measured in terms of watt and its multiples (such as kW and MW) or its fraction (such as mW). It is the average number of photons $(\tilde{N})$ in the beam multiplied by the energy of a photon $(h\nu)$ flowing across a plane per second. Thus, the power of the beam $P = \tilde{N}\,h\nu/second$ (electron volt per second). Flow of electronic charge (Coloumb) per second constitutes current (ampere). Hence the product of current and volt gives watt. Power density = Power/cm^2.

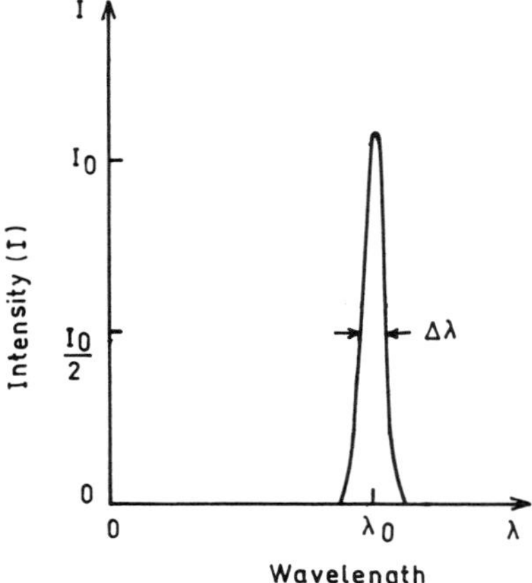

Figure 6. Shape of the spectral line.

1.6   OPTICAL COHERENCE LENGTH AND TIME

In equilibrium at temperature T, atoms/molecules of the active medium are distributed among various energy levels E_1, E_2, etc. as given in Figure 4. This distribution is known as the Maxwell-Boltzmann distribution. By the application of external energy, such as in electric bulbs or a fluorescent tube, the atoms from a given equilibrium state are excited to a number of higher but non-equilibrium energy states and the de-excitation that follows in an attempt to reach equilibrium again, give rise to the emission of photons of different energies. De-excitation from these different energy levels are not co-related to each other. This is spontaneous emission and the radiation consisting of these photons may be termed as disordered. The emitted light, therefore, consists of groups of photons each corresponding to a certain number of excited atoms in a given energy state. Each such group represents a *wave train*. The number of photons in the train is referred to as the length of the wave train. Thus, a greater number of photons in a state is represented by a longer wave train. The duration τ (life time of the atomic state) of the wave train is called the *coherent time* and the length of the wave train $c\tau$ (c, the velocity of light) is known as the *coherent length*.

From the uncertainty principle; $\Delta E \Delta t \approx h$; *or* $h\Delta v\Delta t \approx h$; $\Delta v\tau \approx 1$. Hence, the monochromaticity is:

$$\mu = \Delta v/v_o = 1/\tau v_o \tag{4}$$

τ is typically of the order of 10^{-8} to 10^{-10} sec.

From equation 4 it is seen that longer the coherence time, the higher will be the coherence of the beam. In the specific example of laser emission, some particular energy states of photon-distribution are much more populated (i.e., much more probable) than the rest which may be nearly empty.

The interference fringe pattern obtained with ordinary light source is characterized by a small degree of coherence (referred to as the incoherent optics). For photons of the same wave train to meet at a point D on the screen and giving rise to the interference fringes, the condition of path difference L, i.e., $L = (BC + CD - BD) < c\tau$, should be satisfied (see Figure 7.)

For ordinary light source, the coherence length does not exceed few centimeters. Still, it is possible to observe interference pattern in many experimental arrangements, say, Fresnel biprism, Michelson interferometer, Newton's rings, thin films, etc., using ordinary light source because the path difference L, in this case is very small; of the order of a millimeter.

In case of a laser source, the coherence time may be as large as 10^{-3} sec. It implies that the coherence length may be as large as 10^{5} meters.

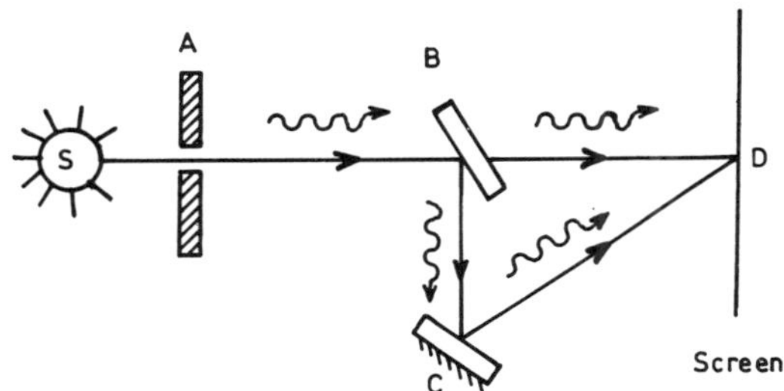

Figure 7.   Experimental arrangement to observe interference between parts of the same wave train. S- light source; B- Partially silvered mirror; C- fully silvered mirror; D- Point of observation of the fringe pattern on the screen.

1.7   INTERACTION OF RADIATION WITH ATOMIC SYSTEM

When an electromagnetic wave is incident on an atomic medium, the following probabilities exist:

(i)   Incident bean of intensity I_o is attenuated to I if the medium (atomic system) is not activated, i.e., the ground state atomic population N is larger than the excited state population N_2. The beam attenuation is given by the equation:

$$I = I_o e^{-\alpha l}$$

where α is the attenuation coefficient (probability of beam attenuation per unit path length traversed in the medium) and l is the total path traversed by the incident beam (thickness of the medium).

(ii)   Incident beam is amplified in accordance with equation 1 if the medium is activated ($N_2 > N_1$).

In 1918, Einstein studied the equilibrium between the incident radiation and the medium. It was proposed that while the spontaneous atomic transition from higher to lower energy state depended only on the internal properties of the atoms; the reverse transition (i.e., from lower to higher energy state) will depend upon the nature of the atoms as well as upon the intensity of the incident radiation. Thus, the two events, on account of mismatch, do not provide for the equilibrium.

To satisfy the requirement of equilibrium at a given intensity of incident radiation it, therefore, calls for the need to have emission transition with a probability that will depend upon the intensity of the incident radiation. These emission transitions are those that are stimulated by the incident radiation. It is for this reason that the emitted light, through this transition process, is called stimulated or induced emission.

Portion of internally emitted photons within the active medium bounded by two perfectly parallel and reflecting dielectric mirrors (this system being called as the cavity) and along the mirror axis indeed serve as the incident stimulating light and survives for sufficiently long time (others are absorbed within the cavity) to bring about stimulated emission and amplification. The photons travelling to and fro between the two mirrors form standing waves and, therefore, constitute the surviving modes whose wavelengths are given by the condition: $L = n\lambda/2$ where L is the distance between the two mirrors and $n = 1,2,3....$ is an integer. The emission process is illustrated in Figure 8.

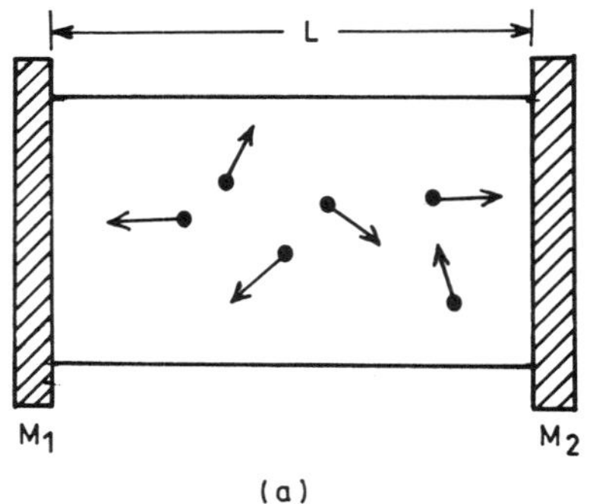

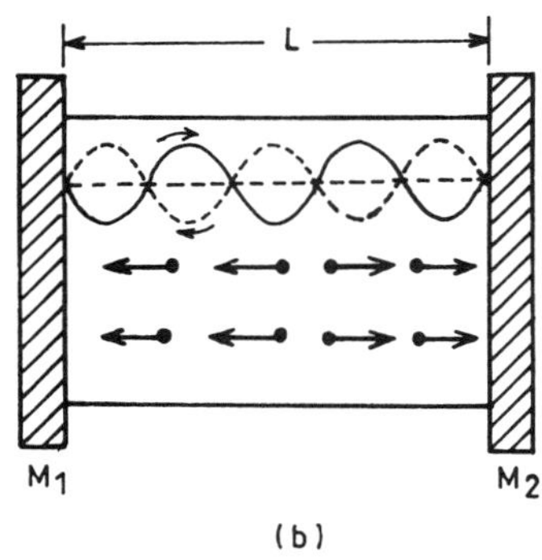

Figure 8.   (a) Spontaneous (random) emission of photons. M_1 and M_2 are mirrors; (b) only axial modes survive in the cavity. The mode wavelength is given by $\lambda = 2L/n$. Number of half-waves or loops $= n = 5$ as shown here.

1.8   EINSTEIN TRANSITION COEFFICIENTS

Einstein had recognized that as electromagnetic radiation field incident on a substance will not only cause excitation of atoms from lower to higher energy state but also induce or stimulate atoms already in the higher energy state to undergo transition to the lower energy state. These transitions were quantified by him in terms of what are known as the transition coefficients. Consider a cavity at temperature $T^{\circ}K$. If $U(\omega,T)$ represents energy density* of the radiation field of frequency ω at temperature $T^{\circ}K$ of the cavity of the substance, the total energy density considering the entire radiation spectrum can be expressed as:

$$U(T) = \int_{0}^{\infty} u(\omega,T)d\omega \tag{6}$$

where $d\omega$ represents an element of frequency width.*

Referring to Figure 9, let P_{21} = probability per unit time of a stimulated transition of an atom from state of energy E_2 to the state of lower energy E_1, and P_{12} = reverse probability; the probability of stimulated transition is evidently proportional to the energy density $u(\omega)$ of radiation field inducing the transition. Thus,

$$P_{21} = B_{21}\, u(\omega) \tag{7}$$

Similarly

$$P_{12} = B_{12}\, u(\omega) \tag{8}$$

B_{21} and B_{12} are known as the Einstein's stimulation transition coefficients. According to Einstein's postulates

$$B_{21} = B_{12} \tag{9}$$

Now while the transition $1 \rightarrow 2$ will occur only under the action of incident radiation because $E_2 > E_1$, the transition $2 \rightarrow 1$ will occur both ways, under stimulation as well as spontaneously. The number of atoms undergoing transition per unit time among the states 1 and 2 is expressed as in equations

---

* Radiation energy per unit volume of cavity per unit frequency interval. If $dn(\omega)$ is the number of photons in the frequency range ω and $\omega+d\omega$ and V is the volume of the cavity; then since each photon has an energy equal to $\hbar\omega$, $u(\omega)=[1/V][dn(\omega)/d\omega][\hbar\omega]$

10 and 11 below.

$$n_{12} = n_{12} \text{ (stimulated)} \tag{10}$$

$$n_{21} = n_{21} \text{ (stimulated)} + n_{21} \text{ (spontaneous)} \tag{11}$$

The frequency of the emitted photon is given by

$$\omega = (E_2 - E_1)/\hbar \tag{12}$$

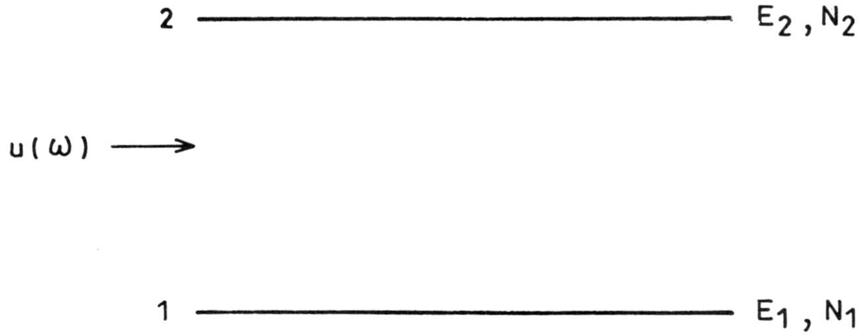

Figure 9. Particle concentrations N_1 and N_2 in energy levels E_1 and E_2 of a substance at temperature $T°K$. $u(\omega)$ = energy density of incident radiation field at frequency ω.

Under equilibrium condition

$$n_{12} = n_{21} \tag{13}$$

This gives

$$n_{12} \text{ (stimulated)} = n_{21} \text{ (stimulated)} + n_{21} \text{ (spontaneous)} \tag{14}$$

where

$$n_{12} \text{ (stimulated)} = P_{12} N_1 = B_{12} u(\omega) N_1 \tag{15}$$

and

$$n_{21} \text{ (stimulated)} = P_{21} N_2 = B_{21} u(\omega) N_2 \tag{16}$$

Let A_{21} = probability per unit time for spontaneous transition from state 2 to state 1.

$$n_{21} \text{ (spontaneous)} = A_{21} N_2 \tag{17}$$

Hence, using equations 14-17; $B_{21}\, u(\omega)\, N_1 = B_{21}\, u(\omega)\, N_2 + A_{21}\, N_2$. This gives:

$$u(\omega) = A_{21}\, N_2/(B_{12}\, N_1 - B_{21}\, N_2) = (A_{21}/B_{21})[1/(N_1/N_2) - 1] \qquad (18)$$

where the equality in equation 9 has been used.

If the cavity has been considered as an enclosure of N atoms distributed among energy states 1 and 2, i.e., $N = N_1 + N_2$; this distribution can be given by Maxwell-Boltzmann distribution law:

$$N_1 = N\exp(-\beta E_1); \quad \text{and} \quad N_2 = N\exp(-\beta E_2) \; ; \quad \text{where} \quad \beta = 1/k_B T,$$
and $k_B = 1.38\times10^{-23}\, J/{}^{\circ}K$ is the Boltzmann constant. We can also write :

$$(N_1/N_2) = \exp[\beta(E_2 - E_1)] = \exp(\beta\hbar\omega)$$

Hence, equation 18 can be expressed as:

$$u(\omega,T) = (A_{21}/B_{21})[1/\{\exp(\beta\hbar\omega) - 1\}] \qquad (19)$$

Comparing this description with the parallel case of black body radiation in a metal cavity at temperature T , and where the energy density of black body radiation is expressed by the Planck's formula, i.e.,

$$u(\omega,T) = (\hbar/\pi^2)(\omega/c)^3[1/\{\exp(\beta\hbar\omega) - 1\}] \qquad (20)$$

We find, matching equations 19 and 20:

$$(A_{21}/B_{21}) = (\hbar/\pi^2)(\omega/c)^3 \qquad (21)$$

where c is the velocity of light.

1.9   LIGHT AMPLIFICATION

Consider a medium suitable to perform as a laser source. In normal circumstances the number of atoms N_1 in lower energy state 1 is considerably larger than the number N_2 in higher energy state 2. If, however, by some external means, a large fraction of N_1 is *pumped* on to level 2, then it is possible that $N_2 > N_1$. When this happens in a medium, the latter is known as the *active* or *inverted* medium. The act of pumping is known as the *inversion process*. Such a medium can amplify the incident light.

Referring to Figure 10, let,

I = Irradiance of a collimated beam of light. This is defined as the energy of light beam per unit area per unit time (Joules $m^{-2} s^{-1}$).

η = photon density of the beam

v = velocity of light in the medium = (c/μ); where c is the velocity of light in vacuum and μ is the refractive index of the medium, then

$$I = \hbar\omega\eta v \tag{22}$$

where $\omega = (E_2 - E_1)/\hbar$. If we denote by ε the light energy generated per unit volume of the medium per unit time and having frequency ω, then we can write,

$$\varepsilon = N_2\, P_{21}\, \hbar\omega - N_1\, P_{12}\, \hbar\omega \tag{23}$$

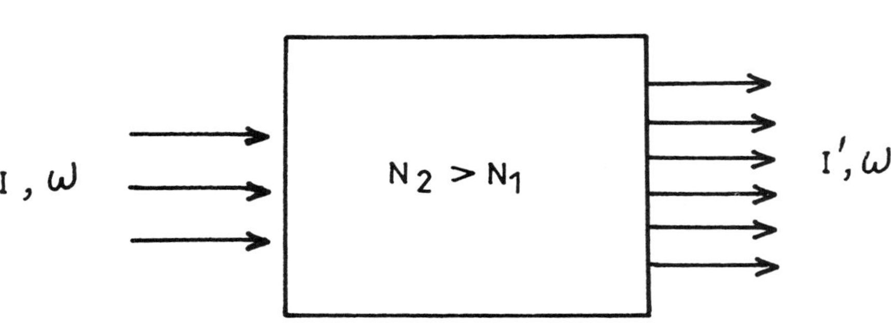

Figure 10. Light amplification by active medium.

Using equations 7 and 8;

$$\varepsilon = N_2\, B_{21}\, u(\omega)\hbar\omega - N_1\, B_{12}\, u(\omega)\hbar\omega \tag{24}$$

Since both the transitions represented by the parameter B_{21} and B_{12} are stimulated, i.e., $B_{21} = B_{12} = B$ (say), this gives: $\varepsilon = (N_2 - N_1)B\, u(\omega)\hbar\omega$. Since the amplification factor χ is defined as the ratio (ε / I), thus:

$$\begin{aligned}
\chi = \varepsilon / I &= (N_2 - N_1)Bu(\omega)\hbar\omega / \eta v\, \hbar\omega \\
&= [Bu(\omega) / \eta v](N_2 - N_1), \\
&= \sigma(N_2 - N_1)
\end{aligned} \tag{25}$$

where $\sigma = Bu(\omega) / \eta v$ is known as the stimulated emission cross section, or the probability of induced transition from higher to lower level as mentioned in equation 1.

1.10 LASER EFFICIENCY OF A MEDIUM

The nature of the medium and the method of pumping (population inversion) have a considerable effect on the laser efficiency of the medium. For instance, in a ruby laser where Cr^{3+} acts as an active center in the ruby crystal (Al_2O_3:Cr^{3+}), the energy levels of the trivalent chromium ions play an important role in determining the laser efficiency of the ruby as a medium.

Suppose, in some given medium, an active center can be characterized by a four level energy diagram as shown in Figure 11. Consider an ideal case in which the level transitions as shown in Figure 11 only take place while the transitions $3 \rightarrow 0$, $3 \rightarrow 1$ and $2 \rightarrow 0$ (known as the parasitic transitions) do not occur. In such an ideal case, the laser emission efficiency (laser yield) of the medium is maximum. If we denote this efficiency by the symbol γ, and $\hbar\omega$ is the energy of an emitted photon, then

$$\gamma = \hbar\omega / E_{exc} \tag{26}$$

γ is also called the quantum yield of the medium for laser emission.

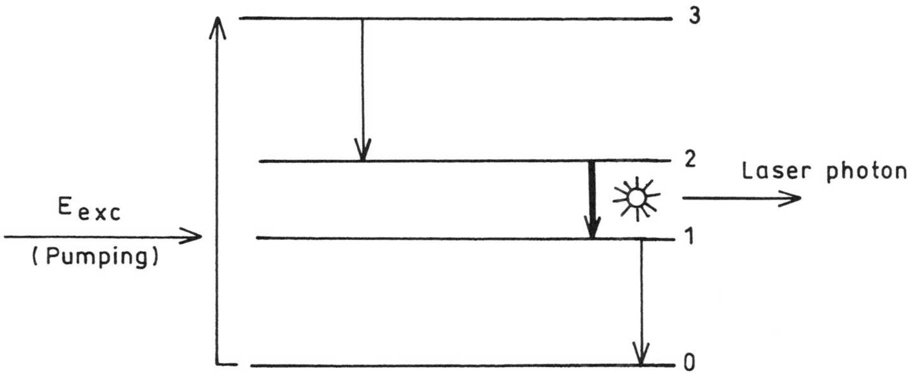

Figure 11. Energy-level diagram of a ficticious active center doped in a medium. E_{exc}-excitation energy; O- ground state; 1,2 – lasing levels (metastable states); 3 – pumping or excitation level.

Actually, not all the pumping energy is absorbed by the active center. A part is dissipated as heat and a part is absorbed by the inactive centers which are always present in the medium. Let f represents the fraction of energy actually absorbed by the active center only; then

$$\gamma_f = (f\,\hbar\omega / E_{exc}); \qquad f < 1 \tag{27}$$

Further, not all the excited centers decay to level 2. They may decay directly to level 0 or 1 leading to a loss of laser events. Let v denotes the fraction of useful excitation (i.e., those decaying to level 2); then

$$\gamma_{fv} = (fv\hbar\omega / E_{exc}); \quad v < 1 \tag{28}$$

Also, not all the centers ariving at level 2 may come to level 1 but, instead, a part of them may go directly to level 0. Let β denotes the fraction of active centers at 2 decaying to level 1 giving , thereby, the desired laser transition; then

$$\gamma_{fv\beta} = (fv\beta\hbar\omega / E_{exc}); \quad \beta < 1 \tag{29}$$

Evidently, in the absence of parasitic transitions, γ will be maximum.

1.11 LASER GAIN

A beam of light of intensity I_o incident on an inactive medium and traversing along the length l of the medium suffers beam attenuation which is expressed by the well known exponential law;

$$I = I_o\, e^{-\alpha l} \tag{30}$$

where I is the emergent intensity of the beam and α is called the attenuation coefficient.

For laser emission to occur, population inversion is needed, Thus, in such an active medium, a photon of energy $(E_2 - E_1)$ will have a proportionately higher probability to interact with and stimulate emission from the excited state than to interact with and get absorbed by the atom in the ground state. This will result in a net increase in the number of photons. This is laser gain. Gain (g) is measured in terms of the number of photons, each of energy $(E_2 - E_1)$, generated per centimeter of the laser medium. Gain can also be expressed by a similar exponential law as equation 30 but with a positive sign, i.e.,

$$I = I_o\, e^{gl} \tag{31}$$

where g is called the gain constant. Thus, intensity grows exponentially in an inverted medium.

1.12 *Q*-SWITCHED LASER

A laser system consisting of two reflecting mirrors (concave mirrors, rather than plane mirrors, are preferred as the alignment with concave mirrors is much easier than with plane mirrors) within which is incorporated the active medium is called optical cavity. As mentioned in Section 1.7, the laser device acts as a source which emits light of wavelength λ satisfying the condition : $L = n\lambda/2$; where L is the length of the resonant cavity and $n = 1, 2, 3 \ldots.$ is an integer.

Just as an electrical oscillator* emits electrical pulses, the optical cavity emits light. Thus, a laser device can also be called an optical oscillator which emits light of wavelength λ. Waves of wavelength λ and subjected to multiple reflections from mirrors get in phase and their amplitudes add up.

Like an electrical oscillator, the optical cavity is also associated with the Q-factor which determines the quality of the oscillator in terms of the wavelength-selectivity. Only those waves reinforce which are travelling along the axis perpendicular to the mirrors and have wavelength given by $\lambda = 2L/n$. A large Q-factor gives greater selectivity of the desired resonant wavelength among many other close-by wavelengths which are also associated with. For instance, a radio receiver with its oscillator having a low value of Q-factor $(=\omega L/R)$, will not be able to separate two closely transmitting stations (i.e., two close frequencies) and will catch both the stations together affecting the reception quality badly.

The power loss in a resonant cavity arising from the attenuation of radiation field is due to transmission, absorption, and diffraction by the mirrors and dielectric absorption in the laser materials. This power loss is related to the Q-value of the cavity. Q-factor signifies the ability of the cavity to store energy. A cavity whose resonance frequency is set equal to the energy level transition value, i.e., equal to $(E_2 - E_1)/\hbar$ can emit power. The rate of loss of energy W is expressed as:

$$- (\mathrm{d}W / \mathrm{d}t) \propto W$$

---

* Current flowing in an LCR circuit makes an oscillator which emits an electromagne-tic wave as in radio transmission. The radio receiver has a similar LCR circuit with a variable capacitor. The value of the capacity C is varied and, thus, when the oscillator frequency of the receiver matches with the transmitted frequency, strong absorption, known as the resonance absorption, of the incoming electrical pulses by the radio receiver takes place. These pulses are then processed further by the electronic circuit and the speaker of the radio receiver to produce sound that we hear from a radio set.

or $$- (dW / dt) = W/\tau \tag{32}$$

where τ is known as the damping time of the cavity. It is the time in which the incident radiation field energy in the cavity declines to $(1/e)$ of the incident value. The Q-value of the cavity is given by:

$$Q = \omega\tau \tag{33}$$

All the losses can be characterized by the single parameter Q or τ.

Laser devices that deliver high power, e.g., Nd^{3+}-YAG and Nd^{3+}-glass, are in the form of rods, typically, 1 meter long. Lasers of this type are Q-switched.

In this mode of operation[*] one mirror of the pair is rotated at high speed and oscillation is only possible when the two mirrors are nearly parallel. During the portion of time (comparatively long) when the two mirrors are not aligned parallel, a very substantial population inversion is built up without oscillation occurring. At the instant of the two mirrors getting aligned during the cycle of their rotation, oscillation sets in and a large burst of radiation is emitted. Using Nd^{3+}-glass laser device, large powers in the range of, say, $10^8 - 10^{10}$ watts for a few nanoseconds can be obtained. If the beam is focussed , power densities upto 10^{14} Wcm^{-2} can be reached.

There are other techniques also for producing large power pulses of laser by using dye-solutions. In this process a small cell containing a solution of a metal-organic compound, say, cryptocyanine in methanol solution is placed in between the end of a ruby rod (Al_2O_3:Cr^{3+}) and one of its mirrors. This device, having Cr^{3+} as the active ions, emits laser of wavelength 6943 nm . The solution in the cell strogly absorbs this light. This absorption prevents the occurrence of net amplification of light and hence a large population of Cr^{3+} ions is built up at the upper energy level in the absence of enough photons which could otherwise cause simultaneous stimulation to the lower lasing level.

This built-up finally becomes large enough causing the amplification in ruby device to overcome absorption in the cell. A small amount of this coherent laser light bleaches the solution in the cell so as to render it fully transparent to the ruby laser. At this instant there is suddenly a large net amplification and a giant pulse is delivered. After this pulse, the solution again returns to its absorbing state and the process of next giant laser pulse-formation starts.

---

[*]See for instance: Elliot RJ and Gibson AF., An Introduction to Solid State Physics and its Applications; MacMillan Press Ltd., London, 1974, page 252.

1.13 RUBY LASER

This laser device was the first to be made and continues to be used widely on account of certain desirable features such as high mechanical strength and thermal conductivity of ruby crystals. These crystals can be grown to high optical quality. Ruby laser device therefore belongs to the class of solid state lasers which consists of some impurity (occurring naturally) or dopant (an impurity added to the crystal) in a crystalline or glass insulator.

The crystal atoms do not participate directly in the lasing action but serve as a host lattice to the impurity/dopant. Today, some 300 dielectric crystals doped by transition element ions are available which can serve as solid state laser devices. Oxide crystals of regular structure are most widely used. Apart from the popular ruby device, which is Al_2O_3 crystal (corundum) doped with Cr^{3+} ions, we have equally popular $Y_3Al_5O_{12}$ (yttrium aluminum garnet; YAG) in which some of the Y^{3+} ions are replaced by neodymium ions, Nd^{+3} Another popular laser device is Nd:Glass.

A ruby laser system, typically, consists of a ruby rod of some 4 cm length and 0.5 cm diameter surrounded by a neon/xenon flash lamp tube which provides the optical pumping to Cr-ions. The two ends of the ruby rod are fixed with mirrors. The unit is enclosed in a vessel having arrangement for cooling. As shown in Figure 12(c), optical pumping raises an electron in the Cr-ion to the broad upper levels denoted as $^4F_1$ and $^4F_2$ in spectroscopic notation. The pumping source which is a cylindrical xenon flash discharge tube is placed parallel and adjacent to the ruby rod. The arrangement in Figure 12(a), and illustrated in Figure 12(b), takes advantage of the focussing properties of an ellipse. The laser rod and flash tube are located at the two focuses inside a cylindrical reflector of elliptical cross section. Any light from the flash escaping in any direction will eventually focus onto the laser rod after reflection from the silvered surface of the reflector. Thus, all the pumping radiation is maximally focussed on the active material. Use of two or four ellipses can further enhance the output power of the laser device. The end faces of the laser rod are polished and silvered to act as optical resonator mirrors. Therefore, in this case, the length of the resonant cavity is the length of the rod.

1.14 HELIUM-NEON LASER

Helium-Neon laser is an example of another popular laser source which is relatively inexpensive and is widely used as a student laboratory source of laser light for performing a number of optics experiments. The mixture of helium and neon (helium at 90 to 80 percent and neon at 10 to 20 percent respectively) is contained in a sealed tube (of 1 cm diameter and 100 cm length) and a pressure of about 1 torr (1 mm of Hg). The He-Ne laser is excited by a glow discharge in the tube activated by dc current at about 10^3 volts. Excitation in helium atoms in the discharge tube is caused by the atomic collision. The helium component subsequently causes excitation of the Ne-gas atoms. Excited Ne-gas atoms, which contain the meta-stable lasing levels at 632.8 nm, give rise to laser emission process.

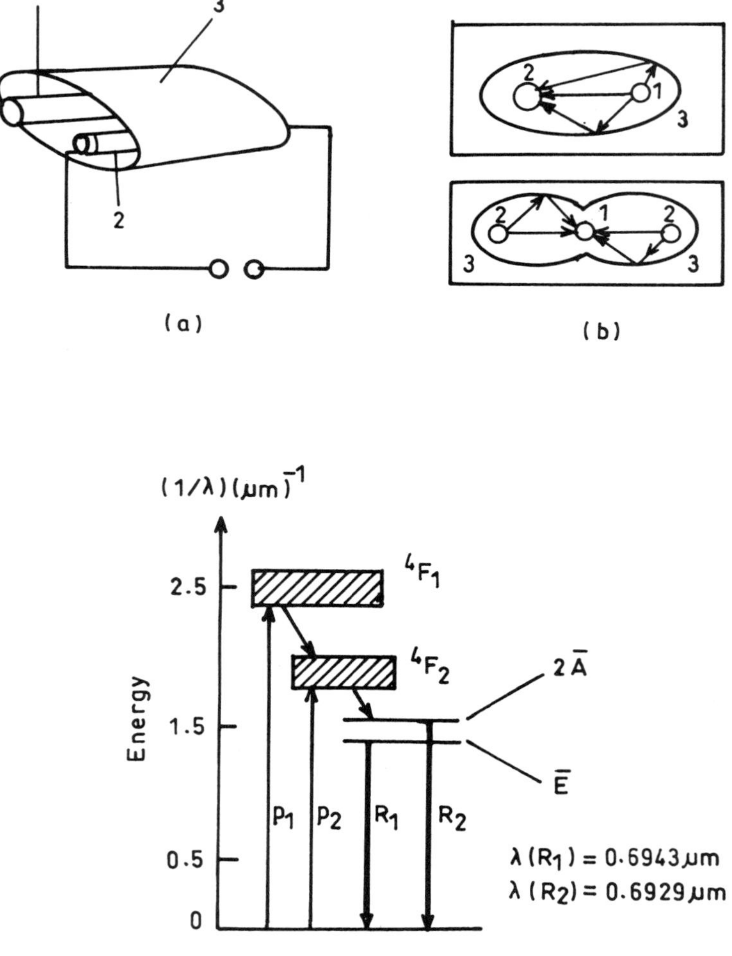

Figure 12. (a) and (b) – configurations of discharge flash tube(2) and solid state laser rod(1) enclosed in an elliptical reflector(3); (c) – energy levels (in units of $1/\lambda$) of chromium ion in ruby and the lasing levels. p_1,p_2 denote optical pumping by gas discharge xenon flash lamp.

1.15 LASERS IN MEDICINE

A brief view of how lasers are being used in physical medicine is presented. Müller* has very succinctly explained various such features. The present section in fact draws strongly from this article. This section, therefore, attempts to explain only the basic features. Various subsequent chapters in this book address this topic at a current and advanced level. Main features of laser-tissue interactions are summarized in Table 1. Table 2 indicates some of the medical uses of various laser devices.

Table 1. Main features of Laser-tissue *interaction.*

Laser Light							
Effects	Photochemical Effects		Thermal Effects			Ionizing Effects	
Process	Photo-induction	Photo-Radiation	Photo-Coagulation	Photo Evaporization	Photo-Carbonization	Photo-ablation	Photo-disruption
Medical Use	Bio-stimulation	Photo-Synthesized Cyto-toxicity	Cauteri-zation (searing of tissue)	Incision	Incision	Incision	Incision

Table 2. Some of the medical uses of various laser devices.

Medical Discipline	Laser Devices
Dermatology	He-Ne, GaAs, Nd:YAG
Rheumatology (rheumatoid, Arthritis, osteoarthritis)	He-Ne, GaAs (λ between 630 and 1300 nm)
Traumatology	He-Ne, GaAs
Dentistry	He-Ne, GaAs
Oncology	Dye lasers; Cu and Au vapor lasers
Ophthalmology	Argon laser, Nd:YAG
Gynaecology	CO_2
Otolaryngology (ENT surgery)	CO_2
Gastroenterology	Nd:YAG
Urology	Nd:YAG

---

*G.J. Müller, Development Trends and Market Potential of Biomedical Laser Applications; SPIE, **658** (1986);Washington (U.S.A.)

Figure 13 illustrates some medical disciplines that are being covered by lasers for diagnostics and therapy.

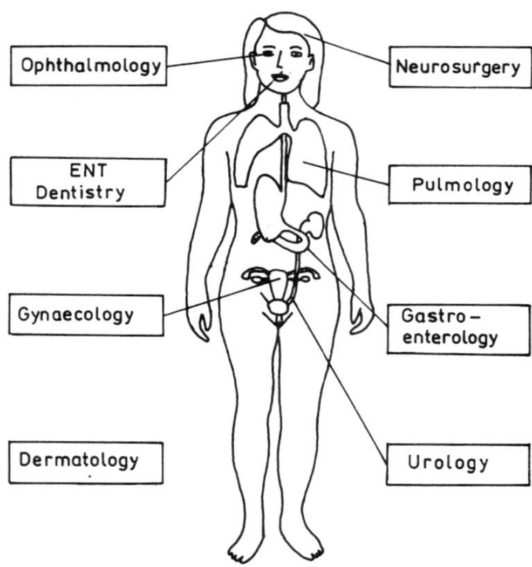

Figure 13 Some laser addressed disciplines and the female human body.

BIBLIOGRAPHY

1. Gibson K.F. and Kernohen W.G., *Lasers in Medicine- a review.* J. Med. Engg. & Tech. 1993; **17**, 51-57.
2. Absten G.T. and Joffe S.N., *Lasers in Medicine: An Introductory Guide.* Cambridge University Press, Cambridge (U.K.), 1985.
3. Wilson J. and Hankes J.F.B. *Lasers: Principles and Applications,* Prentice Hall, London, 1987.
4. Treat M.R., Oz M.C. and Bass L.S., New Technologies and Future Applications of Surgical Lasers, *Lasers in General Surgery,* 1992; **72**:705-742.
5. Tarasov L.V., *Laser Physics,* Mir Publications, Moscow (Russia), 1983.
6. Sharupich L. and Tugov N., *Optoelectronics,* Mir Publishers, Moscow (Russia), 1987.
7. *Endoscopic Therapy Applications of Advanced Solid State Lasers* (1991). A review, Commercially available from JGM Associates Inc., 6 New England Executive Park, Suite 400, Burlington, Massachussetts 01803, U.S.A.

Chapter 2

LASER-TISSUE INTERACTION

Cameron H. G. Wright,[1] Steven F. Barrett,[2] and Ashley J. Welch[3]
[1]Department of Electrical Engineering, U.S. Air Force Academy, Colorado, U.S.A.
[2]Department of Electrical and Computer Engineering, University of Wyoming, U.S.A.
[3]Department of Electrical and Computer Engineering, University of Texas at Austin, U.S.A.

2.1 INTRODUCTION

There are many uses of lasers for medical purposes, including both diagnostic and therapeutic procedures. In order to effectively select, and predict the result of laser energy that is to be applied to living tissue, one must have a basic understanding of laser-tissue interaction. For example, how does a clinician choose the appropriate wavelength, power, and spot size to achieve a particular effect? The mechanisms of tissue optics and the ramifications of photon absorption, scattering, and propagation all contribute to the result. This chapter provides a basic overview of these considerations, and provides brief descriptions of some of the more common modeling techniques used to predict laser-tissue interaction. The reader is referred to sources such as [1–5] for more extensive background information and theory. Note that while some equations describing aspects of laser-tissue interaction will appear in this chapter, the level of discussion is such that the reader can gain much useful information without necessarily having an extensive background in physics or engineering. This chapter is an overview only; it should *not* be considered a rigorous mathematical treatment.

2.1.1 Notation Used

Throughout this chapter, we endeavor to use the most commonly accepted notations but the reader should be aware that there are many conflicting naming conventions among the areas of physics, optics, thermodynamics, biomedical engineering, and other disciplines which apply to lasers in medicine. Similarly, we use the most commonly used units of measure, but many variations exist in the literature. Watts versus milliwatts, meters versus centimeters, Kelvin versus Celsius are all examples of this variety in units.

When laser propagation is described in three dimensional Cartesian coordinates (x,y,z), the beam is assumed to be traveling in the positive z direction and the beam cross section is thus in the x and y directions. Typically $z = 0$ is located at the tissue surface. A particular point (x,y,z) in space is designated **r**. Note this is different from r, which is used in one section to depict the radial distance $r = \sqrt{x^2 + y^2}$ from the center of the laser beam. The "strength" of laser light is usually described in terms of the power density, which is called irradiance (E) at the tissue surface or the fluence rate (ϕ) within the tissue, with the units for both being power per unit area (typically in mW/cm^2). Another commonly used term is radiance (L), which is the power density per unit solid angle (typically in mW/cm$^2 \cdot$ sr) where "sr" is the abbreviation for one steradian of solid angle (see the chapter Appendix for a brief review of solid angles). The relationship between fluence rate and radiance at point **r** is

$$\phi(\mathbf{r}) = \int\limits_{4\pi} L(\mathbf{r},\hat{\mathbf{s}})\, d\omega \tag{1}$$

where **s** is a unit vector pointing in the direction of photon movement, and $d\omega$ represents an infinitesimal solid angle swept around direction $\hat{\mathbf{s}}$. The fluence rate $\phi(\mathbf{r})$ can be thought of as all the power incident upon a tiny sphere centered at point **r**, divided by the cross sectional area of the sphere. Recall that power (W) is energy per unit time (i.e., J/s); often the term laser energy density in tissue refers to the fluence (ψ), with the units being energy per unit area (typically mJ/cm^2). Obviously $\psi = \int \phi\, dt$. Note that the symbol ψ, as used in Section 2.5, may also stand for the azimuth angle of photon scattering. The usage will be clear from the context of the discussion.

2.2 GENERAL CONSIDERATIONS OF LASER-TISSUE INTERACTION

2.2.1 Coherent Light

Lasers produce light that is unlike other light sources such as the sun, electric room lights, or a candle. Since its invention by Theodore H. Maiman at Hughes Aircraft Company in 1960,[1] the laser has been recognized for two primary characteristics which set it apart from other light sources: (a) the laser emits a highly collimated beam of light, which means a narrow beam tends to stay narrow; and (b) the laser light is nearly monochromatic (i.e., it consists primarily of only one color or wavelength). These two characteristics mean that laser light is highly ordered in space and correlated in time – which by definition means a laser produces *coherent* light. This coherent light from a laser can be focused to a much smaller spot (on the order of a wavelength in diameter) than incoherent light can be, resulting in extremely high energy or power densities (incident energy or power divided by the area irradiated). The study of laser physics is an entire category in itself, and it is assumed the reader is already somewhat familiar with the topic. For a refresher, some good references are [6–10].

2.2.2 Laser Parameters

The coherent nature of laser light makes it particularly useful for medical applications. By adjusting laser parameters appropriately, the clinician can control the effect the laser has on biological tissue. The wavelength of the laser light is always important, as we shall see that this parameter has a profound effect on how light interacts with tissue. The wavelength (λ) produced by a laser is primarily determined by the substance used to produce the lasing effect, which is generally classified into the categories of solid state, liquid dye, or gaseous. Maiman's original ruby laser ($\lambda = 694$ nm), the Nd:YAG laser (yttrium aluminum garnet doped with neodymium, $\lambda = 1064$ nm), and the increasingly common laser diodes (various λ based on material, typically in the range of 532–830 nm) are all solid state lasers. Liquid dye lasers use a mixture of dye to produce a "tunable" laser which can provide various wavelengths (from $\lambda = 400$–1000 nm for example). The CO_2 laser (carbon dioxide, $\lambda = 10.6$ μm), the Ar^+ laser (argon ion, $\lambda = 488$, 514.5 nm), and the commonly available He-Ne laser (helium neon, $\lambda = 632.5$ nm) are typical gas lasers. Note that each category of laser has specific advantages and disadvantages independent of wavelength such as available power, stability of output, beam characteristics, or laser lifetime.

Other laser parameters depend upon the laser type: CW or pulsed. Depending upon the design, a laser can emit either a constant beam (called CW for continuous wave), or it can emit pulses of laser light. For CW lasers, parameters which must be considered in addition to wavelength are power, irradiation time, and spot size. Note that as the spot size decreases for a given power, the power density (irradiance, typically in mW/cm^2) increases. For pulsed lasers, the parameters of interest are energy per pulse, irradiation time, spot size, and the pulse repetition rate. In the case of very short duration pulses, peak power per pulse may be of equal or greater interest than energy per pulse.

Note that very short duration pulses from a laser capable of producing moderate energy per pulse or low average power can still generate a very high value of peak power per pulse. This can be illustrated by Figure 1, where P is

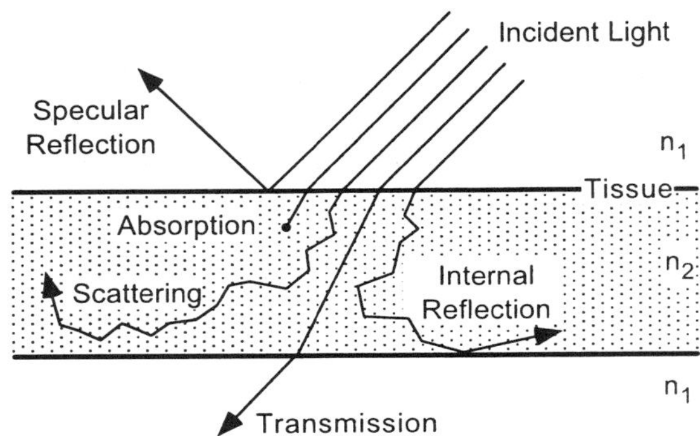

Figure 1. An example of the power output of a pulsed laser. When τ is very short, peak power P can be quite high even if average power is low.

power (W), ε is the energy (J) per pulse, τ is the pulse duration (s), and T is the time between pulses (s). Note that $f = 1/T$ is the pulse repetition rate (Hz), and the *duty cycle* is defined as τ/T. Instantaneous power is $P = d\varepsilon/dt$; the average power output of the laser is

$$P_{\text{avg}} = \frac{1}{T} \int_{t_0}^{t_0+T} P \, dt = \frac{\varepsilon}{T} \tag{2}$$

and the peak power is

$$P_{\text{pk}} = \frac{\varepsilon}{\tau}. \tag{3}$$

In recent years, advances in pulse compression techniques have enabled researchers to produce ultra short pulses of less than 100 femtoseconds (note 1 fs = 10^{-15} seconds) in duration [11]. Suppose a given pulsed laser is capable of only 1 mJ (0.001 J) per pulse and a maximum repetition rate of 100 Hz (100 pulses per second). From Equation 2, this translates to a maximum average power output of 100 mW (i.e., 100 mJ/s), which seems rather moderate. But suppose this laser was delivering the 100 mW average power via pulses only 100 fs in duration; from Equation 3 we can see that the peak power per pulse is 10 GW (1×10^{10} watts). If the laser beam spot size is 3 mm in diameter, then the peak power density per pulse is 141.5 GW/cm^2. Peak power density of this magnitude is well beyond the normal limit for ionization of 10^8 W/cm^2, and has a significant effect on tissue, as discussed in Section 2.6.2.

Discussion on the proper selection of the various laser parameters for a given medical application is discussed in other chapters.

2.2.3 Laser Effects on Tissue

In the years since the introduction of the laser, there has been a steady increase in the use of lasers for medical purposes. As far back as 1963, dermatologists used a CO_2 laser for cancerous tissue removal, and in 1964 a ruby laser was used for the first "noninvasive" surgery of the eye [2]. Today, thousands of medical laser procedures are performed each day around the world. These procedures rely upon predictable effects of laser energy on tissue, which are based upon the laser-tissue interactions discussed in this chapter. The clinician can control the laser effects on tissue by appropriate selection of the various laser parameters discussed above in Section 2.2.2. These effects can be grouped into general categories as shown below.[2]

- Diagnosis: causes no long-term change to the tissue. Low-intensity lasers are used to illuminate difficult to reach areas or to interact with tissue to produce a characteristic fluorescence or other luminescence that provides information about the tissue [12]. For example, blood flow, oxygen content, and pH can be ascertained with a diagnostic laser, as can certain cancerous or precancerous conditions.

- Therapy: causes long-term change to the tissue, usually using higher power lasers than those for diagnostic use. This category of laser effects can be further grouped as follows, listed in order of increasing laser power typically used.

  - Photochemotherapy: laser light is used to trigger chemical reactions in the body for therapeutic purposes. For example, the increasingly popular *photodynamic therapy* (PDT) uses an injected chemical which, when irradiated with the proper wavelength, undergoes the desired chemical change which produces a beneficial effect on tissue [13]. Also called photochemical effects.

  - Heating: laser irradiation is used to heat the tissue, resulting in *coagulation* or *welding* [14]. For example, blood is easily coagulated by laser energy thus allowing blood vessels to be

> "sealed" during surgery to control bleeding. Two sections of tissue can be heated such that they "weld" together, often eliminating the need for sutures.

- Ablation: laser irradiation is used to cause even greater heating of the tissue, resulting in vaporization, vacuolization, and pyrolysis of the tissue itself [15, 16]. This effect is useful for cutting through tissue or for removing certain areas of diseased tissue.

- Photoablation and Photodisruption: typically pulsed lasers are used to produce intentional removal or mechanical damage to tissue, such as the breaking up of gallbladder or kidney stones. Little thermal damage is observed in the surrounding tissue. This effect is possible when using lasers that produce very short time duration pulses that have extremely high peak power (e.g., in the megawatt or gigawatt range) per pulse [11, 17, 18].

When the desired effect of the laser energy does not match the actual result, it can be usually attributed to a less than complete understanding of the many variables related to laser-tissue interaction [19]. For example, in ophthalmology lasers are used extensively to produce therapeutic lesions on the retina to treat conditions such as diabetic retinopathy or detached retina. Despite years of experience, an ophthalmologist will sometimes encounter a lesion which has unexpected characteristics [20]. Typically this has little or no detrimental effect, but the danger of unexpected results from lasers is always present. While our current understanding has enabled us to make great strides in applying lasers to clinical needs, the reader should keep in mind that this field is still in its infancy [1].

Given the increasing use of lasers for both diagnostic and therapeutic purposes in a broad range of medical specialties, understanding the fundamentals of laser-tissue interaction becomes increasingly important. These fundamentals make up the remainder of this chapter.

2.3   OVERVIEW OF LASER PROPAGATION IN TISSUE

2.3.1 Basic Optical Considerations

Laser-tissue interactions follow the well-known rules of optics. When laser light strikes tissue (or passes from one type of tissue to another) it can be reflected, transmitted, absorbed, scattered, internally reflected, or some combination thereof [21–24].[3] This is shown graphically in Figure 2. Note that when dealing with the propagation of light, various methods are used based upon the situation. Ray tracing is perhaps the simplest method, while solving Maxwell's equations of electromagnetics provides the most complete, albeit almost impossible analysis.

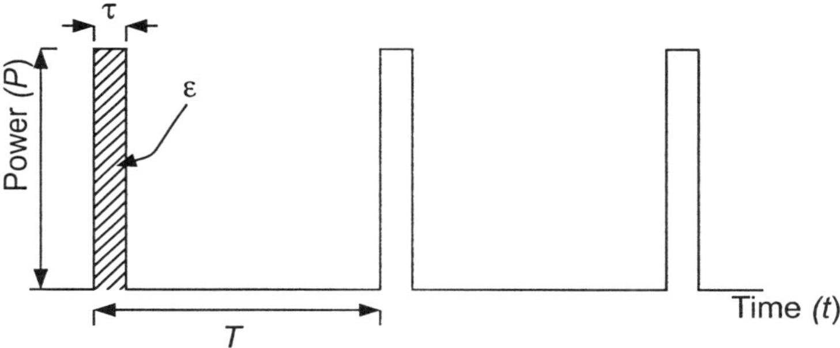

Figure 2. Propagation of laser generated photons in a thin section of tissue, assuming that $n_1 < n_2$. The photons may be reflected, transmitted, absorbed, scattered, internally reflected, or some combination thereof.

Since tissue is a highly scattering multilayer medium, with random absorbing and scattering sites and with many of its properties only known in terms of lumped estimates, Maxwell's equations are seldom used explicitly. One common technique is to consider the laser light in terms of photon paths; this method is called *photon transport*. A higher power laser would emit a greater number of photons in a given amount of time. Recall from quantum physics that the energy of an individual photon is *not* a function of the laser power but rather is a function of the frequency[4] and hence the wavelength of the laser light. When the mean free path of a photon is relatively short as is typical in tissue, this method of discussing light propagation in terms of short linear photon paths is quite useful, and is similar in its ease of use to the ray tracing model. In the discussion to follow, it will be evident which type of model is being used. While a specific polarization of laser light is sometimes employed that would affect the propagation in tissue, it is a specialized technique that is beyond the scope of this chapter. Normally, tissue is so highly scattering that light becomes randomly polarized in only a short penetration depth; the discussion in this chapter assumes random polarization of light. To illustrate the main points in a highly simplified but useful example, we shall "follow" a typical laser beam as it passes from air into tissue.

2.3.2 Optical Properties of Tissue

There are many factors that determine how light will behave in a given type of tissue [1–3, 25]. Some of the more important parameters, collectively called the optical properties, are functions of wavelength, so two lasers of different wavelengths may behave quite differently in the same region of tissue. See Table 1 for a comparison of typical penetration depths of some commonly used lasers.

Table 1. Approximate depth of penetration in soft tissue for various types of lasers. Adapted from [1, 3]. Note some lasers are capable of producing additional wavelengths.

Laser Type	Wavelength	Typical Penetration Depth (δ')
ArF excimer	193 nm	1 μm
KrF excimer	248 nm	5 μm
XeCl excimer	308 nm	40 μm
XeF excimer	351 nm	150 μm
dye	465 nm	250 μm
Ar^+	514.5 nm	330 μm
HeNe	632.5 nm	700 μm
diode	830 nm	1.3 mm
Nd:YAG	1.064 μm	1.4 mm
Tm:YAG	2.01 μm	180 μm
Ho:YAG	2.12 μm	400 μm
Er:YAG	2.94 μm	1 μm
CO_2	10.6 μm	20 μm

To complicate matters further, these properties are not static: they may change dynamically with changes in tissue temperature or hydration, for example. Furthermore, while we can assume the permeability of tissue to be constant for particular optical wavelengths, the permittivity can vary considerably both temporally and spatially as the dielectric constant changes.

The four primary optical properties for a given material are:

Index of refraction (n) is the ratio of the velocity of light in a vacuum to the velocity of light in the given material (dimensionless, $n \geq 1.0$).

Coefficient of absorption (μ_a) is the reciprocal of the mean free path length of a photon before an absorption event occurs (units are length^{-1}). The probability of photon absorption in an infinitesimal path length ds is $\mu_a ds$.

Coefficient of scattering (μ_s) is the reciprocal of the mean free path length of a photon before a scattering event occurs (units are length^{-1}). The probability of photon scattering in an infinitesimal path length ds is $\mu_s ds$.

Anisotropy factor (g) characterizes the angular distribution of light after a scattering event occurs (dimensionless, $-1 \leq g \leq 1$). If light scatters equally in all directions (called *isotropic* scattering) then $g = 0$; fully backward scattering would be described by $g = -1$; fully forward scattering is when $g = 1$. Many types of tissue have been found to be highly forward scattering for most laser wavelengths; typical values of g for tissue range from 0.3 to 0.98 with $g \approx 0.9$ in the visible spectrum being common.

These properties appear in most literature regarding propagation of electromagnetic fields in a scattering medium [1, 3, 26, 27]. Other optical parameters, such as the total attenuation coefficient $\mu_t = \mu_a + \mu_s$, the reduced scattering coefficient $\mu_s' = [1 - g]\mu_s$, the reduced attenuation coefficient $\mu_{tr} = \mu_a + \mu_s'$, and the albedo $a = \mu_s / \mu_t$, can be derived from the four basic optical properties. Note that penetration depth δ is usually defined as $\delta = 1/\mu_t$; it is the depth at which we expect the value of the laser light to have dropped to 37% of the value transmitted into the surface of the tissue. The values shown in Table 1 use the slightly different δ', which is defined as $\delta' = 1/\mu_{tr}$.

There are considerable differences in the optical properties of various types of tissue and even more significant differences in the same tissue at different wavelengths. Some representative examples of optical properties for selected tissue types, presented in Section 2.7, will illustrate this point. We now continue our discussion of "following" a laser beam as it encounters the tissue boundary.

2.3.3 Reflection and Transmission

When light encounters an interface where n changes, such as the air-tissue boundary (or a boundary between two types of tissue), reflectance occurs. The remaining fraction of the light that is not reflected is transmitted. In tissue optics, we consider two types of reflectance: specular and diffuse. In specular reflection, light is always reflected at an angle equal to the incoming angle. In the case of totally diffuse reflection, light from a given incoming angle will be reflected equally at all angles. We consider the specular case first as it tends to be associated with tissue boundaries. While diffuse reflection tends to be associated with scattering "inside" tissue, some diffuse reflection may occur at the boundary if the surface "roughness" is on the order of a wavelength.

Specular reflectance occurs when the object or "smooth" region encountered by the light is very large compared to the wavelength, such as the initial air-tissue interface of a laser shining on skin. When light encounters such an interface where the index of refraction changes, the path of light changes as illustrated in Figure 3.

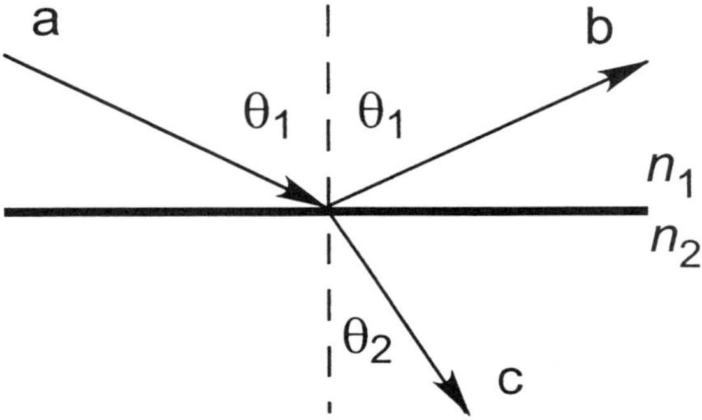

Figure 3. Snell's law depicted as a light ray model where it encounters a change in the index of refraction. The rays are drawn assuming that $n_1 < n_2$. Rays a, b and c all lie in the same plane. For clarity, the interface is shown as planar.

Some portion of the incoming light will be specularly reflected at an equal angle to the normal depicted as θ_1 in Figure 3. The remaining fraction of light will be transmitted, albeit with a change in direction (called refraction) according to Snell's Law,

$$n_1 \sin\theta_1 = n_2 \sin\theta_2 \quad \text{or} \quad \theta_2 = \arcsin\left(\frac{n_1}{n_2}\sin\theta_1\right). \tag{4}$$

We ignore the possibility of absorption or the effect on polarization. The fraction R of the total incoming light which is reflected is given by Fresnel's relation:

$$R = \frac{1}{2}\left[\frac{\tan^2(\theta_1 - \theta_2)}{\tan^2(\theta_1 + \theta_2)} + \frac{\sin^2(\theta_1 - \theta_2)}{\sin^2(\theta_1 + \theta_2)}\right] \tag{5}$$

where the angles are measured as shown in Figure 3. If the light is normal to the interface, Equation 5 can be simplified to

$$R = \frac{(n_1 - n_2)^2}{(n_1 + n_2)^2} \quad \text{for } \theta_1 = 0. \tag{6}$$

The fraction of light which is not specularly reflected is given by $T = 1 - R$, and it is this amount of light which enters the tissue.

In Figure 3, if the condition is changed such that $n_1 > n_2$, then there exists a critical angle $\theta_c = \arcsin(n_2 / n_1)$ where if $\theta_1 \geq \theta_c$, then $R = 1$ and *all* the light is reflected. This is known as *total internal reflection*. Thus light traveling from tissue toward air may encounter total internal reflection. This condition is illustrated in Figure 2. Note that if $n_1 > n_2$ and $\theta_1 < \theta_c$, then the transmitted ray would have an angle such that $\theta_2 > \theta_1$.

We ignore for the moment the reflected light, and continue to "follow" that portion T of the incident light which is transmitted into the tissue in a new direction θ_2.

2.3.4 Scattering and Absorption

Light which passes through the boundary into the tissue finds itself in an environment which is often highly scattering (also called *turbid*) and contains many potential absorption sites. Scattering tends to dominate the propagation of light in tissue because inhomogeneities of the cellular structure and the various particle sizes are all on the order of the wavelength of the light [26]. These potential scattering sites are randomly distributed in the tissue. A greater overall concentration of scattering sites yields a larger μ_s and thus results in a shorter photon path before the probability of a scattering event approaches certainty.[5] When scattering does occur, the expected new direction taken by the scattered light is characterized by the anisotropy factor g discussed above. Thus scattering doesn't result in an actual attenuation of the light—it just changes its direction. For example, Figure 4 depicts a photon encountering a scattering event. However, if one is interested in the propagation of light along a specific intended direction, then this scattering into other directions can alter the amount of light in the intended direction. Scattered photons are no longer part of the collimated beam; turbid tissue has the effect of "spreading out" or decollimating the laser beam.

Also randomly distributed throughout the tissue are absorption sites, made up of particles called *chromophores* (e.g., water, blood, or melanin). The chromophores transform the energy of the light into heat energy; this is the primary mechanism (discussed in Section 2.6.1) for the thermal effects of laser-irradiated tissue. A greater overall concentration of absorption sites yields a larger μ_a and thus results in a shorter photon path before the probability of an absorption event approaches certainty. Absorption results in an actual attenuation of light energy available to continue its propagation through the tissue, and generates heat at the absorption site.

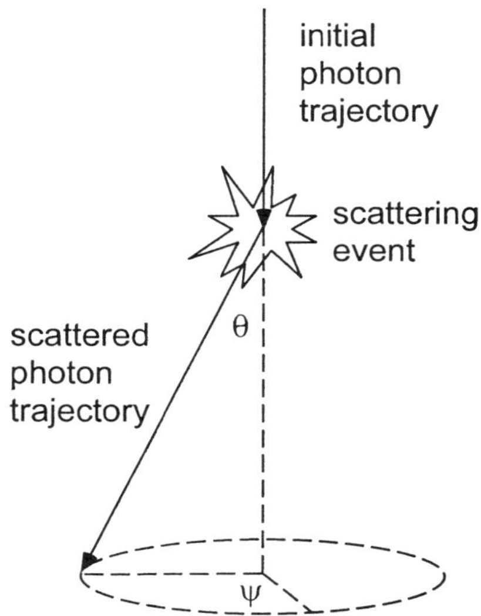

Figure 4. A photon encountering a scattering event.

2.3.5 Light Propagation Versus Tissue Depth

While not common, some tissue consists of only homogeneously distributed absorption sites. For example, researchers examining the absorption characteristics of *in vitro* hemoglobin (Hb) often rupture the erythrocyte membrane and release the Hb into solution yielding *hemolyzed blood*, which is a homogeneous absorbing medium [26]. In such a medium, the direction of light is unchanged since little or no scattering occurs, and the attenuation of light through this tissue can be described by Beer's law:[6]

$$\phi(z) = (1-R)E_0 e^{-\mu_a z} \tag{7}$$

where $\phi(z)$ is the fluence rate (in mW/cm^2) of collimated light at some depth z (measured in cm) in the tissue along the intended path (along the z-axis), E_0 is the collimated irradiance (in mW/cm^2) that "hits" the surface of the tissue, μ_a is the absorption coefficient (in cm^{-1}), and R is the specular reflection term from Equation 5.

If all tissues were purely absorbing media at optical wavelengths, then Equation 7 and knowledge of the beam profile (discussed below) would be sufficient to completely describe the spatial light distribution in tissue. Unfortunately, that is not the case. In most tissue, where scattering is significant, Beer's law can be modified to:

$$\phi(z) = (1-R)E_0 e^{-(\mu_a+\mu_s)z} = (1-R)E_0 e^{-\mu_t z} \tag{8}$$

where μ_s is the scattering coefficient and μ_t is the total attenuation coefficient (both in cm^{-1}). It is important to keep in mind that Equation 8 describes the fluence rate distribution of *collimated* light versus depth regardless of how complex the tissue. However, the collimated light alone is not the whole picture. While photons are scattered out of the main beam path, multiple scattering events can just as easily bring various photons back into the main beam path. These photons, although no longer part of the collimated beam, add to the fluence rate at a given point along the z-axis. This can result, for example, in the nonintuitive situation of having a fluence rate just below the tissue surface that is actually *greater* than the incident irradiance [1]. We also must be cognizant of how laser energy scattered out of the collimated beam affects surrounding tissue which is not on the intended beam path. This constitutes a much more complicated situation than Equation 8 describes, and requires correspondingly more complicated modeling techniques to allow reasonable predictions of the overall spatial light distribution in turbid tissue. Some of the more commonly used models (see Section 2.4) and simulations (see Section 2.5) will be discussed subsequently.

2.3.6 Laser Delivery Issues

Laser-tissue interaction predictions generally require some knowledge of the distribution of laser energy incident on the tissue surface. The two most common distributions are Gaussian and uniform. The distribution of energy (and hence power) in the beam cross section produced by most lasers is a circularly symmetric Gaussian profile beam, shown in Figure 5. In this profile, the irradiance is greatest at the center of the beam and falls off rapidly as the distance from the beam center increases. The Gaussian beam irradiance E (in mW/cm^2) is described by the equation

$$E(r) = E_0 e^{-2\left(\frac{r}{w_0}\right)^2} \tag{9}$$

where r is the distance from the center of the beam, E_0 is the peak irradiance (in mW/cm^2) at the center of the beam, and w_0 is called the *beam radius*. At

$r = w_0$, the irradiance has fallen to $1/e^2 \approx 13.5\%$ of the peak value; the quantity $2w_0$ is called the *beam diameter* or the *spot size*. Thus while Equation 9 describes a beam that tapers off radially to infinity, the diameter $2w_0$ is considered to be the "size" of the beam, and roughly 86.5% of the total beam power[7] is contained within this beam diameter. Not all laser sources produce a circularly symmetric Gaussian beam. Laser diodes in particular produce a highly elliptical beam, where the beam diameter along the x-axis is much larger than the beam diameter along the y-axis. There are also differences in the divergence, or level of collimation, of the beam depending upon the laser source. It is straightforward, as discussed in [7, 10] for example, to modify the beam as needed with simple optics to yield the desired beam profile. Note also that the beam characteristics affect how small a spot size can be achieved with a focusing lens [10]; details of beam manipulation are beyond the scope of this chapter.

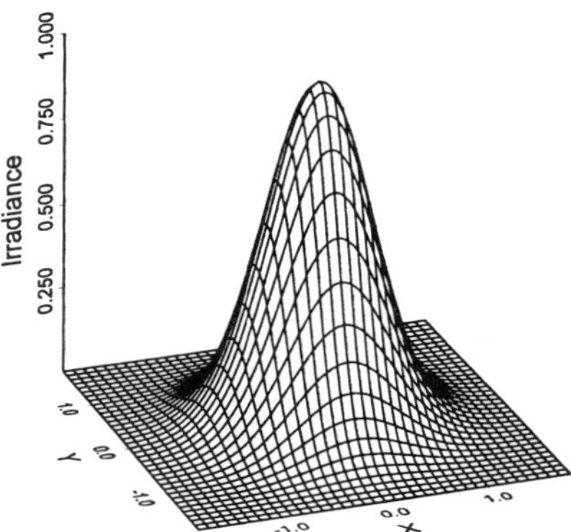

Figure 5. Irradiance of a circularly symmetric Gaussian beam. The beam radius is $w_0 = 1.0$ for this example.

It is often not possible to deliver laser energy directly into tissue from the laser. Whether dictated by the available equipment or the tissue location, it is increasingly common to use an optical fiber to couple energy from the laser source to the tissue location. In this case, the beam profile may not be Gaussian. For small diameter fibers ($d < 10$ μm), also called *single mode* fibers, the irradiance profile of the beam is preserved. However, these small diameter fibers are useful only for low-power applications. For higher power lasers, fibers with larger diameters ($d > 80$ μm), also called *multimode* fibers, are used. It can be shown [1] that for most multimode fibers, the beam irradiance distribution exiting the fiber end is a uniform distribution, often called the "tophat" profile as shown in Figure 6. In this profile, the irradiance is constant from the center of the beam to the edge of the beam radius. The uniform beam irradiance E (in mW/cm^2) is described by the equation:

$$E(r) = \begin{cases} E_0 & \text{for } 0 \le r \le w_0 \\ 0 & \text{for } r > w_0 \end{cases} \tag{10}$$

where r is the distance from the center of the beam, E_0 is the irradiance (in mW/cm^2) at the center of the beam, and w_0 is the beam radius. The quantity $2w_0$ is the beam diameter or the spot size. Obviously, 100% of the total beam power is contained within this beam diameter. The uniform distribution is only true at or very near the distal end of the fiber, where *near field* conditions exist. Further away from the end of the fiber, in the *far field* (i.e., at some distance much greater than the fiber diameter away from the end of the fiber), the irradiance distribution reverts to a Gaussian profile [1].

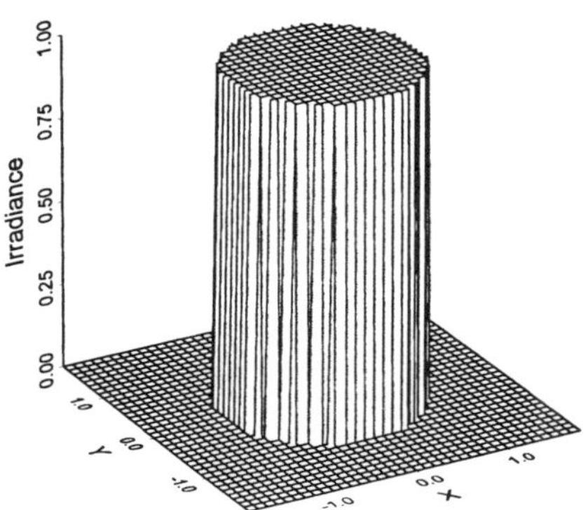

Figure 6. Irradiance of a circularly symmetric tophat beam. The beam radius is $w_0 = 1.0$ for this example.

When the beam profile $E(r)$ is known, the distribution of *collimated* light in tissue would then be given by

$$\phi(r,z) = (1-R)E(r)e^{-(\mu_a+\mu_s)z} = (1-R)E(r)e^{-\mu_t z} \tag{11}$$

which is just a modification of Equation 8. As discussed above, the collimated light alone is not the whole picture; the effect of scattered photons must also be taken into account. Thus Equation 11 is still not sufficient for our needs.

The preceding discussion assumed a single flat cleaved or polished fiber end cut perpendicular to the z-axis. It is becoming increasingly common for clinicians to employ special fiber tips and fiber bundles that optically modify the distribution of the laser energy incident on the tissue. Different tip materials such as sapphire, having a preferred refractive index and thermal conductivity, are also used to "tailor" the coupling of laser energy into the tissue. Some tips are intended to be in contact with the tissue or even submerged in some liquid between the tip and the target tissue. It is beyond the scope of this chapter to discuss delivery issues in further detail. Regarding laser-tissue interaction, one merely needs to know the distribution of laser energy incident on the tissue surface. For more information on fiber modes and beam characteristics, see [2, 9]. For more information on fiber tips and many other delivery issues, see [1, 2].

2.4   MODELS OF LASER-TISSUE PROPAGATION

As previously mentioned, the nature of tissue makes it very difficult to calculate a solution to Maxwell's equations of electromagnetics to predict light propagation inside a volume of tissue. A common approach has been to concentrate instead upon the energy transfer due to light interaction in a turbid medium. Called *photon transport*, the technique takes advantage of the known statistical behavior related to movement of an electrically neutral particle in the presence of multiple scattering sites. This approach usually ignores wave-like phenomena such as diffraction, interference, and polarization.[8] While the foundation of this technique was developed to predict neutron behavior in a nuclear reactor, its application to laser-tissue interaction has been well validated [1].

2.4.1   Transport Theory

The general equation used to describe photon transport is called the *transport equation*, which is given as

$$\frac{dL(\mathbf{r},\hat{\mathbf{s}})}{ds} = -\mu_a L(\mathbf{r},\hat{\mathbf{s}}) - \mu_s L(\mathbf{r},\hat{\mathbf{s}})$$
$$+ \int_{4\pi} p(\hat{\mathbf{s}},\hat{\mathbf{s}}')L(\mathbf{r},\hat{\mathbf{s}}')\,d\omega' + S(\mathbf{r},\hat{\mathbf{s}}) \tag{12}$$

where L is the radiance (mW/cm^2 · sr) in unit direction s at position $\mathbf{r}$, p is the phase function related to g, and S is the light source term (mW/cm^3 · sr) for power generated at position $\mathbf{r}$ in direction $\hat{s}$. In the notation above, an infinitesimal solid angle swept around direction $\hat{s}'$ is represented by $d\omega'$. Note that time as a variable is implicitly present in Equation 12, since L and S are defined in terms of power, which is energy per unit time. Some authors refer to Equation 12 as the *time-dependent radiative transport equation*.

Basically, Equation 12 predicts the spatial gradient of the radiance at position $\mathbf{r}$ in direction $\square$, which in compact vector calculus notation (see the chapter Appendix) would be $\left[\hat{s}\cdot\nabla L(\mathbf{r},\hat{s})\right]$. A reduction in radiance due to absorption and scattering is shown by the first two terms of the equation; the third and fourth terms show any increase in the radiance, all at position $\mathbf{r}$ in direction s. Specifically, the third term includes light scattered from all other directions s' into direction s, and the fourth term includes any primary irradiance, internal fluorescence, or other internal light source which might be present. The scattering phase function $p(\hat{s},\hat{s}')$ is a normalized probability density function. The probability weighted (i.e., "expected") cosine of the scattering angle is defined as g, the anisotropy factor. That is,

$$g = \int\limits_{4\pi} p(\hat{s},\hat{s}')(\hat{s}\cdot\hat{s}')\,d\omega \qquad (13)$$

which predicts the forward scattering found in tissue. Some commonly used phase functions used for the prediction of scattering in tissue are the Henyey-Greenstein, modified Henyey-Greenstein, and delta-Eddington [1].

While the transport equation describes the light distribution in tissue effectively, it is difficult to use in practical applications. Thus simpler models have been devised.

2.4.2 Simplified Models

If one is primarily interested in predicting reflection or transmission of laser light through tissue, simplified models may be used that are derived from transport theory. Two examples are the one-dimensional *Adding-Doubling Method* and the *Diffusion Approximation*.

Adding-Doubling Method. The *adding-doubling method* provides an analytical one-dimensional solution to the transport equation (Equation 12), and is based upon single scattering through thin layers that are added together. This model is characterized by restrictions on the time-dependent radiative transport equation which include:

- no time dependence,
- a geometry limited to uniform parallel layers of tissue with finite thickness in the z direction and infinite size in the x and y directions,
- each tissue layer has constant absorption and scattering coefficients, and
- uniform illumination by collimated or diffuse light.

While these restrictions limit the situations in which this method may be used, it is the most accurate model available.

Half of this technique, the *doubling* method, was first proposed by van de Hulst [27] and assumes knowledge of the reflection and transmission properties of an optically thin slab of tissue. For a slab twice as thick, two of the thin slabs are "stacked" one on top of the other and the contributions from each layer are summed. By adding an arbitrary number of thin slabs on top of one another and summing the contributions, a layer of any thickness can be modeled. The *adding* half of the technique extends the doubling method for use with dissimilar layers, allowing more complex tissue models and taking into account the possibility of reflections at layer boundaries [1].

This is the model of choice for evaluation of the optical properties such as μ_a and μ_s' of a thin tissue sample, based upon measurements of reflectance and transmittance.

Diffusion Approximation Model.   The search to find a useful approximation to the transport equation (Equation 12) that could be used to calculate fluences inside the tissue volume led researchers to the topic of diffusion. It can be shown that diffusion theory can be derived as an approximate solution to the transport equation [1]. This model provides a reasonably accurate prediction of light propagation in turbid media such as tissue where $\mu_s \gg \mu_a$. When the geometry involved is simple, such as a layered tissue geometry similar to that described in Section 2.4.2, the diffusion approximation yields an exact closed-form solution that provides not only reflection and transmission but also internal fluences. For more complicated tissue geometries, the diffusion approximation model can be solved using iterative numerical techniques. Both time-dependent and steady-state solutions are available. In this chapter, we describe the steady-state solution [1].

This useful model makes use of the first two moments of the transport equation to yield the diffusion approximation, which is given as:

$$\nabla^2 \phi_s(\mathbf{r}) - 3\mu_a \mu_{tr} \phi_s(\mathbf{r}) \\ + 3\mu_s \mu_{tr} E(\mathbf{r}, \hat{\mathbf{s}}_0) - 3\mu_s g \nabla \cdot \left[E(\mathbf{r}, \hat{\mathbf{s}}_0) \hat{\mathbf{s}}_0 \right] = 0 \tag{14}$$

using the shorthand notation of vector calculus (see the chapter Appendix for a brief review). In Equation 14, $\phi_s\,(\mathbf{r})$ is the fluence rate of scattered light at point $\mathbf{r}$ in the tissue, μ_a is the absorption coefficient, μ_{tr} is the reduced attenuation coefficient (sometimes called the transport attenuation coefficient) where $\mu_{tr} = \mu_a + (1 - g)\mu_s$, μ_s is the scattering coefficient, $E(\mathbf{r},\hat{\mathbf{s}}_0)$ is the nonscattered and nonabsorbed primary irradiance at point $\mathbf{r}$ in the tissue, g is the anisotropy factor, and $\hat{\mathbf{s}}_0$ is the direction of propagation for unscattered light.

The solution for the one-dimensional form of the diffusion approximation is typically expressed in terms of μ_{eff}, called the *effective attenuation coefficient*, which describes the expected far field decrease of light in a typical scattering medium. If the diffusion approximation is valid for the given tissue geometry, then $\mu_{eff} = \sqrt{3\mu_a\mu_{tr}}$. See [1] for solutions of specific one-dimensional geometries.

As stated above, the diffusion approximation can be solved for many useful tissue geometries, providing a good description of light propagation in tissue. While it is sometimes a poor approximation of the transport equation at points very close to tissue boundaries or light sources, and is difficult to apply to complex geometries, researchers are still exploring variations on the technique to improve its fidelity and ease of use [1].

2.5   MONTE CARLO SIMULATION OF LASER-TISSUE INTERACTION

In this section we discuss a method which can be used to model nearly any type of tissue geometry and laser beam characteristics. It can provide information about reflection, transmission, and fluences at any point in tissue.

2.5.1   The Probabilistic Approach

When trying to predict the results of laser-tissue interaction, we have previously discussed the fact that some method of calculating the associated light distribution in tissue is needed. Relying on Maxwell's equations is exceedingly cumbersome [1], and the uncertainty of known tissue properties makes the effort toward an exact solution in this manner less motivating. As discussed in Section 2.4, there has been impressive research to date creating analytical approximations to the solution, such as the diffusion approximation. While considerably more tractable than the exact solution, they are still relatively difficult to implement and solve in closed form on a general purpose computer, especially when complex geometry such as a buried blood vessel must be taken into account. See [1, 28] for additional background.

A different approach relies on the Monte Carlo technique [29] to create a probabilistic model of light propagation in tissue [30]. This method simulates the "random walk" of photons in a turbid medium that contains absorption and scattering sites, using the known rules that govern photon movement in tissue.

Controlling parameters such as the mean free path length s of the photon, whether or not a scattering event or absorbing event occurs, and the scattering angle can all be determined probabilistically using the known optical properties discussed in Section 2.3.1 and the predicted probability distribution of the event. The Monte Carlo method maps the probability of the various photon events to uniform probability distributions which are easily generated by computer. This mapping is shown graphically in Figure 7, where $p(s)$ represents the known probability density function of a photon event (and $F(s)$ is the associated probability distribution function), and where $p(\zeta)$ is the uniform probability density function of computer generated random numbers between zero and one (and $F(\zeta)$ is the associated probability distribution function). By setting the value of $F(\zeta)$ equal to the random number ζ_1, a value s_1 is selected by the inverse solution of $F(s)$. In effect, the computer "rolls the dice" (i.e., generates a pseudorandom number ζ in the range of 0 to 1) for each decision which must be made regarding photon propagation.

The probability distribution for various events which may occur to a photon traveling through tissue can be estimated from the assumptions we made about light propagation [31]. For example, in Equation 8 the attenuation of light (as it passes through tissue) is described in terms of the total attenuation coefficient μ_t. It can be shown that evaluation of the probability density function $p(s)$ for a particular path length s_1 that a photon would traverse before a scattering or absorption event occurs has the form of

$$p(s_1) = \mu_t e^{-\mu_t s_1} \tag{15}$$

where $p(s)$ is similar to that shown in Figure 7. The probability $P(s < s_1)$ that the path length s for a given photon is *less than* some value s_1 is found by evaluating the probability distribution function $F(s)$ for a particular value s_1 which has the form of

$$F(s_1) = P(s < s_1) = \int_0^{s_1} \mu_t e^{-\mu_t s}\, ds = 1 - e^{-\mu_t s_1} \tag{16}$$

where $F(s)$ is as shown in Figure 7. Since we are equating the $F(\zeta)$ plot to what would be the value from the $F(s)$ plot in Figure 7, we can relate some path length s_1 to the computer generated pseudorandom number ζ_1.

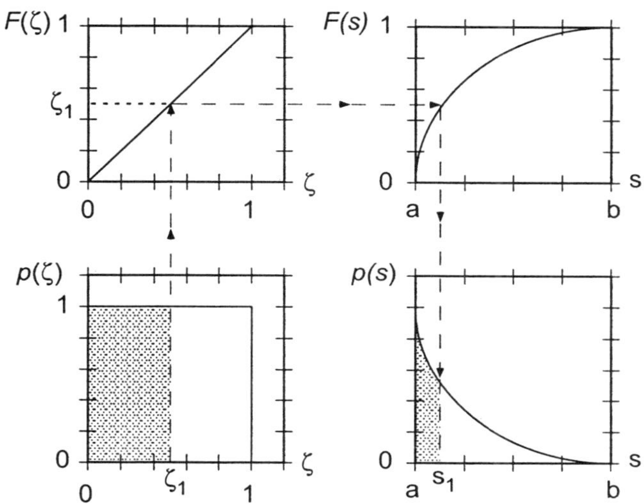

Figure 7. Monte Carlo method of mapping a computer generated pseudorandom number, having probability density $p(\zeta)$, to the actual probability density $p(s)$ of a photon event in tissue (adapted from [31]).

As shown in Figure 7, we can now conclude that to find a probabilistic path length s_1 we use

$$\zeta_1 = 1 - e^{-\mu_t s_1} \tag{17}$$

which can be rearranged to yield

$$s_1 = -\frac{\ln(1-\zeta_1)}{\mu_t} \tag{18}$$

for the desired path length.[9] Note that each time a new ζ_1 is generated, a new path length s_1 is found.

Using a similar logic, it can be shown [31] that we can use two new random numbers (both called ζ) to generate the probabilistic angle θ and azimuth ψ after a scattering event as depicted in Figure 4.

Without derivation, we state that

$$\theta = \arccos\left(\left\{\begin{array}{ll} \dfrac{1}{2g}\left[1+g^2-\left(\dfrac{1-g^2}{1-g+2g\zeta}\right)^2\right] & \text{for } |g|>0 \\ \\ 2\zeta-1 & \text{for } g=0 \end{array}\right.\right) \tag{19}$$

based upon the Henyey-Greenstein probability density function for Mie scattering (where the size of scattering particles are on the order of a wavelength), and where g is the anisotropy factor. Also without derivation, we find that

$$\psi = 2\pi\zeta \tag{20}$$

which is not dependent upon g.

2.5.2 Simulating Photon Propagation in Tissue

The computer simulates photons propagating through tissue by "following" each photon until it is either absorbed or it exits the tissue. Let us briefly examine this procedure, starting with a "new" photon being initialized (i.e., the computer simulates that a new photon was sent out of the laser source along the direction of the laser beam). It's typical in simulations of this type to assume the z-axis is normal (i.e., perpendicular) to the tissue surface, and that the origin point $(x,y,z) = (0,0,0)$ is where the center of the beam meets the tissue surface. The actual direction of a given photon at any place in the simulation is tracked by what are called the *direction cosines* designated μ_x, μ_y, and μ_z, (new direction cosines after scattering are calculated from θ, ψ, and from the previous direction cosines) which, taken together with the magnitude s_1 of the photon path, yield the complete photon path vector **s**. The direction, location, and number of photons launched depend upon the beam characteristics; see [31] for specific techniques to account for a variety of situations. The reader may find the example flowchart shown in Figure 8 to be of some help in following the discussion below which describes the simulation procedure.

At a tissue boundary (where the index of refraction n changes), the photon is either reflected at angle θ_1 or it moves across the boundary in a new direction θ_2 as depicted in Figure 3. The decision regarding reflection or transmission is made by comparing a new pseudorandom number ζ to the reflection coefficient R calculated from Equation 5. If $\zeta \leq R$, then this particular photon reflected from the surface; otherwise the photon must have transmitted through the boundary. For the boundary at the air-tissue interface, if the photon reflects back into air the computer is finished with this photon and a new photon is initialized. When a photon passes into tissue, the simulated path length s in the new medium is determined by generating a new ζ and calculating the value s_1 from Equation 18. The new direction for this path **s** is determined by Snell's law (Equation 4), and μ_x, μ_y, and μ_z, are updated accordingly. The photon is "moved" along this path by updating its position to a point at distance s_1 in the appropriate direction from the current position. If another boundary is crossed due to this path, the preceding logic is repeated at the new boundary. Otherwise, the computer must decide whether the photon is absorbed or scattered at this new location. This decision is made by comparing a new ζ to the albedo $a = \mu_s / \mu_t$; if $\zeta \le a$, then the photon must scatter, otherwise it is absorbed. If scattered, new values for s_1, θ, and ψ are generated using Equations 18, 19, and 20, which are then used to update the direction cosines μ_x, μ_y and μ_z determine a new path vector **s**, and to "move" the photon to the new location. If absorbed, the computer increments the absorption counter for that location in the tissue and starts over with a new photon. This type of logic keeps repeating until every photon is either absorbed or exits the tissue.

2.5.3 Algorithm Considerations

As described above, the computer makes various decisions as to the photon path based upon the underlying probabilities, and keeps track of the location and number of absorption events in the tissue. The overall program logic for this Monte Carlo simulation is shown in Figure 8. Note that there are six places in the flow chart where a new pseudorandom number ζ must be generated by the computer each and every time the logic flow encounters that item. A high quality pseudorandom number generator algorithm is thus vital to a good simulation.

The specific simulation program details are beyond the scope of this introductory treatment. See [31, 32] for an excellent discussion of all the implementation issues. The Monte Carlo technique is rigorous yet statistical in nature, and therefore provides a useful simulation only for a large sample size of photons. For example, 3000 photons can yield an acceptable result when seeking only the expected reflection from tissue, but in order to map the three dimensional spatial light distributions inside tissue can require 10,000–100,000 photons or more [1]. Some researchers regularly use 1,000,000 photons per simulation for particularly complex sensor geometries and fiber delivery systems. Given the power of today's desktop computers, this is not an obstacle.

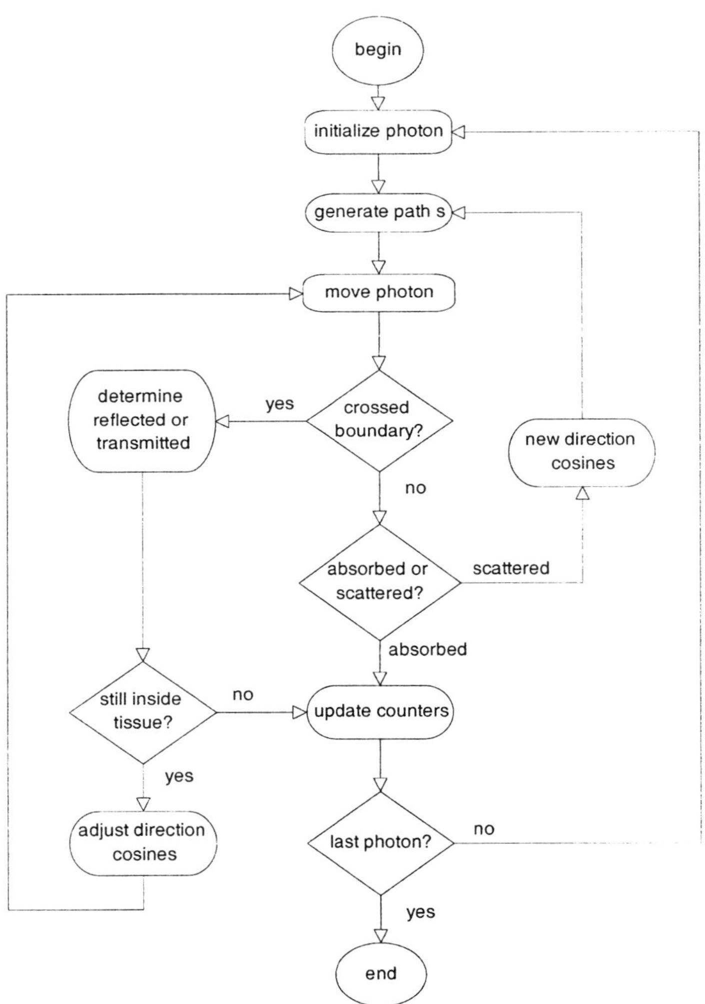

Figure 8. Simplified flow chart of computer-based decisions for a fixed-weight variable-distance Monte Carlo simulation of laser-tissue interaction.

Rest assured the reader does not need to program these algorithms from scratch; programs which implement this type of simulation have been made available to the public. Arguably the best Monte Carlo software for laser-tissue interaction can be found at Dr. Lihong Wang's Web site [33].

2.5.4 Time-Resolved Photon Propagation

Note that in the above description of the Monte Carlo simulation technique, no direct mention was made of time. Each photon is treated as a neutral particle, with the more wave-like phenomena such as polarization and interference ignored in favor of energy transport. This approach has proven to be quite useful, and is based upon the large body of work describing neutron transport in nuclear reactors [1].

If a time-resolved simulation is needed, the key is to apply the implicitly known photon velocity to the Monte Carlo simulation method. Recall that the tissue index of refraction n is simply the ratio of the velocity of light in a vacuum to the velocity of light in the tissue. Therefore, the photon velocity in tissue is $v = c/n$, where $c = 3 \times 10^8$ m/s (or 3×10^{10} cm/s) is the speed of light in a vacuum. For example, given some typical soft tissue with $n = 1.37$, the reader should verify that $v = 2.2 \times 10^{10}$ cm/s.

If a path length s_1 is assumed, then the time to traverse this linear path is just $t_1 = s_1/v$. The most common technique of making a time-resolved simulation is to use fixed time increments Δt. As the simulation runs each photon through the various paths of randomly generated length s, the simulation determines how much time would have transpired. When the time increment Δt is reached, the current path length is truncated and any absorption events that occurred in the last time increment are stored with a time tag. How the halted photon is treated depends upon the specifics of the simulation code; some programs resume the photon and others give it a weighted absorption at the halted location. See [1] for more detail. Time-resolved modifications can also be made in a similar way to analytical models such as the diffusion approximation.

Note that time-resolved simulations are generating more interest as photonic instrumentation limits are being pushed back [34]. For a known tissue thickness and index of refraction, the travel time for a photon to traverse a direct path through the tissue with no scattering events can be calculated. A photon taking longer must have been scattered. Using a sensitive photon detector, a fast stable clock, and a short time pulse laser, the detector could be "gated" such that it only detects photons which have path lengths no longer than the direct, or unscattered, path length. A clear image of inside the tissue can be assembled given that the scattered photons having path lengths significantly longer than the direct path length have been "removed" from the image.

2.6 THERMAL AND MECHANICAL DAMAGE OF TISSUE

As stated earlier, the two primary purposes for irradiating tissue with a laser are (1) diagnostic and (2) therapeutic. While no permanent change to tissue occurs in the diagnostic realm, the ultimate objective of the therapeutic use of lasers is to cause some sort of damage to tissue in a controlled manner that is ultimately beneficial to the patient. The amount and type of damage is dependent primarily upon the power density and the irradiation time; a generalized relationship between the two is shown graphically in Figure 9 for typical soft tissue. This section introduces the basics of the two primary types of tissue damage due to lasers: thermal and mechanical. Ablation (tissue removal) is discussed in both categories, referred to as thermal ablation versus photoablation. While the latter shows little or no evidence of thermal effects in surrounding tissue, most researchers agree that thermal effects also play a significant role in photoablation. Its treatment as a separate category is for clarity of the discussion.

2.6.1 Laser Induced Thermal Effects on Tissue

In general, predicting thermal damage to tissue due to laser irradiation involves three steps: (1) modeling the propagation and distribution of light within the tissue, (2) estimating the temperature rise and distribution in the tissue, and (3) predicting the thermal damage that would result. The first step is covered in previous sections. Steps two and three will be discussed here.

Estimating Temperature Rise.   As previously noted, heat is generated in tissue when photons are absorbed. The larger the absorption coefficient (μ_a), the greater the number of photons that will be absorbed for a given fluence rate, with consequently greater heat generation in the tissue. The basic relationship is

$$S(\mathbf{r}) = \mu_a(\mathbf{r})\phi(\mathbf{r}) \tag{21}$$

where $S(\mathbf{r})$ is the heat source term (mW/cm^3), which should not be confused with the light source term from Equation 12, $\mu_a(\mathbf{r})$ is the absorption coefficient (cm^{-1}), and $\phi(\mathbf{r})$ is the fluence rate (mW/cm^2), all at point $\mathbf{r}$ in the tissue.

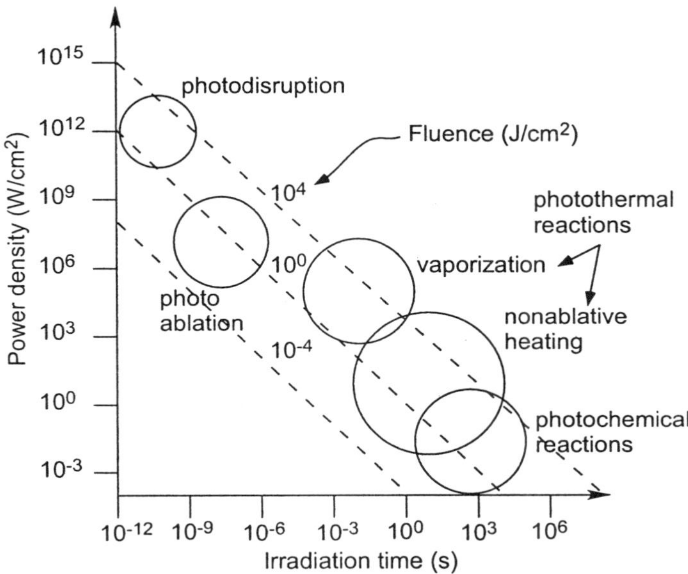

Figure 9. Laser-tissue interaction regimes for various power densities and irradiation times in typical soft tissue. Adapted from [2].

In most cases of laser-tissue irradiation, a reasonable assumption is that convection, radiation, vaporization, and metabolic heat effects are negligible. Given that and the known rate of heat generation from the source term, the change in temperature can be calculated by using energy balance of the traditional *bioheat equation*:

$$\rho c \frac{\partial T(\mathbf{r},t)}{\partial t} = \nabla \cdot \left[k_m \nabla T(\mathbf{r},t)\right] + S(\mathbf{r}) + \rho c w (T_a - T_v) \qquad (22)$$

where ρ is the tissue density (g/cm^3), c is the tissue specific heat (mJ/g · °C), $T(\mathbf{r},t)$ is the tissue temperature (°C) at time t, k_m is the thermal conductivity (mW/cm · °C), $S(\mathbf{r})$ is the heat source term (mW/cm^3), w is the tissue perfusion[10] rate (g/cm^3 · s), T_a is the inlet arterial temperature (°C), and T_v is the outlet venus temperature (°C), all at point $\mathbf{r}$ in the tissue. Note that we assume the source term is stationary over the time interval of heating. Some authors write Equation 22 using the factor $\alpha_m = k_m / \rho c$, which is the thermal diffusivity (cm^2/s). The term on the left of the equal sign of Equation 22 is obviously the change in temperature over time at point **r** in the tissue, the first term to the right of the equal sign describes any heat conduction (typically away from point **r**), and the source term accounts for heat generated due to photon absorption. In most cases of laser tissue heating, the heat transfer due to perfusion as indicated by the right most term is negligible and can be ignored.

The bioheat equation must be solved subject to appropriate initial and boundary conditions. The initial condition is the tissue temperature which exists at time $t = 0$. The boundary conditions depend upon many factors and may take linear or nonlinear forms. Methods of solving Equation 22 are somewhat complex and beyond the scope of this chapter. See [1] for an extensive treatment.

Predicting Thermal Damage.   When tissue is exposed to a high temperature for a prolonged period of time, damage results. It can be shown that this damage may be described mathematically by a rate process equation that defines a damage function Ω [1,35]. This damage function is expressed in terms of an Arrhenius integral:

$$\Omega(\tau) = \ln\left(\frac{C(0)}{C(\tau)}\right) = A\int_0^\tau e^{-\frac{E_a}{RT(t)}}\, dt \tag{23}$$

where τ is the total heating time (s), $C(0)$ is original concentration of undamaged tissue, $C(\tau)$ is the remaining concentration of undamaged tissue after time τ, A is an empirically determined constant (s^{-1}), E_a is an empirically determined activation energy barrier (J/mole), R is the universal gas constant (8.32 J/mole $\cdot$ K), and T is the absolute temperature (K).

Below a certain threshold temperature, called the critical temperature T_{crit}, the rate of damage accumulation is negligible. Diagnostic and photochemical uses of medical lasers keep tissue below T_{crit}. Researchers have found it convenient to define T_{crit} as the temperature where the damage accumulation rate, $d\Omega/dt$, is equal to 1.0:

$$\frac{d\Omega}{dt} = Ae^{-\frac{E_a}{RT_{\mathrm{crit}}}} = 1 \quad \text{thus} \quad T_{\mathrm{crit}} = \frac{E_a}{R\ln(A)}. \tag{24}$$

Different researchers refer to the damage function Ω in slightly different ways. Several authors assume complete tissue necrosis for $\Omega \geq 1$ and no damage for $\Omega < 0.5$; the reader should be aware of these variations. This treatment likely results from an often used method for experimental determination of A and E_a. In this method, several trials are performed where tissue is exposed to a constant temperature, and then those trials are identified for which $C(\tau) = 36.8\%$ of $C(0)$, which means that $\Omega = 1$. The constants A and E_a can then be easily calculated [1]. Using this method for pig skin, researchers determined that $A = 3.1 \times 10^{98}$ and $E_a = 6.28 \times 10^5$, yielding the value $T_{\text{crit}} = 59.7\ ^\circ\text{C}$ [36].

With CW lasers, energy is constantly applied to the tissue. Heat is generated as photons are absorbed and the temperature rises. As the temperature differential between the irradiated and the surrounding tissue increases, conduction of heat away from the absorption point and into the surrounding tissue increases. With pulsed lasers, little heat is usually lost during the time duration of each pulse since absorption is a fast process while conduction is relatively slow.

Depending upon the fluence rate that creates the source term and the tissue properties, equilibrium may be reached at some temperature. If the fluence rate is high enough, temperature will continue to rise until vaporization begins. This requires modifications to Equation 22 to account for enthalpy and latent heat of vaporization.

Categories of Thermal Damage. As tissue temperature rises past T_{crit}, the first form of irreversible damage often observed is *coagulation*, caused primarily by the denaturization of cellular and tissue proteins. Blood, for example, coagulates at $T \approx 60\ ^\circ\text{C}$. Coagulation is visually apparent; most soft tissue tends to "whiten" as the denaturization causes μ_s to increase and more light of all wavelengths is scattered back out of the tissue. A familiar example of this is what happens to egg white when it is cooked. On the other hand, coagulation of collagen-rich tissue such as tendon and skin seems to lower μ_s and they become more transparent. A coagulation bond between tissues is the basis for *tissue welding* used as a replacement for suturing. The regime in which coagulation occurs is depicted as "nonablative heating" in Figure 9.

If the fluence rate causes temperature to continue to rise beyond the range for coagulation, vaporization results. Most tissue has a high water content; at approximately $100\ ^\circ\text{C}$, water vapor is generated and for high fluence rates more vapor is produced than can exit by diffusion. The excess vapor is trapped between tissue layers and begins exerting mechanical stress on the tissue. At this point the tissue temperature hovers around $100\ ^\circ\text{C}$ due to the vapor phase equilibrium. For sufficiently high fluence rates, the trapped vapor becomes superheated, expanding vacuoles are created (called vapor bubbles by many authors), the walls of the vacuoles rupture, and holes are created in the tissue. In the case of slow heating, tissue compression and desiccation result; rapid heating produces explosive ruptures that typically eject tissue fragments via the "popcorn effect" [19]. The now desiccated tissue temperature continues rising to approximately 350–450 °C, and pyrolysis of the tissue results. The combination of intense vaporization, vacuolization, and pyrolysis combine to produce thermal ablation; this phenomenon forms the basis of laser surgical tissue removal. The regime discussed here is depicted as "vaporization" in Figure 9.

2.6.2 Laser Induced Mechanical Effects on Tissue

While mechanical effects can be induced from CW lasers (such as the "popcorn effect" mentioned above), it tends to be more common when using pulsed lasers. Thus this section concentrates on pulsed lasers. We include acoustic damage in the discussion below.

Photoablation.   A disadvantage of thermal ablation with CW lasers is the unintended damage to surrounding tissue. Coagulum around the edge of an ablation crater is known to impede the healing process, for example. Clinicians wish to minimize the collateral damage and to have precise cutting control. Pulsed lasers can deliver in each pulse sufficient energy to ablate tissue, but in a short enough time period that the tissue is removed before any heat is transferred to the surrounding tissue. Thus the resulting tissue removal would appear to be primarily mechanical, although thermal effects are a part of the process. Some pulsed lasers, such as the eximers in the UV range, may involve a photochemical process that causes molecular bonds to be broken and ultimately results in ablation, but other researchers believe even these lasers depend upon photothermal mechanisms.

In general, mechanical effects include thermoelastic expansion of tissue and recoil caused by ejection of ablated material, both of which cause stress waves and shock waves [1]. These waves, along with the vacuole explosions of rapidly expanding vapor bubbles, may aid the ablation process but may also damage surrounding tissue if they are too intense. The recoil effect is significant since, despite the small mass of ejected matter, the process involves a short expulsion time and a high ablation velocity (sometimes greater than twice the speed of sound in air).

To achieve precise cutting control, a laser with a very short penetration depth is used (recall Table 1). An example of extremely precise tissue removal without any thermal damage is the use of the ArF excimer laser (where $\lambda = 193$ nm) for corneal reshaping. The photoablation regime is shown in Figure 9.

Photodisruption.   Another reason clinicians use pulsed lasers is that they provide the ability to ablate or fracture dense tissue such as bone or tooth.

Recall from Section 2.2.2 that lasers which produce very short pulses (typically $\tau < 1$ μs) are capable of extremely high peak power per pulse. In this situation, dielectric breakdown can occur in tissue leading to the formation of high-pressure plasma and large-amplitude stress waves. This effect is used, for example, in laser lithotripsy to fragment urinary calculi (kidney stones), and in ophthalmology to destroy the clouded posterior capsule membrane that often remains after cataract surgery. The photodisruption regime, as depicted in Figure 9, actually extends to shorter pulse times than shown in the figure.

2.7 EXAMPLES OF TISSUE PROPERTIES

2.7.1 Importance of Tissue Properties

It is obvious from the preceding discussions that some knowledge of the optical and thermal properties of tissue are required in order to predict the outcome of laser-tissue interaction. From the simple expression of Beer's Law to the more complex analytical models and Monte Carlo simulations, we need to know optical properties such as index of refraction n, absorption coefficient μ_a, scattering coefficient μ_s, anisotropy factor g, and the quantities derived from these in order to predict the light distribution in laser irradiated tissue. To predict the effect on tissue from the absorption of this distributed light energy, we also need to know something about the thermal properties of tissue such as thermal conductivity k_m, thermal diffusivity α_m, perfusion w (when that effect is nonnegligible), and the constants A and E_a for the damage integral. Reliable estimates of these optical and thermal values are exceedingly hard to measure, but researchers have created many innovative techniques to gather this needed data. The reader should keep in mind three things: (1) the known database of tissue properties is still small but growing, (2) many properties are highly dependent on wavelength, and (3) the properties can vary both spatially within the tissue and temporally due to changes in aspects such as water concentration and temperature.

2.7.2 Optical Properties

Researchers have devised a variety of methods to measure the optical properties of tissue. Techniques may be classified in various ways, such as *in vivo* versus *in vitro*, where the former can be invasive or noninvasive and the latter is usually performed on thin tissue sections. There are *direct* versus *indirect* methods, where the former is independent of any one propagation model, while the latter infers the optical property by solving an "inverse solution" of one of the propagation models. There are photometric techniques (measuring light, which is the most common method) and the less common photothermal or photoacoustic methods.

Actual measurement techniques are well beyond the scope of this chapter, but a brief list of some representative tissue optical properties (shown in Table 2) may give the reader some insight. For more detail, see [1].

Table 2. Approximate optical properties of human tissue. Adapted from [1].

Tissue	λ (nm)	μ_a (cm^{-1})	μ_s (cm^{-1})	g
aorta	632.5	0.52	316	0.87
	1064	0.5	239	0.90
intima	580	8.9	183	0.81
	632.5	3.6	171	0.85
adventitia	580	11.3	217	0.77
	632.5	5.8	195	0.81
brain (white matter)	632.5	2.2	532	0.82
	1064	3.2	469	0.87
brain (gray matter)	632.5	2.7	354	0.94
	1064	5.0	134	0.90
liver	632.5	3.2	414	0.95
myocardium	1064	0.3	178	0.96
dermis	632.5	2.7	187	0.81
uterus	632.5	0.35	394	0.69

Note that, as mentioned before, most tissue is highly forward scattering. While index of refraction n is not given in the table, it has been found that most soft tissue is in the range of $1.3 \leq n \leq 1.5$ at visible and near infrared wavelengths.

2.7.3 Thermal Properties

Thermal properties of tissue used for temperature calculations such as thermal conductivity k_m, thermal diffusivity α_m, and perfusion w, are also challenging to determine. Normally, thermal probe techniques are used [1]. The constants A and E_a needed to evaluate the damage integral are somewhat easier to find as discussed in Section 6.1, but as with optical properties the available database of all thermal properties of tissue is limited but growing.

A brief list of some representative tissue thermal properties may give the reader some insight. While thermal properties are not wavelength dependent, they do change with temperature. Table 3 illustrates the temperature dependence of thermal conductivity k_m and thermal diffusivity α_m. Table 4 shows some typical values for constants A and E_a, and the associated T_{crit} for the damage integral. Values for perfusion are not shown. For more detail, see [1].

Table 3. Approximate thermal properties of human tissue for the bioheat equation. Solve for $k_m = k_0 + k_1 T$ and $\alpha_m = \alpha_0 + \alpha_1 T$, for T in °C. Adapted from [1].

Tissue	k_0 (mW/cm · °C)	k_1 (mW/cm · °C)	α_0 (cm²/s)	α_1 (cm²/s)
cerebral cortex	5.043	0.00296	0.001283	0.000050
liver	4.692	0.01161	0.001279	0.000036
lung	3.080	0.02395	0.001071	0.000082
myocardium	4.925	0.01195	0.001289	0.000050
aorta	3.895	0.02472	0.001085	0.000053

Table 4. Approximate thermal properties of human tissue for the damage integral. Adapted from [1].

Tissue	A (s⁻¹)	E_a (J/mole)	T_{crit} (°C)
skin	3.1×10^{98}	6.28×10^5	59.7
retina	3.1×10^{99}	6.28×10^5	56.0
aorta	5.6×10^{63}	4.30×10^5	78.9

2.8   SUMMARY

This chapter has provided an introductory overview of the rather broad subject of laser-tissue interaction. The field is still in its infancy, as the fine details of many of the controlling mechanisms and processes are still being investigated. However, with the basic understanding provided by this chapter the reader may better appreciate and put in context the information in the following chapters. The authors highly recommend more comprehensive sources [1–5, 37] for a fuller understanding of this topic.

ACKNOWLEDGMENTS

The authors wish to thank the faculty and students associated with the Biomedical Engineering Laser Laboratory (BELL) at The University of Texas at Austin for many fruitful discussions. For more information, please see http://www.ece.utexas.edu/bell/index1.htm.

Appendix: Helpful Mathematical Relations

Solid Angles. Recall that a solid angle ω is defined as an arbitrarily shaped area on the surface of sphere that has unit radius. The total surface area A_T of a sphere with an arbitrary radius r is $A_T = 4\pi r^2$. Thus for any area A on the surface of a sphere with radius r, the associated solid angle ω is given by the expression $\omega = A/r^2$ with the units of ω being steradians (sr). The maximum possible solid angle is obviously 4π steradians.

An infinitesimal solid angle around the direction of unit vector $\hat{s}$ is depicted as $d\omega$. We can express $\hat{s}$ in Cartesian or spherical coordinates, depending upon which is more convenient. Conversion from spherical coordinates to Cartesian coordinates follows the relationship

$$x = r \sin\theta \cos\varphi$$
$$y = r \sin\theta \sin\varphi \qquad (1)$$
$$z = r \cos\theta$$

where r is the magnitude of vector $\mathbf{r}$ which points in the direction of $\hat{s}$, θ is the angle between vector $\mathbf{r}$ and the positive z-axis, and φ is the angle between vector $\mathbf{r}$ and the positive x-axis, assuming the standard right-hand coordinate system. See [1, p. 44] for an excellent illustration. Given the above, we can see that the infinitesimal solid angle $d\omega$ around direction $\hat{s}$, which sweeps over an infinitesimal area $r\,d\theta\,r\sin\theta\,d\varphi$ on the surface of a sphere with radius r, must be as shown below.

$$d\omega = \frac{r\,d\theta\,r\sin\theta\,d\varphi}{r^2} = \sin\theta\,d\theta\,d\varphi \qquad (2)$$

Conversion from Cartesian to spherical coordinates is shown below.

$$r = \sqrt{x^2 + y^2 + z^2} \qquad\qquad (r \geq 0)$$

$$\theta = \arccos\left(\frac{z}{\sqrt{x^2 + y^2 + z^2}}\right) \qquad (0° \leq \theta \leq 180°) \qquad (3)$$

$$\varphi = \arctan\left(\frac{y}{x}\right)$$

Vector Calculus.   Some of the compact notation of vector calculus is used in the preceding sections. For this discussion, we assume right-hand Cartesian coordinates with unit vectors $\hat{\mathbf{x}}$, $\hat{\mathbf{y}}$ and $\hat{\mathbf{z}}$. The unit vector $\hat{\mathbf{s}}$ points in some arbitrary direction. Useful vector calculus relations are given below using an arbitrary scalar function $A(x,y,z)$, abbreviated as simply A, and arbitrary three-dimensional vector $\mathbf{B}$.

The gradient of scalar A is

$$\nabla A = \frac{\partial A}{\partial x}\hat{\mathbf{x}} + \frac{\partial A}{\partial y}\hat{\mathbf{y}} + \frac{\partial A}{\partial z}\hat{\mathbf{z}} \qquad (4)$$

The component of the gradient in the direction of $\hat{\mathbf{s}}$ is simply $\hat{\mathbf{s}} \cdot \nabla A$.

The Laplacian of scalar A is

$$\nabla^2 A = \nabla \cdot \nabla A = \frac{\partial^2 A}{\partial x^2} + \frac{\partial^2 A}{\partial y^2} + \frac{\partial^2 A}{\partial z^2}. \qquad (5)$$

The divergence of vector $\mathbf{B}$ is

$$\nabla \cdot \mathbf{B} = \frac{\partial B_x}{\partial x} + \frac{\partial B_y}{\partial y} + \frac{\partial B_z}{\partial z} \qquad (6)$$

where $B_x = \hat{\mathbf{x}} \cdot \mathbf{B}$, $B_y = \hat{\mathbf{y}} \cdot \mathbf{B}$, and $B_z = \hat{\mathbf{z}} \cdot \mathbf{B}$ are the x, y, and z components of vector $\mathbf{B}$.

Most introductory electromagnetics texts, such as [38], give excellent summaries of vector calculus in more detail than above.

NOTES

1. The first theoretical analysis predicting that a laser could be built was made in 1958 by Arthur L. Schawlow of Stanford University and Charles T. Townes of Columbia University, who called their prediction an *optical maser.*
2. The references given as examples for each category of laser effects on tissue is by no means meant to be complete, only to give a representation of that effect as cited in the literature. See other chapters of this book for more complete references specific to a particular medical application.
3. We will not discuss the arguments of terminology that spring from the fact that reflection, scattering, diffraction, etc., are all manifestations of the same phenomenon. For historical reasons they are traditionally given these different names. See [24, pp. 6.3–6.5] for an interesting discussion.
4. The energy of a photon in Joules is equal to $E = hf$, where $h = 6.626 \times 10^{-34}$ J·s is Planck's constant and f is the frequency of the light in Hz.
5. The "scattering" has also been called a form of diffuse reflection by some authors (since light "reflects" from the scattering site in a variety of directions) and an instance of diffraction by other authors. All are correct in their own interpretation; however, the majority of authors refer to this phenomenon as scattering and we shall do the same.
6. Depending upon one's original training (e.g., optics, physical chemistry, analytical chemistry, etc.), Beer's law may be known as the "Beer-Lambert," the "Lambert-Beer," the "Beer-Lambert-Bouguer," or the "Bouguer-Lambert-Beer," law [40].
7. For a circularly symmetric Gaussian laser beam, the total power contained within a circle of radius r_1 is $\int_0^{r_1} E(r)\, 2\pi r\, dr = P\left[1 - \exp\left(-2\left(r_1 / w_0\right)^2\right)\right]$, where P is the total beam power.
8. Transport theory can include wave-like effects such as polarization [26].
9. With ζ being a uniformly distributed random variable in the range (0,1), we can save computing time by realizing that $\ln(1-\zeta) = \ln(\zeta)$ for the purpose of the simulation.
10. Another common unit of measure for perfusion is mL/100g · min.

REFERENCES

1. A. J. Welch and M. J. C. van Gemert, eds., *Optical-Thermal Response of Laser Irradiated Tissue.* Plenum Press, 1995.
2. A. Katzir, *Lasers and Optical Fibers in Medicine.* Academic Press, 1993.
3. A. J. Welch and M. J. C. van Gemert, "Lasers in Medicine," in Waynant and Ediger [39], ch. 24.
4. S. L. Jacques, ed., *Laser-Tissue Interaction*, vol. I – XI, SPIE Press, 1990–2000. Annual collection of SPIE papers.
5. G. P. Delacretaz *et al.*, eds., *Laser-Tissue Interaction and Tissue Optics*, vol. I – III, SPIE Press, 1996–1998. Annual collection of SPIE papers.
6. J. T. Verdeyen, *Laser Electronics.* Prentice Hall, 3rd ed., 1995.
7. J. Hecht, *Understanding Lasers: An Entry-Level Guide.* IEEE Press, 1992.
8. A. E. Siegman, *Lasers.* University Science Books, 1986.
9. A. Yariv, *Optical Electronics.* Saunders, 4th ed., 1991.
10. B. E. A. Saleh and M. C. Teich, *Fundamentals of Photonics.* John Wiley & Sons, 1991.

11. B. A. Rockwell, D. X. Hammer, R. A. Hopkins, D. J. Payne, C. A. Toth, W. P. Roach, J. J. Druessel, P. K. Kennedy, R. E. Amnotte, B. Eilert, S. Phillips, G. D. Noojin, D. J. Stolarski, and C. P. Cain, "Ultrashort laser pulse bioeffects and safety," *Jour. Laser Appl.*, vol. 11, pp. 42–44, 1999.

12. R. R. Richards-Kortum, R. Rava, M. Fitzmaurice, L. Tong, N. B. Ratcliff, J. R. Kramer, and M. S. Feld, "A one-layer model of laser induced fluorescence for diagnosis of disease in human tissue: Applications to atherosclerosis," *IEEE Trans. Biomed. Eng.*, vol. 36, pp. 1222–1232, 1989.

13. T. J. Dougherty, "Photodynamic therapy: Status and potential," *Oncology*, vol. 3, pp. 67–73, 1989.

14. A. J. Welch, J. A. Pearce, K. R. Diller, G. Yoon, and W. F. Cheong, "Heat generation in laser irradiated tissue," *Trans. ASME*, vol. 111, pp. 62–68, 1989.

15. A. J. Welch, M. Motamedi, S. Rastegar, G. LeCarpentier, and D. Jansen, "Laser thermal ablation," *Photochem. Photobiol.*, vol. 53, no. 6, pp. 815–823, 1991.

16. G. L. LeCarpentier, M. Motamedi, L. P. McMath, S. Rastegar, and A. J. Welch, "Continuous wave laser ablation of tissue: Analysis of thermal and mechanical events," *IEEE Trans. Biomed. Eng.*, vol. 40, pp. 188–201, Feb. 1993.

17. S. F. Cleary, "Laser pulses and the generation of acoustic transients in biological material," in *Laser Applications in Medicine and Biology* (M. L. Wohlbarst, ed.), ch. 3, pp. 175–219, Plenum Press, 1977.

18. A. A. Oraevsky, "Laser-induced acoustic and shock waves in ocular tissues," Tech. Rep. AL/OE-TR-1995-0044, Armstrong Laboratory, Brooks AFB, TX, May 1995.

19. S. Thomsen, "Pathologic analysis of photothermal and photomechanical effects of laser-tissue interactions," *Photochem. Photobiol.*, vol. 53, no. 6, pp. 825–835, 1991.

20. C. H. G. Wright, J. K. Barton, D. E. Protsenko, H. G. Rylander III, and A. J. Welch, "Anomalous reflectance of laser-induced retinal lesions," *IEEE J. Special Topics Quant. Elect.*, vol. 2, pp. 1035–1040, Dec. 1996.

21. E. Hecht, *Optics.* Addison-Wesley, 2nd ed., 1987.

22. M. Born and E. Wolf, *Principles of Optics: Electromagnetic Theory of Propagation, Interference, and Diffraction of Light.* Pergamon Press, 6th (corrected) ed., 1986.

23. F. L. Pedrotti and L. S. Pedrotti, *Introduction to Optics.* Prentice Hall, 2nd ed., 1993.

24. M. Bass, ed., *Handbook of Optics*, vol. 1. McGraw-Hill, 2nd ed., 1995.

25. J. D. Enderle, S. M. Blanchard, and J. D. Bronzino, *Introduction to Biomedical Engineering.* Academic Press, 2000.

26. A. Ishimaru, *Wave Propagation and Scattering in Random Media*, vol. 1. Academic Press, 1978.

27. H. C. van de Hulst, *Light Scattering by Small Particles.* Dover, 1981.

28. S. A. Prahl, *Light Transport in Tissue.* Ph.D. dissertation, The University of Texas at Austin, 1988.

29. J. M. Hammersley and D. C. Handscomb, *Monte Carlo Methods.* London: Methuen, 1964.

30. M. Keijzer, S. L. Jacques, S. A. Prahl, and A. J. Welch, "Light distributions in artery tissue: Monte Carlo simulations for finite diameter laser beams," *Lasers Surg. Med.*, pp. 148–154, 1989.

31. S. L. Jacques and L. Wang, "Monte Carlo modeling of light transport in tissues," in Welch and van Gemert [1], ch. 4, pp. 73–100.

32. L. Wang, S. L. Jacques, and L.-Q. Zheng, "MCML: Monte Carlo modeling of photon transport in multi-layered tissues," *Computer Methods and Programs in Biomedicine*, vol. 47, pp. 131–146, 1995.

33. L. Wang, "Monte Carlo simulation package: Software for laser-tissue interaction studies." URL: `http://oilab.tamu.edu/mc.html`, 2000. Texas A&M University Optical Imaging Laboratory.

34. P. C. Jackson, H. Key, and P. N. T. Wells, "Transillumination imaging," in *Optronic Techniques in Diagnostic and Therapeutic Medicine* (R. Pratesi, ed.), pp. 101–115, Plenum Press, 1991.

35. F. C. Henriques, "Studies of thermal injury V: The predicability and significance of thermally induced rate processes leading to irreversible epidermal injury," *Arch. Pathology*, vol. 43, no. 12, pp. 489–502, 1947.

36. J. A. Pearce and S. Thomsen, "Rate process analysis of thermal damage," in Welch and van Gemert [1], ch. 17, pp. 561–606.

37. S. A. Prahl and S. L. Jacques, "Oregon Medical Laser Center website." URL: `http://omlc.ogi.edu`, 2000. Oregon Graduate Institute of Science and Technology.

38. J. D. Kraus, *Electromagnetics*. McGraw-Hill, 4th ed., 1992.

39. R. W. Waynant and M. N. Ediger, eds., *Electro-Optics Handbook*. McGraw-Hill, 1994.

40. D. N. Lapedes, ed., *Dictionary of Scientific and Technical Terms*. McGraw-Hill, 1976.

Chapter 3

LASER OPHTHALMOLOGY

Steven F. Barrett[1], Cameron H. G. Wright[2] and Ashley J. Welch[3]
[1]Department of Electrical and Computer Engineering, University of Wyoming, U.S.A.
[2]Department of Electrical Engineering, U.S. Air Force Academy, Colorado, U.S.A.
[3]Department of Electrical and Computer Engineering, University of Texas at Austin, U.S.A.

3.1   INTRODUCTION

Lasers have been employed in ophthalmology since their inception over four decades ago. In this chapter we will investigate many of these exciting applications. The chapter begins with a brief review of the characteristics of the human eye including eye anatomy and movements, visual refractive errors, and fixation capability. We will then briefly review laser interaction with eye tissue followed by a detailed look at therapeutic and diagnostic applications of lasers in ophthalmology. The chapter concludes with new laser technologies now on the horizon.

3.2   CHARACTERISTICS OF THE HUMAN EYE

In this section we will investigate the anatomy and characteristics of the human eye pertinent to laser applications. We will begin with a review of the gross anatomy of the eye followed by a detailed look at both the cornea and the retina. We will then discuss eye movements and fixation capability followed by characteristics of the aging eye.

3.2.1 Gross Anatomical Structure

Eyes are the complex sense organs of the visual system. The adult eye is somewhat like a fluid filled globe approximating a spherical shape measuring 24 mm long by 22 mm across [1], as shown in Figure 1. The shell includes the cornea and the sclera, with the semi-spherical optically clear cornea being

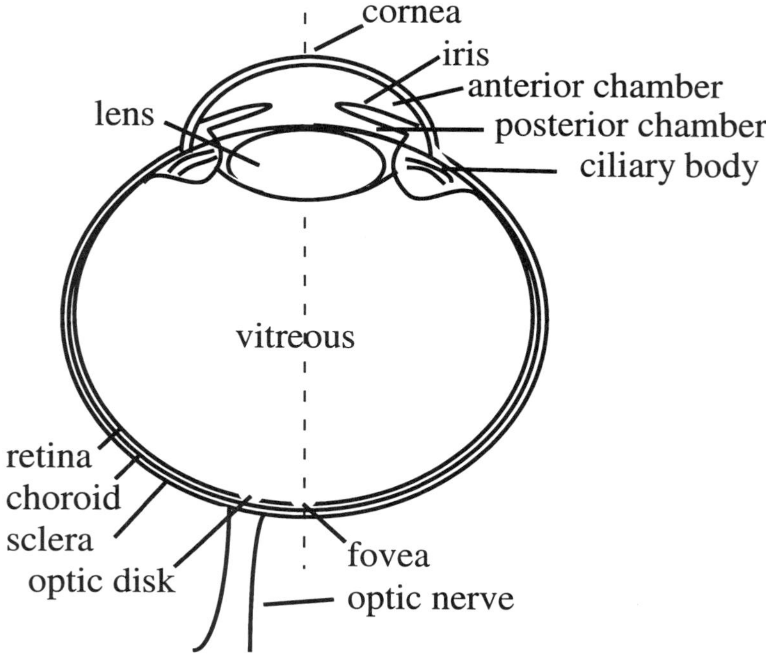

Figure 1. Horizontal section of the right eye. Adapted from [2].

joined to the white sclera. The firm, acellular sclera protects the eye and anchors the muscles that move the eye. The posterior of the eye consists of the sclera, choroid, pigment epithelium (**PE**), and the retina. The choroid provides structural support and contains blood vessels. The black pigment of the **PE** minimizes light reflection that would distort vision. The retina makes up part of the eye's inner wall. It is the layer upon which a light image is focused. Light sensitive cells in the retina, the rods and cones, translate light energy into nerve impulses [2]. The cones which are responsible for acute vision are densely concentrated in the fovea and the rods are dispersed through out the remaining retina.

There are three main fluid-filled chambers in the eye. The anterior and posterior chambers are separated by the iris, and are filled with a watery fluid called the aqueous humor. This fluid is derived from blood plasma. The vitreous body (also called the vitreous humor) is the gel that fills the cavity between the lens and the retina. This gel has an electrolyte composition similar to that of the aqueous humor and contains protein fibers [2].

A small portion of light striking the eye is reflected and the remaining light is refracted because of the mismatch in index of refraction of the air and cornea. After light passes through the cornea and the iris (which controls the amount of light reaching the retina) it passes through the lens. The lens contributes to the focusing of the light on the retina. The lens which consists of a membrane sac filled with a gel is biconvex and transparent. Its shape is changed by a group of ring-shaped muscles in the ciliary body. Relaxation of the ciliary muscles increases tension on the lens by tightening the zonular fibers, causing it to flatten [2].

3.2.1.1 The Cornea

The cornea accounts for 70 percent of the refractive power of the eye (45 diopters). The different eye structures have similar refraction indices. The largest difference in refraction index n that light encounters is when it passes from the air outside the eye $n = 1$ to the cornea n = 1.38 [3].

The cornea in a normal eye is transparent and perfectly curved. As shown in Figure 2, it has a convex, external surface and a concave internal surface.

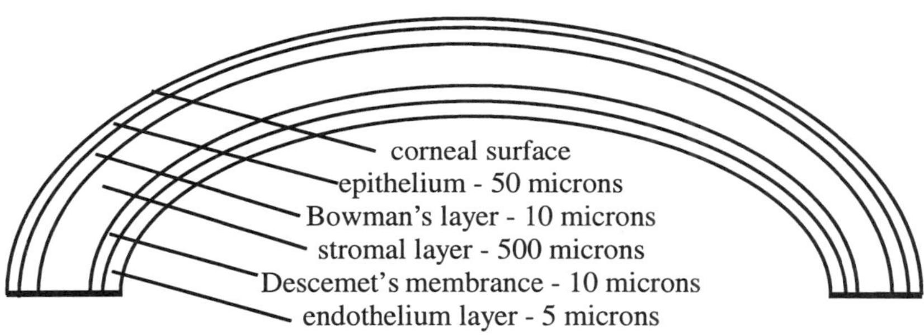

Figure 2. Corneal layers [4].

The epithelium, 50 microns thick, is the most anterior layer of the cornea. Bowman's layer, 8-14 µm thick, lies between the epithelium and the stroma, which comprises 90 percent of the cornea's thickness. The stroma is optically clear and contains collagen fibers. Decemet's membrane and the endolthelium are the two most posterior layers of the cornea. Decemet's membrane is a tough layer that helps protect the endothelium. Although the cells of the epithelium, Bowman's layer and stroma are renewable, the cells of the endothelium are not. Destruction of the endothelium causes loss of transparency and must be avoided during ophthalmic procedures [3,4].

3.2.1.2 The Retina

The retina consists of ten layers. The posterior layer contains the rods and the cones. Other retinal layers contain four types of neurons: bipolar cells, ganglion cells, horizontal cells, and amacrine cells. The rods and cones coupled with the neurons provide a matrix of receptors with converging links to the optic nerve. The rods and cones synapse with bipolar cells, the bipolars cells synapse with the ganglion cells, and the ganglion cells converge to form the optic nerve. The optic nerve routes the visual information from the eye to the occipital cortex of the brain [2].

The retinal features visible by a fundus camera form distinct visible landmarks as shown in Figure 3. The most visible feature on the retinal surface is

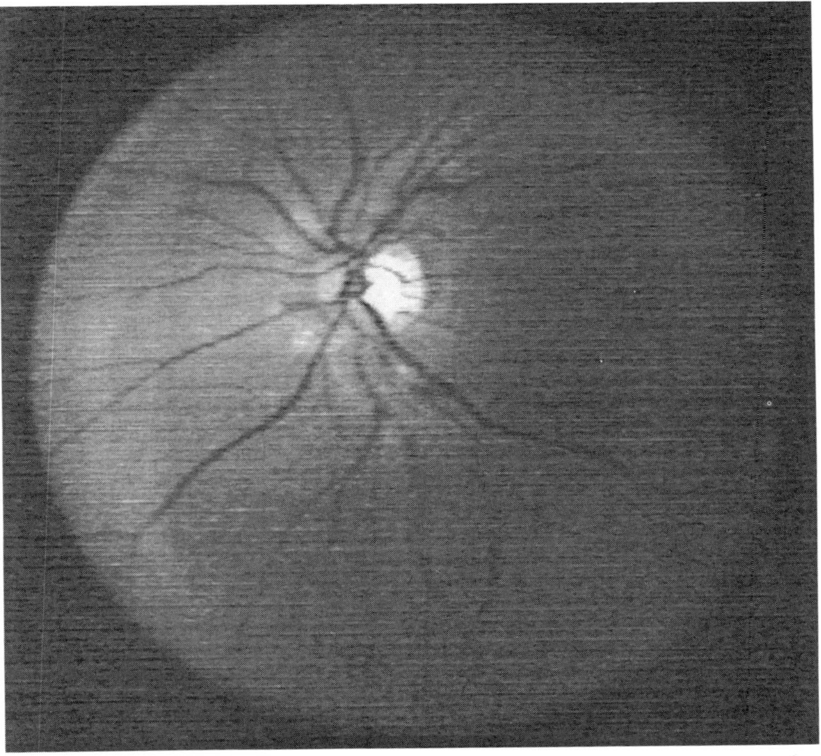

Figure 3. The visible retinal surface as viewed from a fundus camera. Retinal vessels were enhanced by illuminating the retina with narrowband green light.

the optic disk. The optic disk is the point at which blood vessels enter the eye and spread over the surface of the retina. It is also the point where nerves from the retina meet and exit the eye as the optic nerve as discussed above. The exact dimensions of the optic disk vary slightly by race, eye, and sex. The mean horizontal axis of the left optic disk is 1.88 mm (standard deviation 0.18) with a mean vertical axis of 1.77 mm (standard deviation 0.19). The right optic disk has similar dimensions [5,6].

Near the optic disk is the fovea which is the area of acute vision due to its high concentration of cone photoreceptors. The fovea is approximately 300~ µm in diameter and it must be protected from damage. A single laser pulse to the fovea can result in permanent degradation of acute vision or even blindness. The center of the fovea, the foveola, is located 3.42 mm ± 0.34 mm) temporally and inferiorly to the horizontal axis of the optic disk [7]. The macula, with a 5000 µm diameter, surrounds the fovea. The retinal vessel network surrounding the optic disk and fovea is called the arcades. It is also visible from the retinal surface. Retinal vessels range in size from 50 µm to 250 µm [8].

3.2.2 Eye Movements

Eye movement is controlled by external ocular muscles. These muscles include the lateral rectus muscles for looking to the side, the medial rectus muscles for looking toward the nose, the superior rectus muscle for looking up, the inferior rectus muscle for looking down and the superior and inferior oblique muscle for depressing and elevating the gaze respectively. These muscles act in a coordinated fashion to affect the different types of eye movement. Certain eye movements suffer age related degradation. Generally, eye movements slow with advancing age. The following paragraphs detail the different types of eye movements [2].

3.2.2.1 Saccades

Saccadic eye movements are rapid with velocities of up to 800 degrees per second for visual target acquisition. These movements rapidly propel the point of visual fixation from one target to another in the visual field. They are typically of short duration, lasting from 20 to 200 milliseconds, and are ballistic in nature. Most naturally occurring saccades are less than 15 degrees. For larger eye movements the head may also move [9].

3.2.2.2 Smooth Pursuit and Vergence Movements

Smooth pursuit and vergence movements are for tracking movements to follow a slowly moving object. These movements maintain the image of moving object on the fovea of each eye. The vergence system maintains the image on the fovea as an object moves toward or away from the observer and the smooth pursuit system tracks objects with horizontal or vertical movement. Both of these systems are slow compared to the saccadic system. The smooth pursuit system can accurately track up to approximately 50 degrees per second [9].

3.2.2.3   Optokinetic and Vestibular-Ocular Movements

The optokinetic and the vestibular-ocular systems are used to compensate for observer motion. These systems maintain stable vision as a person moves. These systems work together to provide accurate compensation for head movement over a wide range [9].

3.2.2.4   Micro-saccades and Micronystagmus Movements

Micro-saccadic movements are required to maintain visibility of stationary objects due to image fading. These small movements occur approximately every second and shift the gaze by 5 to 10 minutes of arc. These movements are difficult to suppress. Micronystagmus are oscillatory movements at rates of approximately 0.02 Hertz and amplitudes up to approximately 1 minute of arc. From an engineering point of view these movements may be regarded as system noise [3].

3.2.2.5   Eye Fixation Capability

Human visual fixation is provided by a negative feedback mechanism. This mechanism prevents the point of visual fixation from leaving the area of the fovea on the retinal surface. When a spot of light is focused on the fovea micronystagmus movements cause the spot to move back and forth across the cones. Each time the spot reaches the edge of the fovea a micro-saccade occurs bringing the spot back to the central foveal region. Studies conducted by Kosnik, Fikre, and Sekuler with untrained psychophysical observers indicate that fixation stability does not degrade significantly with age. They define fixation stability using a contour ellipse of the scatter of eye positions about its mean position. The area of the ellipses is expressed in minutes of arc squared. The young group (mean age = 22 years) have a mean ellipse area of 165 min of arc^2 (standard deviation 90.2) while the older group (mean age = 70 years) have a mean ellipse area of 198 min of arc^2 (standard deviation 90.4) [10].

3.2.3 The Aging Eye

It is important to review the effects of aging on the eye since many of the techniques described later in this chapter may be effected by age related eye degradation. Weale has carefully documented the effects of aging on different eye structures [11]. The effects include:

- The cornea yellows in advanced age. Also, the older cornea tends to scatter more light.
- There is a marked decrease in pupil area. Weale notes the ratio of maximum to minimum pupillary area slowly decreases with age.
- The crystalline lens tends to scatter more light.
- The vitreous body usually has a clear, gel consistency. With advanced age the collagen fibrillar network within the gel tends to agglomerate and form a floating ``powder".
- The retina may experience the appearance of blood vessels, yellowish-white spots, and drusen. Drusen is hyaline excresences in the eye due to aging.
- The gel in the lens sac becomes hard, reducing the accomodation of the lens.

3.3 VISUAL REFRACTIVE ERRORS

Ideally, a light image should come to a focus directly on the retinal surface in the region of the fovea. This is what occurs in the emmetropic eye. The primary mechanisms of focusing an image on the retina is the cornea and the lens. Due to refractive errors, this does not always occur and results in a blurred image on an object. The three main visual refractive errors are myopia, hyperopia, and astigmatism as shown in Figure 4 [3].

A myopic eye focuses an image in front of the retina. Myopia is caused by an abnormally long eye or a steep curvature of the cornea. This condition is also called nearsightedness. This condition is corrected by introducing a concave lens in the vision path or by surgically flattening the curvature of the cornea which causes the cornea to focus an image on the retina [3].

A hyperopic eye has a focal length longer than the distance to the surface. It is caused by an abnormally short eye or an excessively flat cornea. This condition is called farsightedness. Hyperopia is corrected by steepening the curvature of the cornea which causes the cornea to focus an image on the retina. This may be accomplished by inserting a convex lens in the vision path or by a surgical procedure to steepen the cornea [3].

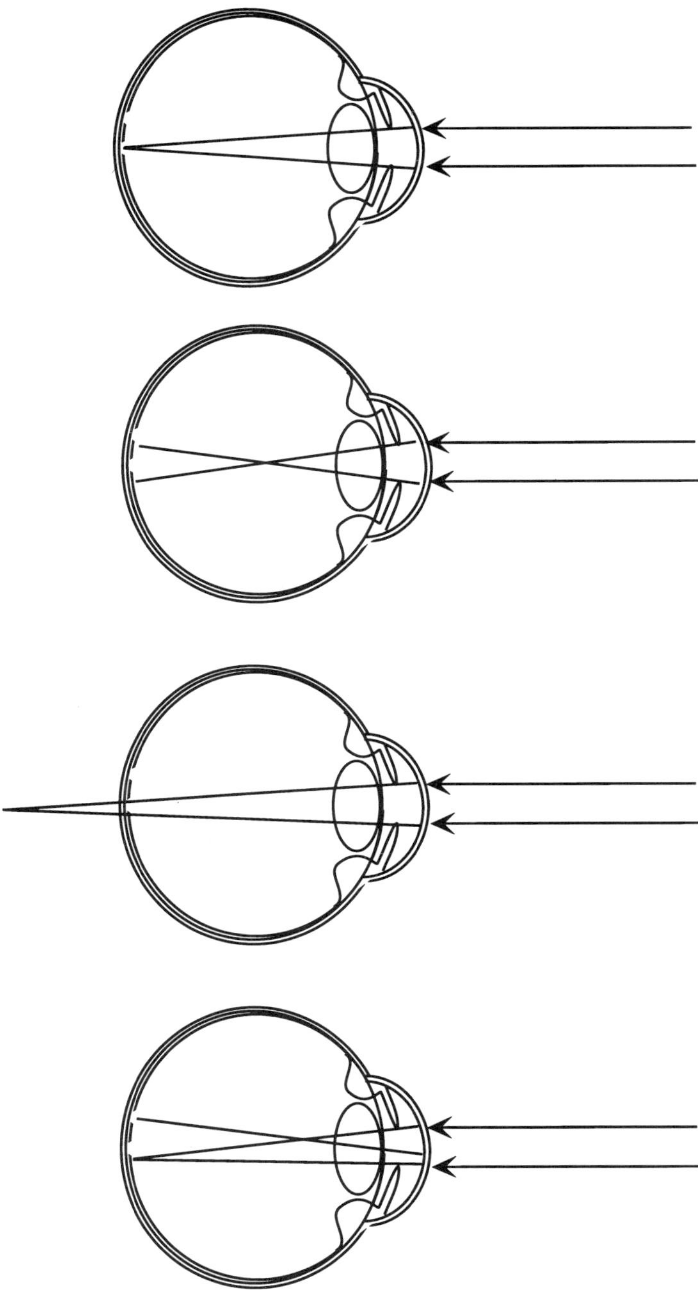

Figure 4. Visual refractive errors. From top to bottom: normal (emmetropic) eye, myopic eye, hyperopic eye, astigmatic eye.

When some parts of the image are in focus, but others are not in focus, the visual diffraction error is called astigmatism. This condition is caused by an oblong shaped cornea as opposed to a normally round cornea. The result is an image that focuses on different parts of the retina. Astigmatism is corrected by making the cornea more spherical. This may be accomplished by placing a cylindrical lens in the vision path or by a surgical procedure to make the cornea more spherical [3].

A related, but non-refractive visual error, is presbyopia. It is a normal effect of aging. The lens within the ocular globe is normally flexible. Muscles within the eye causes the flexible lens to change shape and hence helps to focus an image on the retinal surface. As a normal, age-related degradation the lens loses its elasticity and hence the ability to focus an image on to the retinal surface [3].

There are several different non-surgical methods of correcting the visual refractive errors. The most common are corrective lenses in the form of eye glasses or contacts. Recently, surgical techniques, known as refractive keratoplasty, have been developed to correct some of these errors. These techniques will be discussed later in the chapter.

3.4 LASER INTERACTION WITH EYE TISSUES

The clinical use of lasers is based on a confluence of four related factors [12].

- laser-tissue interaction mechanisms,
- the penetration depth of laser light in tissue,
- laser availability at a desired wavelength, and
- the availability of fibers to transmit the desired wavelengths.

3.4.1 Laser-tissue Interaction Mechanisms

Laser-tissue interaction mechanisms are a function of laser wavelength and other laser parameters. Chapter 2 provided a detailed discussion of these mechanisms. Mainster provided a thorough discussion of laser effects for ophthalmic photosurgery. As a brief review, ophthalmic laser applications may be placed in one of four categories: 1) thermal effects, 2) ionizing effects, 3) photochemical effects, and 4) illumination [13]. The first three categories relate to therapeutic applications, while the fourth category is used for diagnostic purposes.

3.4.1.1   Thermal Effects

Thermal effects elevate the temperature of the target tissue. This is brought about by absorption of laser energy by light in the target tissue. The surrounding tissue also experiences a temperature elevation due to heat conduction. Depending on how quickly light energy is deposited in the target tissue, either photocoagulation or photovaporization will result. Photocoagulation occurs when light absorption produces a temperature rise in the target tissue sufficient to produce protein denaturation. Photovaporization occurs when sufficient light energy is deposited in the target tissue to elevate its temperature to the vaporization temperature of water [13]. Note: in certain cases temperatures higher than 100 degrees centigrade are required to reach vaporization conditions.

3.4.1.2   Ionizing Effects

Ionization, also called optical breakdown or photodisruption, occurs when a focused laser beam produces sufficient irradiance to strip molecules from the target tissue. A plasma results which creates acoustic shock waves to incise the target tissue via a process called photodisruption. The high irradiance required for photodisruption is achieved by a combination of high fluence, small spot size, and a short pulse such that fluence rates on the order of 10^8 W/cm^2 are reached [13].

3.4.1.3   Photochemical Effects

A photochemical reaction occurs when photon absorption by a molucule's outer shell electron provides sufficient energy to induce a chemical reaction. A good example of a laser induced photochemical effect is photoablation provided by the 193 nm Argon Flouride (ArF) excimer laser. The excimer laser irradiation can be used to break strong intramolecular bonds which produce precise incisions [13].

3.4.1.4   Illumination

In illumination laser illumination applications, wavelengths are chosen to image specific features of the eye. For example, the scanning laser ophthalmoscope (SLO) using a low intensity laser beam to map the retina. Different wavelengths may be employed with the SLO to image a specific retinal layer or feature.

3.4.2 Laser Availability

The availability of laser systems and fiber optic delivery systems is governed by technological advances and by national regulatory agencies. Currently, the following lasers are commonly used in ophthalmology applications: Argon (Ar), Krypton (Kr), pulsed:Yttrium-Aluminum-Garnet (Nd:YAG), and the ArF excimer. Details on how these lasers are employed in specific applications will be covered later in the chapter [12].

3.4.3 Penetration Depth of Laser Light

The penetration depth of the laser light in the eye is wavelength dependent. Light entering the eye for therapeutic or diagnostic applications may be transmitted, absorbed, reflected, or scattered. A laser wavelength must be carefully chosen such that it passes through the intervening tissue layers and then is absorbed in the target tissue. The transmittance and absorbance properties of ophthalmic tissues have been analyzed and measured by many researchers.

A milestone study was conducted by Boettner *et al.* for the United States Air Force School of Aerospace Medicine from 1966 to 1967. The goal of the study was to determine the spectral transmittance of the human eye. In the study the spectral transmittance of ultraviolet, visible, and near infrared light through the human eye and primates was measured. The transmittance for each major eye tissue was determined: cornea, aqueous humor, lens, vitreous humor, retina, and choroid from 220 nm to 2.8 μm. The results are summarized in Figure 5.

Once light passes through the intervening tissue it must be absorbed in the target tissue of interest. The absorption property of ocular tissues is determined by its constituent chromophores. A chromophore is a molecule that absorbs light. Each chromophore has its own distinctive, wavelength specific absorbance properties. The primary chromophores in eye tissue include melanin, hemoglobin, and xanthophylls. As previously mentioned, the absorption in the cornea can be approximated by the absorption properties of water [12].

3.4.3.1 Fundus Chromatic Studies

Closely related to the optical properties of tissue, is the monochromatic imaging of selected retinal tissues. A detailed analysis of retinal monochromatic response was conducted by Delori *et al.* in 1976. Delori found that specific features of the fundus could be imaged with increased contrast when appropriate monochromatic illumination was used. Delori illuminated the

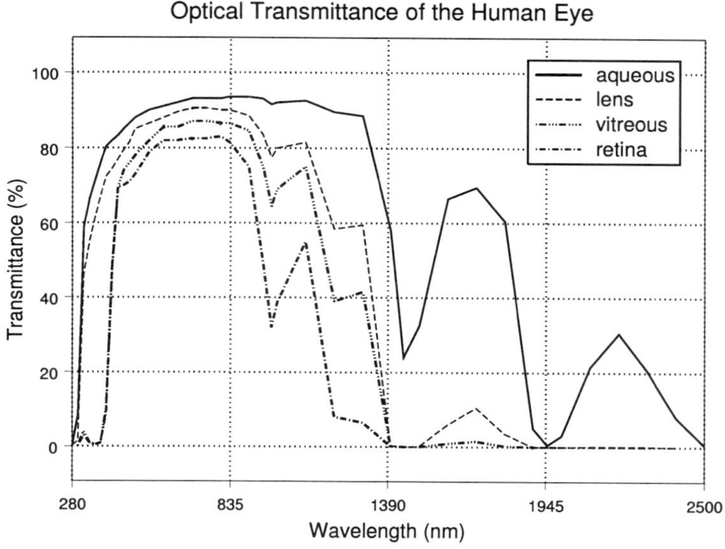

Figure 5. Total transmittance of the human eye. Adapted from data extracted from [14]

Retinal Structure	Wavelength [nm]		
	450 nm	550 nm	650 nm
physiological cupping	▨▨▨▨ ⧄⧄	⧄	
macular pigmentation	⧄▨⧄		
surface reflections	⧄⧄		
arcuate fiber bundles		⧄⧄	
papillo-macular bundle		⧄⧄	
small vessels in macula		⧄▨⧄	
small vessels on disk	⧄⧄	⧄	
large retinal arteries		⧄▨⧄	
large retinal veins		⧄▨⧄	
choroidal vessels (albinotic)		▨⧄	
RPE granularity: macula		⧄▨⧄	
RPE granularity: nasal to disk		▨▨▨	
choroidal vessels (pigmented)			⧄▨▨▨

▨▨▨▨ : range of optimum contrast in more than half the observations

⧄⧄⧄ : range of optimum contrast in more than one sixth the observations

Figure 6. Spectral ranges for optimal visibility of fundus structures. Adapted from [15].

retina with different bands of narrow-band spectral illumination. This technique enhanced the contrast of various retinal features at the different wavelength bands by enhancing the retinal feature contrast. Delori found that short wavelengths (470 nm) were predominantly reflected by the retina layers. At longer wavelengths (510 to 570 nm) the retina appeared transparent. The retinal vessels become clearly visible in the 510 to 570 nm band. Delori noted that the optical wavelength for observing large retinal vessels is 570 nanometers, but their visibility is generally excellent between 540 and 580 nanometers. The vessels appear dark and well defined with a central irregular streak of light along the larger vessels." The improved visibility of vessels in the region is due to the peak of hemoglobin absorption near 570 nm. At wavelengths above 580 nm light penetrates deeper into the fundus. Results of Delori's study are summarized in Figure 6. This landmark study is important to choosing the correct wavelengths to image or target specific layers of the retina for treatment [15].

3.5 LASER APPLICATIONS IN OPHTHALMOLOGY – DIAGNOSTIC

Lasers have been employed in a wide variety of applications to image the retina using several different technologies, measure visual acuity, measure absolute dimensions on the retina, measure retinal blood flow, and track eye movement via monitoring pupil position. Some of these applications are discussed in this section. Those still under development are covered in the "future applications" section.

3.5.1 Scanning Laser Ophthalmoscope (SLO)

The SLO technique of retinal imaging uses a low power 568.2 nm krypton laser beam to scan the retina, as shown in Figure 7. Recall from Delori's study that 568.2 nm is close to the peak absorption of hemoglobin. There are two main optical paths in the SLO system: 1) the raster path, and 2) the light collection path. The raster optical path provides the vertical and horizontal sweeps of the laser light source. The sweeps are accomplished using acousto-optical modulators (AOM) and mirrors connected to galvanometers. Basically, the beam from the AOM is swept vertically in a sawtooth waveform by a mirror mounted on a galvanometer. A second mirror mounted to a tuned resonant galvanometer sweeps the beam horizontally with a sinusoidal waveform. The vertical and the horizontal sweeps of the beam by the mirror galvanometers produce a raster pattern of parallel horizontal lines directly on the retina. The returned light from a specific point on the retina is captured by a photomultiplier tube and displayed as the intensity of the spot on a television monitor. This is accomplished via a small mirror optically conjugate with the eye's pupil and brought to a focus on the retina by an aspheric ophthalmoscopic lens. The laser moves over the retina synchronously with the spot on the monitor such that there is a one-to-one correspondence between a specific point on the retina and a specific point on the television screen. Thus, a video image is built up point-by-point. Figure 8 provides a sample of the fine resolution available with the SLO technique [17,18].

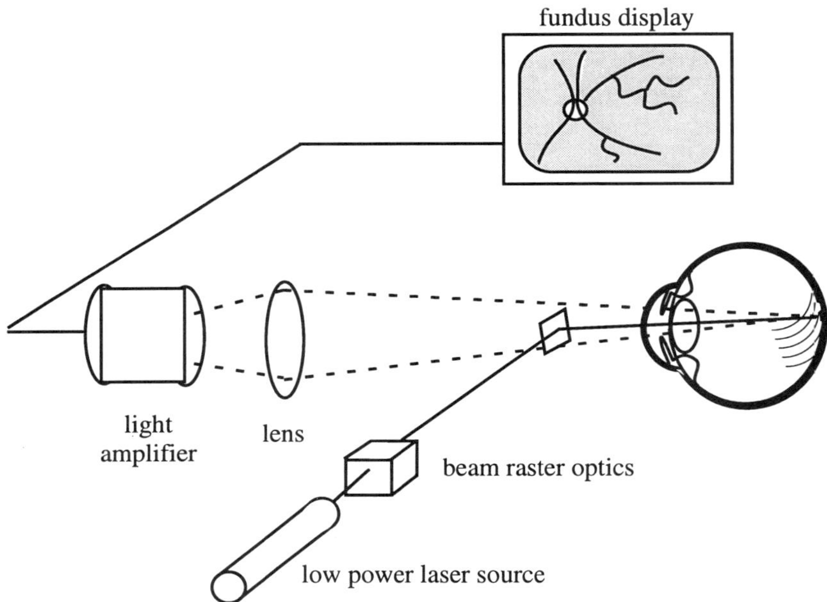

Figure 7. Scanning Laser Ophthalmoscope. Adapted from [16,17,18].

3.5.1.1   Advantages/Disadvantages of the SLO

The SLO imaging technique has many advantages including:

- The retinal illumination required for SLO imaging is on the order of 1000 times less than standard fundus imaging and 10,000 times less than the amount of light required for a standard fluorescein angiogram [18].
- The SLO uses only a 0.9 millimeter diameter entrance pupil leaving the rest of the pupil for the image. Thus, pupil dilation is not required [18,19].
- The laser source may be steered around opacities such as cataracts [18].

- The SLO fluorescein angiography with many orders of magnitude less light and one-tenth the dye dosage allows the examination of both eyes and repetitive examinations during a single clinical visit [18].
- As a patient ages, the lens and the vitreous humor tend to scatter and absorb light in greater quantities. The scattering is seen as a glare by the patient and as a cloudiness by the clinician. The cloudiness reduces image contrast. Increasing the level of retinal illumination in a standard fundus camera further increases the scattering and degrades image contrast. SLO reduces these scattering effects since retinal illumination is provided through a smaller portion of the scattering medium [18].
- Color images are possible by using the illuminating laser in a "white light mode". In this case there is a simultaneous emission of 647, 568, and 502 or 496 nm light. Three separate detectors are required [18,19].
- Any graphical material that can be displayed on a computer monitor can also be impressed on the retinal pattern formed by the sweeping laser beam. This capability allows an adaptive feedback patient fixation device. This technique has been used to investigate how patients with macular scotomas (area of depressed vision) use residual functional retinal areas to inspect visual detail [18].
- The SLO imaging system has a large depth of field which permits the iris, vitreous humor structures, and the retinal surface to be in focus simultaneously. It also has the capability to be used in the confocal mode where a single retinal plane is in focus [18,19].

The primary disadvantage of the SLO is its limited availability due to high cost.

Some researchers have taken the video image produced with the SLO as an input to an eye tracking algorithm. The algorithm plots the movement of the retina under different conditions. This technique has also been used to measure development of a pseudo-fovea following vocation related laser retinal injury [21].

3.5.2 Optical Coherence Tomography (OCT)

Optical Coherence Tomography (OCT) is a fairly new advancement in the ophthalmology field. It provides a noninvasive cross-sectional imaging capability of ophthalmic structures. The groundbreaking work in this technology was performed in the early 1990's. In the mid-1990's the OCT was proposed for use in a number of ophthalmic applications. OCT devices are now readily available for the ophthalmology clinic [22].

OCT is similar to ultrasound pulse-echo imaging (ultrasound B-mode). However, instead of using ultrasonic sound energy, OCT employs a low (μW) level optical signal to illuminate the target tissue. The coherence properties of light reflected from the tissue provides information on time-of-flight delay from reflective boundaries. The delay information is then processed to yield the longitudinal location of the reflection sites and hence information about tissue microstructure. The OCT beam may be scanned to provide a two-dimensional (cross-sectional) image of the target tissue [22].

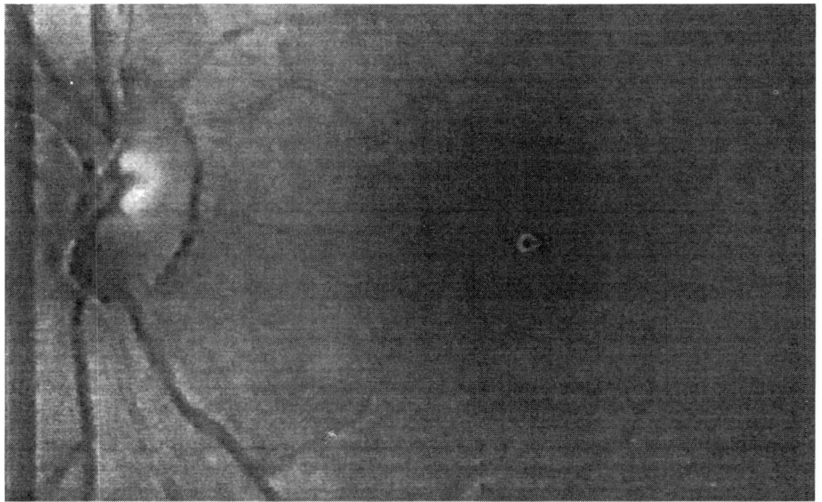

Figure 8. SLO image of retina. Note that the letter "C" has been imaged directly on the patient's retina by the SLO. Image provided courtesy of H.S. Zwick, B. Stuck, and D.J. Lund [20].

Illustrated in Figure 9 is the schematic of the OCT scanner. The OCT is an application of the Michelson interferometer. The Michelson interferometer is an optical configuration developed by A.A. Michelson in 1881. It is used to measure lengths or changes in lengths with great accuracy [23]. A super luminance diode (SLD), wavelength: 830 nm, can be used as the optical source in the Michelson OCT configuration.

Recall from Delori's work, that good light penetration into eye tissues is possible at this wavelength. The output from the SLD is passed into a 50/50 coupler where it is split to form the sample and reference arms of the interferometer. In the sample arm a piezoelectric transducer provides modulation of the signal. Reflection from the two interferometer arms are recombined at the 50/50 coupler. The signal is then fed to an optical detector. Demodulation of the signal is then performed to extract the interferometer signal from noise. The signal is then digitized for further processing by a host computer [22].

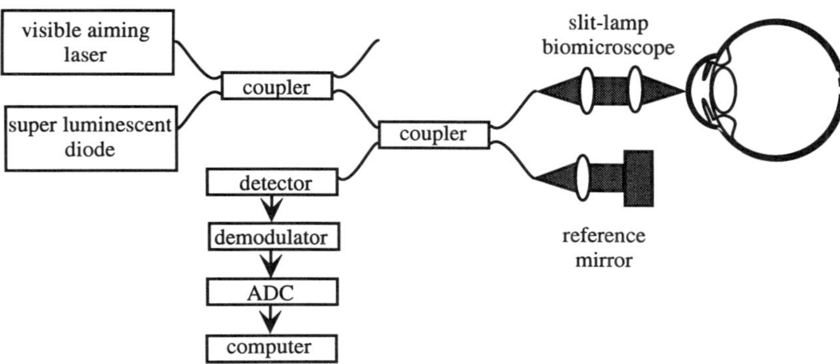

Figure 9. OCT scanner schematic. Adapted from [22].

Many ophthalmic applications have been proposed for the OCT. Hee *et al.* [24] proposed that the micron scale resolution of the OCT could be used as a powerful diagnostic tool for the anterior and posterior portions of the eye. Specifically the OCT can provide a quantitative evaluation of ocular microstructure and hence early diagnosis and treatment of ophthalmic related diseases prior to vision loss.

In the anterior portion of the eye, Hee proposes using OCT to image pathologies of the cornea, iris, lens, and anterior chamber. Specifically, high resolution (3-4 μm) OCT could be used for contact lens fitting, intraocular lens implant power calculation required for lens replacement after cataract removal, and real-time monitoring of corneal refractive surgery [24].

In the posterior portion of the eye, Hee indicates that tomographic imaging of the retina including the retinal tissue layers and the optic nerve head would allow quantitative assessment and treatment of degenerative retinal diseases.

OCT has become a clinical reality. Shown in Figure 10 is an OCT image of the retina [20]. There is considerable ongoing research to extend the capabilities and features of OCT. Researchers have recently reported advances in providing: *in vivo* video rate OCT capable of imaging cataracts, employing different wavelengths with the OCT system to achieve better tissue resolution, different scanning mechanisms to image the target tissue, and different methods to increase the contrast of the OCT image. Four new imaging modes have been developed to enhance image contrast: 1)polarization, 2) Doppler, 3) absorption, and 4) elasticity [25-30].

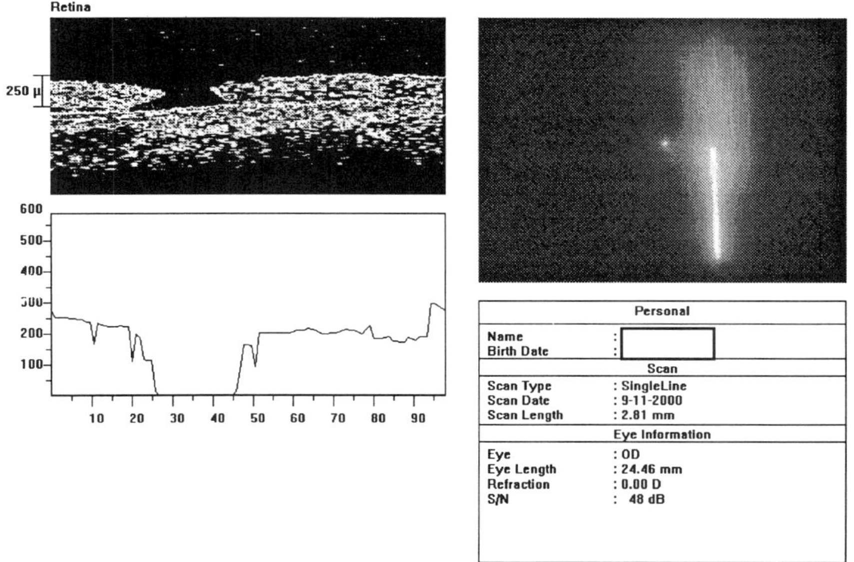

Figure 10. OCT image of the retina. The OCT scan is through a macula hole induced by blunt trauma. The individual received blunt ocular trauma from a spring-loaded packaging cable. The OCT shows the retinal thickness in the macula hole is zero. Image provided courtesy of H.S. Zwick and J. Brown, Jr. [20].

3.5.3 Double-Purkinje Image Eyetracker

Crane and Steele have developed an optical system to track the movement of the retina using a double-Purkinje image method. This system, called the Double-Purkinje Image eyetracker, detects the reflections of an near infrared (0.93 μms) beam projected into the eye from four optical surfaces of the eye: the anterior and posterior surfaces of the cornea and the anterior and posterior surfaces of the crytalline lens. These four reflected images are called the Purkinje-Sanson images I, II, III, and IV. The tracker monitors the movement of the I and IV images to derive information on retinal rotation and translation. This system requires a dental-impression bite board and a 2-point forehead rest to stabilize the patient's head against movement. Recent improvements in this design have resulted in tracking capability to a maximum of 100 degrees per second with a response time of 0.13 seconds [3,31,32].

3.5.4 Multiple-Beam Interference Fringe Measurements Applications

Laser interference fringes may be used for a variety of tests in the ophthalmology clinic including measuring visual acuity, measuring the retina's contrast sensitivity function, and measuring absolute ocular fundus dimensions. In these applications a low level Helium Neon (He-Ne) laser is used to produce interference fringes. These fringes are projected on to the patient's retina. The fringe spacing and contrast may be adjusted to facilitate different tests.

3.6 LASER APPLICATIONS IN OPHTHALMOLOGY – THERAPEUTIC

Lasers have been employed in the treatment of cataracts, glaucoma, retinal disorders, and in refractive keratoplasty. These applications are covered in this section.

3.6.1 Cataract Surgery

A condition in which some portion of the intraocular lens becomes clouded is called a cataract. The clouded areas reduce vision and may cause blindness. Cataracts are treated by removing the clouded lens and replacing it with a plastic intraocular prosthetic lens. A number of methods have been developed to remove and replace the lens. The United States Food and Drug Administration has recently approved a laser based cataract-removal system. The system manufactured by Laser Corp, called Dodick Laser PhotoLysis System, employs a Nd:YAG laser to quickly remove the cataract through a smaller incision than required for other techniques [33].

3.6.2 Glaucoma Surgery

The aqueous humor in the anterior chamber between the cornea and the lens provides nourishment to the cornea and the lens. The aqueous humor is formed in the ciliary body. After it is formed it flows into the anterior chamber due to a temperature gradient set up by the cooler cornea. Drainage channels for the aqueous humor are the trabecular meshwork between the junction of the sclera and the cornea.

Normally the intraocular pressure is maintained about 15-20 mm Hg above atmospheric pressure. This pressure may be elevated if anything interrupts the normal flow of the aqueous humor. The disruption of flow is called glaucoma. If this condition is not treated in a timely manner, the optic nerve head may be severely damaged [34].

There are two major types of glaucoma: open-angle glaucoma and narrow-angle glaucoma. In open-angle glaucoma, also called chronic glaucoma, vision to the side gradually narrows and total blindness may eventually result. This condition is normally treated with medication to reduce intraocular pressure and hence relieve the pressure on the optic nerve head [34].

Narrow-angle glaucoma or acute glaucoma may occur suddenly. It is characterized by extreme pain in the eye and forehead region, seeing rainbow-like rings of light, and redness of the eye. If not treated with surgery blindness will result [34].

Since glaucoma is due to excess intraocular pressure, surgical techniques to treat glaucoma concentrate on either decreasing the inflow or increasing the outflow of the aqueous humor. Laser iridectomy is a surgical procedure in which a laser is used to make a drainage hole for the aqueous humor in the iris. On the other hand, laser trabeculoplasty decreases the production of aqueous humor by sealing off some of the fluid-generating trabecular meshwork. The Argon and Nd:YAG lasers have been used for this procedure [34].

3.6.3 Diabetic Retinopathy

Diabetic retinopathy is a disease of the retina that begins in a non-inflammatory role and progresses through increasingly severe stages. The non-inflammatory stage is characterized by small aneurysms and hemmorhages along the retinal surface. The preproliferative stage is characterized by blood vessel obstruction. The final and most severe stage is called the proliferative stage. The key feature of the proliferative stage is the rapid formation of new, poor quality blood vessels. This characteristic is called neovascularization. These new vessels grow into the vitreous portion of the eye and may obstruct the visual path. Also, these poorly formed vessels leak blood into the vitreous chamber further obstructing vision.

The precise stimulus for neovascularization is unknown. In 1956, Wise hypothesized a retinal hypoxic condition stimulated the new vessel growth [35]. His hypothesis has yet to be confirmed. However, work by Stefansson *et al.* [36] support Wise's hypothesis. Their experiments demonstrate that oxygen tension is significantly higher over retinal areas treated with panretinal photocoagulation than untreated areas of the same retina.

To better understand the treatment protocol for diabetic retinopathy a closer examination of the retinal oxygen supply is required. The retinal oxygen supply is provided by two separate systems: 1) the inner retinal supply providing oxygen from the vitreous to the outer plexiform layer, and 2) the outer retinal supply providing the needs of the avascular photoreceptors (the rod and cones). The inner retinal supply is provided by the retinal circulatory system while the outer retinal supply is provided by diffusion from the choroidal circulation [37].

The retinal circulatory system is sensitive to changes in the oxygen supply. A hypoxic condition induces an autoregulatory vasodilation response. The retinal vessels adjust their flow to maintain the tissue oxygen level at a constant level. The retinal circulatory system provides 50 percent of its oxygen to the tissue. The choroidal system does not autoregulate significantly[37].

Homeostasis of oxygen availability in the retina provides a sufficient mechanism to initiate or inhibit vessel growth. Dilation of retinal vessels for any length of time initiates new vessel growth which is proportional to the amount of dilation of retinal vessels. The loss in diabetes of the sphincter-like mural cells may facilitate retinal vessel dilation [37].

Diabetic retinopathy is treated with panretinal photocoagulation. An argon laser at a wavelength of 488 and 514 nm is used to selectively denature peripheral portions of the retina while sparing critical vision anatomy about the fovea and optic disk. The retinal vessel network is also spared. Many different lesion patterns may be used. A pattern of two concentric rings of 200 µm lesions about the critical vision anatomy surrounded by concentric rings of 500 µm lesions out to the far retinal periphery is common. This technique preserves acute vision about the macula at the expense of the peripheral vision. This treatment is based on the hypothesis that the lesions selectively destroy rods and cones by photocoagulation to allow more choroidal oxygen to reach the inner retina and constrict retinal vessels. This selective denaturation improves the oxygen supply to the retina by increasing the oxygen tension. This has recently been verified in human patients. The improved oxygen tension suppresses the neovascularization response. The success of argon laser treatment is roughly proportional to the amount of retinal tissue photocoagulated [36,37].

3.6.4 Macular Degeneration

Macular degeneration is also called senile macular degeneration because it is most common in the elderly population. This disease is the leading cause of blindness in people over 65 years of age. However, the disease may also affect younger people. This disease occurs in two forms: the more common drusenoid or dry form and the neovascularization or exudative form. The neovascularization form occurs in approximately 20 percent of the macular degenerative cases. This is the more active of the two forms. This form can be treated via argon laser photocoagulation techniques while the drusenoid form can not. The neovascularized form is typified by leaky blood vessels and hemmorhaging into the macula and the fovea. Treatment is similar to that prescribed for diabetic retinopathy. In about 10 percent of the neovascularized cases, the bleeding is so close to the fovea that treatment is not currently possible. If untreated, the fovea may become obliterated and destroyed within a month or two resulting in loss of acute vision [38]. Recently, a photodynamic therapy treatment has been approved for treating certain types of macular degeneration. This technique will be discussed later in the chapter.

3.6.5 Retinal Tears

The retina may be subdivided into two main layers: the neural retina and the retinal pigment epithelium. The pigment epithelium provides a nursing role to the rods and the cones. Certain traumatic injuries result in retinal breaks and tears. If left untreated the two layers may separate. This separation is called retinal detachment. If the layer separation is not repaired blindness will result. The retinal breaks and tears may be repaired using photo-coagulation to seal the break. The rods and cones within the trauma site are no longer functional. A common technique is to surround the torn area with two continuous, concentric rings of 200 µm lesions [39].

3.6.6 Refractive Keratoplasty

Surgical techniques for correcting visual refractive errors (procedures known as refractive keratoplasty) include laser *in situ* keratomileusis, lamellar keratoplasty, radial keratotomy, laser thermal keratoplasty, and photo-refractive keratectomy. A brief description of these techniques follows:

Laser In-situ Keratomileusis – LASIK This technique combines the use of an excimer laser and a microkeratome. The keratome is used to produce a flap in the cornea. The flap is then lifted and the cornea is reshaped using an ArF excimer laser. After reshaping the cornea, the flap is replaced.

Lamellar Keratoplasty - LK Lamellar keratoplasty is a procedure that replaces the cornea in a patient with a cornea from a donor eye. Although a laser is not used in this technique, it is included here for completeness.

Radial Keratotomy - RK Radial Keratotomy is used to correct myopia and astigmatism involves making incisions of a certain depth on the cornea, away from the optical zone. In one of the more common forms of keratotomy, radial keratotomy, incisions are made radially away from the optical zone, producing a spoke-like pattern to correct a myopic condition. "T-shaped" incisions have been used to correct astigmatism.

Incisions weaken the cornea, permitting pressure from within the eye to alter the curvature of the cornea, thereby reducing myopia or astigmatism. The incisions are made with a calibrated diamond blade in the periphery portion of the cornea. RK is rarely performed anymore since the change in refractive error is thought to be less predictable than laser surgery [22].

Laser Thermal Keratoplasty - LTK   Laser thermal keratoplasty uses heat to shrink the collagen of the corneal stroma. Lasers with wavelengths in the infrared range are used to produce the heat. By shrinking the collagen, the shape of the cornea and its refractive power is changed. The cornea is comprised of approximately 78% water; therefore, several researchers have used the optical properties of water to model the cornea [40-45].The continuous wave Thulium (λ: 2.01 μm) and the Holmium (λ: 2.09 μm) are good candidates for LTK since water highly absorbs these wavelengths. Other laser wavelengths heavily absorbed by water are the Erbium:YAG (λ: 2.94 μm) and the CO_2 laser (λ: 10.6 μm) [46-50]. There is a 1.87 μm diode laser currently being tested in Germany. The United States Food and Drug Administration recently approved Sunrise Technologies' Holmium laser based Hyperion LTK laser system for the treatment of hyperopia.

Photorefractive keratectomy - PRK Photorefractive keratectomy with an ArF excimer laser changes the curvature of the anterior surface of the cornea to treat myopia, hyperopia, and astigmatism. Some believe that the processes involved are not thermal, but photon-induced molecular decomposition, resulting in the removal of thin layers of tissue. This process has been termed photoablation. The ArF excimer laser (λ: 193 nm) operates in the ultra-violet range and when used on the cornea, virtually all of the energy is absorbed within a few microns of the surface.   Photorefractive keratectomy takes longer to heal than the LASIK technique [49,51-56].

Phototherapeutic Keratectomy – PTK A technique to treat corneal irregularities currently in the development stage is phototherapeutic keratectomy. The technique currently under development uses a liquid collagen-derivative gel, called Biomask. This material is heated to a liquid state, placed on the corneal surface, and then covered with a rigid contact lens. The lens provides a template or mold for the desired shape and curvature of the cornea. Once the Biomask material has solidified, the contact lens is removed. An ArF excimer laser is then applied to the masked cornea for ablation. As the laser ablates the mask, it trims steeper areas of the cornea which break through first. During the ablation process, the curvature on the front of the mask is transferred to the cornea. An ultraviolet light is used during the process to help delineate the

Biomask/cornea boundary. Under the UV light, the cornea fluoresces. The fluorescence can be used as an indicator of corneal elevation. As the surgeon proceeds further into the mask, the area of fluorescence increases. The procedure continues until there is a little fluorescence left. This is an indicator that the laser has processed through the epithelium layer of the cornea. This technique is being developed to treat patients with irregular corneal surfaces such as corneal scars, irregular astigmatisms, overcorrections, undercorrections, and nodules [57,58].

3.7 LASER APPLICATIONS IN OPHTHALMOLOGY - THE FUTURE

This section discusses laser applications of ophthalmology currently in the research stage. Many of them show promise and may result in clinical applications in the near future.

3.7.1 Laser Doppler Flowmetry – LDF

Laser Doppler Flowmetry (LDF) is the term for a noninvasive method that measures red blood cell flux in the microvasculature of tissue. Geiser *et al.* [59] have developed a compact laser doppler system to measure the choroidal blood flow. They have used the system to measure blood flow in the optic nerve head, the retinal microcirculation, and the choriocapillaris in the foveal region of the choroids. These measurements may be key to understanding the pathogenesis of age-related macular degeneration.

The LDF technique is based on the Doppler effect. A low power laser(λ: 785 nm, spot size at cornea: 1.3 mm, power at cornea: 90 μW) is used to illuminate the fovea. The laser beam has a foveal spot size of 12 μm. Light striking moving red blood cells (RBCs) in the choroid are scattered and shifted in frequency by amounts proportional to the speeds of the the RBCs. The shifted light mixes with reflected light from non-moving tissues. A photodetector captures the mixed light and converts it to current. The current is analyzed to obtain the Doppler Shift Power Spectrum (DSPS) of the reflected light. Flow parameters are derived from the DPSS measurements[59].

Although this technique shows promise there are currently considerable differences in measurements between individuals due to the difference in optical tissues between individuals. Geiser *et al.* [59] concluded, "....direct comparison between flow values for different subjects is in general of limited value. However, a comparison of changes in the flow parameters in a given subject is of great interest from a physiological and pathological point of view and valid under the assumption that the properties of the tissue at the site of LDF measurements have not changed between measurements."

3.7.2 Glucose Level Monitoring

Approximately 100 million people worldwide suffer from different forms of diabetes mellitus or diabetes. This is a chronic disease where the body fails to produce or fails to respond to insulin, the glucose regulatory hormone. Insulin is required for cells to take up glucose from the blood. In diabetics, a defect in insulin signaling produces a large fluctuation in blood glucose levels. Therefore, diabetics must routinely sample blood sugar levels using the "finger-stick" method to extract a small blood sample. The blood sample is then applied to glucose level indicators. The information obtained from this technique allows the diabetic to determine the required amount of insulin injections. For over 30 years researchers have worked to develop a painless technique based on optical glucose sensing to replace the "finger-stick" technique [60].

Although blood glucose monitoring is not directly related to ophthalmology, monitoring the glucose level in the eye's aqueous humor provides an indirect but readily available secondary measure of blood glucose level. Researchers have shown that the glucose level in the aqueous humor has an age-dependent, steady-state concentration which is 70 percent of that found in the blood. Furthermore, a time-lag on the order of 30 minutes exists between the blood glucose level and that found in the aqueous humor [60].

Many optical techniques are under development to indirectly measure blood glucose via the aqueous humor. These include: optical absorption spectroscopy, polarimetry, Raman spectroscopy, and fluorescent glucose sensing. The Raman spectroscopy technique and the polarimetry techniques use the aqueous humor as a window into the glucose levels in the blood [60].

3.7.2.1 Raman Spectroscopy

In the Raman spectroscopy technique, excitation light is scattered by molecules within a substance. The loss or gain of photon energy results in a change of incident light frequency during the scattering event. The resulting frequency shifts provide information about the chemical structure of the sample. The Raman signal is much weaker than native fluorescence and requires newly available, extremely sensitive charge-coupled device (CCD) based cameras to capture. Although, the Raman spectroscopy technique shows promise, there are several technical difficulties that need to be solved. First, the laser power required to elicit Raman response poses an eye safety concern. Furthermore, fluorescence signals generated by ocular tissues often overwhelm the Raman response. Many researchers are currently working to overcome these hurdles [60].

3.7.2.2   Optical Polarimetry

Optical polarimetric quantification of glucose is based on the concept of optical rotatory dispersion or ORD. In ORD, a linearly polarized light source is passed through a sample. Molecules within the aqueous sample rotate the plane of polarization due to chirality ("handedness") properties of the constituent molecules. The angle of rotation depends linearly on three factors: the concentration of chiral molecules, the pathlength through the sample, and a specific rotation molecular constant. Therefore, the amount of rotation can be used as an indirect measure of the molecular concentration within the sample [60].

Glucose provides a right hand rotation and has an associated, repeatable, wavelength specific rotation. At physiological concentrations and pathlengths of 1 cm, the glucose optical rotation is approximately 5 millidegrees. A number of techniques are under development to accurately measure this rotation. Although these techniques all show promise, there is much work that needs to be done before a non-invasive, easy-to-use, glucose monitoring device is readily available to the millions of diabetics worldwide [60].

3.7.3   Photodynamic Therapy – PDT

Photodynamic therapy or PDT employs light-activated drugs to treat a wide variety of diseases. Diseases associated with rapidly growing tissue become potential candidates for this treatment protocol. Photodynamic therapy has shown promise for treatment in ophthalmic diseases particularly certain forms of macular degeneration [61].

Photodynamic therapy consists of a two-step process. The first step consists of administering a photosensitizer drug by intravenous injection. The photosensitizer attaches to molecules called lipoproteins in the bloodstream. Concentration of the photosensitizer is greater in cells undergoing rapid cell division and growth. This is because they require a greater amount of lipoproteins than non-dividing cells. When the drug concentrations reaches appropriate levels in the targeted disease cells, it is activated with a low dose of light at a specific wavelength. The activated drug causes the conversion of normal oxygen found in tissue to a form called singlet oxygen. The singlet oxygen causes cell death by disrupting normal cellular functions [61].

Photodynamic therapy is a minimally invasive procedure that can be performed on an out-patient basis. It appears to be a cost-effective alternative to other treatments. The light source used varies depending on the disease being treated. In ophthalmology, diode laser light is shone through the slit lamp of a microscope into the patient's eye. Photodynamic therapy was recently approved for AMD patients [61].

3.7.4 Automated Retinal Lesion Placement

Laser photocoagulation has been used to treat retinal disorders such as diabetic retinopathy, macular degeneration, and retinal tears for several decades. Typical treatment protocols require placement of multiple (often several thousand) therapeutic lesions on the retina in an out-patient environment. Lesion placement is determined by the ophthalmologist, and the patient is fully awake during the procedure. Although the patient's head is supported in a chin cup and the conjugate eye is stabilized with a fixation target, considerable retinal movement may occur. The procedure is currently performed completely manually and suffers from several drawbacks: it often requires many clinical visits, it is very tedious for both patient and ophthalmologist, the laser pointing accuracy and safety margin are limited by a combination of the ophthalmologist's manual dexterity and the patient's ability to hold their eye still, and there is a large variability in lesion size even with identical irradiation parameters.

In the late 1980's, Markow *et al.* at the University of Texas at Austin (UT) proposed an automated system to treat retinal disorders. These researchers investigated the feasibility of digital tracking, lesion parameter control, and Fourier-based optical tracking. Their work demonstrated a feasible concept; however, they were limited by available computer and image processing technology. Through the 1990's, UT researchers worked to transform the conceptual design into a practical, clinical system. Jerath [62,63] and Maharajh [64] extensively studied lesion parameter control while Barrett studied a practical digital tracking system to stabilize an irradiating laser on the moving retina. Wright further improved on this digital tracking system and coupled it with an optical tracking system developed by Ferguson for the first prototype hybrid tracking system known as CALOSOS (Computer Aided Laser Optical System for Ophthalmic Surgery).

Since 1996, Barrett, Wright, and de Graaf have worked toward an improved hybrid prototype for CALOSOS. Their goal has been to develop a clinically significant photocoagulation system to provide a user-friendly interface for the ophthalmologist, to quickly and safely place therapeutic laser-induced lesions of desired parameters at desired retinal coordinates (while compensating for patient retinal movement), and to permit consistent retinal lesion formation (compensating for variations in the retinal absorption coefficient). The requirements for this system are: retinal tracking rates equal to or better than 10 degrees per second (deg/s), laser pointing accuracy better than 100 μms at the retinal surface, uniform lesion formation within 5% of apparent size and depth, and system reaction time of no more than 5 milliseconds. Furthermore, should retinal movement exceed the ability of the system (or other anomalous condition occurs such as patient blinking), the tracking system should register a loss-of-lock condition, immediately close the laser shutter, and attempt to re-establish system lock.

Currently, researchers are working to provide consistent therapeutic lesions across the surface of the non-uniform retina. They are using the reflectance from a forming therapeutic lesion as a visible marker of immeasurable lesion depth. They are also working on a seamless, clinically significant prototype to safely and quickly place therapeutic retinal lesions for the treatment of various disorders [65-69].

REFERENCES

1. Hecht, E., *Optics*. Addison-Wesley Publishing Company,MA..1987, 176-181.
2. Ganong, WF. *Review of Medical Physiology*, Appleton and Lange, Norwalk, CN., 1989, 119-124.
3. Barlow, HB. and JD. Mollon, *The Senses*, Cambridge University Press, London, 1984, 35-37.
4. Beatrice, E. S. and B. E. Stuck. "Occular Effects of Laser Radiation: Cornea and Anterior Chamber."*Agard Lecture Series*, No. 79:**5**, 1975.
5. Quigley, HA., AE. Brown, JD. Morrison, and SM. Drance. "The Size and Shape of the Optic Disk in Normal Human Eyes."Arch Ophthalmol, 108: 451-57.
6. Mansour, AM. "Measuring Fundus Landmarks." *Investigative Ophthalmology and Visual Science*, 31:1:41-42.
7. Straatsma, BR., MB. Landers, AE. Krieger, and L. Apt."Topography of the Human Retina.'"In : *The Retina Morphology, Function, and Clinical Charact-ristics*,University of California Press, Berkeley and Los Angeles, 1969, 379-474.
8. Eaton, A. M. and D. L. Hatchell. "Measurement of Retinal Blood Vessel   Width Using Computerized Image *Analysis.*"*Investigative Ophthalmology* and Visual Science,} 29:**8**: 1258-1264.
9. Engelken, EJ. *Influence of Visual and Auditory Stimuli on Saccadi Eye Movement*, Ph.D. Thesis, The University of Texas at Austin, May 1987.
10. Kosnik, W., J. Fikre, and R. Sekuler. "Visual Fixation Stability in Older Adults." *Investigative Ophthalmology and Visual Science*, 27:12, 1720 - 1725.
11. Weale, RA., *The Aging Eye*, Harper and Row Publishers, 1963.
12. van Gemert, MJ. C. and AJ. Welch."Clinical Use of Laser-Tissue Interactions."IEEE Engineering in Medicine and Biology December 1989,10-13.
13. Mainster, MA. "Finding Your Way in the Photoforest: Laser Effects for Clinicians." *Ophthalmology*. 91:7: 886-888.
14. Boettner, EA. *Spectral Transmission of the Eye*. USAF School of Aerospace Medicine, Brooks Air Force Base, Texas, July 1967, 30.
15. Delori, FC., ES. Evangelos, S. Gragoudas, R. Francisco, and RC. Pruett. "Monochromatic Ophthalmoscopy and Fundus Photography." *Arch Ophthalmol*, May 1977, 861-863.

16. Webb, H. and GW. Hughes. "Scanning Laser Ophthalmoscope." *IEEE Transactions on Biomedical Engineering.* BME-28:7:488-489.

17. Timberlake, GT., MA. Mainster, E. Peli, RA. Augliere, EA. Essock, and LE. Arend. "Reading with a Macular Scotoma - I. Retinal Location of Scotoma and Fixation Area." Invest Oph and Vis Science Volume 27, July 1986, 1137-1139.

18. Mainster, MA., GT. Timberlake, RH. Webb, and GH. Hughes. "Scanning Laser Ophthalmoscopy - Clinical Applications." *American Academy of Ophthalmology.* 89:7:852-857.

19. Elsner, E., AH. Jalkh, and J. J. Weiter. "Retinal Imaging and Function Evaluation", In : *Practical Atlas of Retinal Disease and Therapy*, W. Freeman, (ed). Raven Press, NY.

20. Zwick, H., "Personal Communication."U.S. Army Medical Research Detachment, Walter Reed Army Institute of Research, Brooks Air Force Base, San Antonio, TX.

21. Barrett, SF. and H. Zwick. "Measuring Visual Fixation with a Retinal Tracking Equipped Scanning Laser Ophthalmoscope." *Proceedings of the 37th Annual Rocky Mountain Bioengineering Symposium*, USAF Academy, CO, April 2000, 183-188.

22. Huang, D., EA. Swanson, CP. Lin, JS. Schuman, WG. Stinson, W. Chang, MR. Hee, T. Flotte, K. Gregory, CA. Puliafito, and JG. Fujimoto. "Optical Coherence Tomography." *Science.* November 22, 1991, 1178-1181.

23. Halliday, D. and R. Resnick. *Fundamentals of Physics*, John Wiley and Sons, New York, 1981, 734.

24. Hee, MR., JA. Izatt, EA. Swanson, D. Huang, JS. Schuman, CP. Lin, CA. Puliafito, and J G. Fuijmoto. "Optical Coherence Tomography for Ophthalmic Imaging: New Technique Delivers Micron-Scale Resolution." *IEEE Engineering in Medicine and Biology.* Jan/Feb. 1995, 67-76.

25. DiCarlo, CD., WP. Roach, DA. Gagliano, SA. Boppart, DX. Hammer, AB. Cox, and JG. Fujimoto. "Comparison of Optical Coherence Tomography Imaging of Cataracts with Histopathology." *Journal of Biomedical Optics.* 4:4:450-458.

26. Rollins, AM., MD. Kulkarni, SYazdanfar, R. Ung-arunyawee, and J. A. Izatt. "In vivo Video Rate Optical Coherence Tomography." *Optics Express.* 3:6:219-229.

27. Schmitt, JM., "Optical Coherence Tomography (OCT): A Review." *IEEE Journal of Selected Topics in Quantum Electronics.* 5:4:1205-1215.

28. Podoleanu, AG., JA. Rogers, and DA. Jackson. "OCT En-face Images from the Retina with Adjustable Depth Resolution in Real Time." *IEEE Journal of Selected Topics in Quantum Electronics.* 5:4:1176-1184.

29. Ducros, G., JF. de Boer, H. Huang, LC. Chao, Z. Chen, JS. Nelson, TE. Milner, HG. Rylander III. "Polarization Sensitive Optical Coherence Tomography of the Rabbit Eye." *IEEE Journal of Selected Topics in Quantum Electronics.* 5:4:1159-1167.

30. Tearney, GJ., BE. Bouma, SA. Boppart, B. Golubovic, EA. Swanson, and FG. Fujimoto. "Rapid Acquisition of In Vivo Biological Images by use of Optical Coherence Tomography." *Optics Letters.* 21:**17**:1408-1410.

31. Crane, HD. and CM. Steele. "Accurate Three-Dimensional Eyetracker." *Applied Optics.* 17:**5**: 691-704.

32. Snodderly, DM., WP. Leung, GT. Timberlake, and DPB. Smith. "Mapping Retinal Features in a Freely Moving Eye with Precise Control of Retinal Stimulus Position" 79-91. % need journal name

33. "FDA Approves First Laser for Cataract Removal." *Reuters Health.* July **4**, 2000.

34. Webb, RH. "Manipulating Laser Light for Ophthalmology." *IEEE Engineering in Medicine and Biology.* December 1985, 12-16.

35. Wise, GN., "Retinal Neovascularization"' *Transactions American Ophthalmology Society,* 1956,**54**, 729.

36. Stefansson, E., R. Machemer, E. de Juan, BW. McCuen, and J.Peterson. "Retinal Oxygenation and Laser Treatment in Patients with Diabetic Retinopathy." *American Journal of Ophthalmology.* 1992, **113**, 36-38.

37. Wolbarsht, ML. and MB. Landers. "The Rationale of Photocoagulation Therapy for Proliferative Diabetic Retinopathy: A Review and Model." *Ophthalmic Surgery*.11:4:235-245.

38. Dickman, IR. "Vision Impairment in Later Years: Macular Degenration." *Public Affairs Pamphlet No. 610*. Public Affairs Committee Incorporated, 1982, 1-10.

39. Spaeth,GL.,*Ophthalmic Surgery*.W.B. Saunders Company, Philadelphia, 1982,360-409.

40. Gartry, D., MK. Muir, and J. Marshall. "Excimer Laser Treatment of Corneal Surface Pathology: A Laboratory and clinical Study." *British Journal of Ophthalmology*. 1991,**75**, 258-269.

41. Hale, GM.and MR. Querry. "Optical Constants of Water in the 200 nm to 200 μm Wavelength Region." *Applied Optics*. 12:**3**:555-563.

42. Mainster, MA., TJ. White, and JH. Tips. "Corneal Thermal Response to the CO_2 Laser." *Applied Optics*. 9:**3**:665-667.

43. Mainster, MA., TJ. White, JH. Tips, and PW. Wilson, "Transient Thermal Behavior in Biological Systems." *Bulletin of Mathematical Biophysics*. 1970:**32**: 303-314.

44. Peppers, NA., AVassiliadis, KG. Dedrick, H. Chang, RR. Peabody, H. Rose, and HC. Zweng. "Corneal Damage Threshold for CO_2 Laser Radiation." *Applied Optics*. 8:**2**:377-381.

45. Shepherd, CK. *Experimental CO_2 Laser Thermokeratoplasty* Masters Thesis, The Univ. of Texas at Austin, Decmber 1986, 1-30.

46. Moretti, M."Holmium Laser Challenges CO_2 Lasers for Surgical Applications." *Laser Focus World*. August 1991, 37.

47. Horn, G., KG. Spears, O. Lopez, A. Lewicky, X. Yang, M. Riaz, R. Wang, D. Silva, and J. Serafin. "New Refractive Method for Laser Thermal Keratoplasty with the $Co:MgF_2$ Laser." *J. Cataract Refract Surg*. Volume 16, September 1990, 611-616.

48. Neuman, AC., DR. Sanders, JJ. Salz, DJ. Bessinger, MG. Raanan, M. Van Der Karr. "Effect of Thermokeratoplasty on Corneal Curvature." J. Cataract Refract Surg. lume 16, 1990:16: 727-731.

49. Seiler, T., T. Bende, J. Wollensak, and S. Trokel. "Excimer Laser Keratectomy for Correction of Astigmatism." *American Journal of Ophthalmology*. 105:2:117-124.

50. Cartilage, G., JM. Parel, T. Yokokura, JA. Lowery, K. Kobayashi, I. Nose, W. Lee, G. Simon, and DB. Denham. "A Laser Surgical Unit for Photoablative and Photothermal Keratoplasty." *SPIE Volume 1423 Ophthalmic Technologies* 1991, 167-174.

51. Kerr-Muir, MG., SL. Trokel, J. Marshall, and S. Rothery. "Ultrastructural Comparison of Conventional Surgical and Argon Fluoride Excimer Laser Keratectomy." American J. of Ophthalmology.} Volume 103, March 1987, 448-453.

52. L'Esperance, FA., JW. Warner, WB. Telfair, PR. Yoder, and CA. Martin. "Excimer Laser Instrumentation and Technique for Human Corneal Surgery." *Archives of Ophthalmology*. 1989:**107**:131-139.

53. McDonnell, PJ., H. Moreira, TN. Clapham, J. D'Arcy, CR. Munnerlyn. "Photorefractive Keratectomy for Astigmatism." *Archives of Ophthalmology*. 1991: **109**:1370-1373.

54. Sher, NA., RA. Bowers, RW. Zabel, JM. Frantz, RA. Eiferman, DC. Brown, JJ. Rowsey, P. Parker, V. Chen, and RL. Lindstrom. "Clinical Use of the 193 nm Excimer Laser in the Treatment of Corneal Scars." *Archives of Ophthalmology*. 1991:**109**:491-498.

55. Trokel, SL., R. Srinivasan, B. Braren. "Excimer Laser Surgery of the Cornea." *American Journal of Ophthalmology*. 96:**6**:710-715.

56. Wu, WCS. , WJ. Stark, WR. Green. "Corneal Wound Healing After 193-nm Excimer Laser Keratectomy." *Arch Ophthalmol*. 1991:**109**: 1426-1432.

57. Kornmehl, EW., RF. Steinert, CA.Puliafito. "A Comparative Study of Masking Fluids for Excimer Laser Phototherapeutic Keratectomy." *Arch Ophthalmol*. 1991:**109**: 860-863.

58. Angelucci, D. "Smoothing the Surface – PTK with Biomask." http://www.eyeworld.com/Sep99.

59. Geiser MH., U. Deiermann, and CE. Riva. "Compact Laser Doppler Choroidal Flowmeter." *Journal of Biomedical Optics*. 4:**4**:459-464.
60. McNichols, J. and GL. Cote. "Optical Glucose Sensing in Biological Fluids: an overview." *Journal of Biomedical Optics*. 5:**1**: 5-16.
61. "Visudyne (verteporfin) Therapy." http://www.visudyne.com
62. Jerath, MR., R. Chudru, SF. Barrett, HG. Rylander, and J. Welch. "Reflectance Feedback Control of Photocoagulation In Vivo." *Archives of Ophthalmology*. 1993:**111**:531- 534.
63. Jerath, MR., R. Chundru, SF. Barrett, HG. Rylander, and AJ. Welch, "Preliminary Results on Reflectance Feedback Control of Photocoagulation In Vivo." *IEEE Transactions on Biomedical Engineering*. 1994: **41**:201-203.
64. Maharajh, N. Use of Reflectance for the Real Time Feedback Control of Photocoagulation. Masters Thesis. The University of Texas at Austin, May 1996, 31-42.
65. Barrett, SF., CHG. Wright, MR. Jerath, R. Stephen Lewis II, Bryan C. Dillard, HG. Rylander, and A. J. Welch. "Computer Aided Retinal Photocoagulating System." *J. of Biomedical Optics*. 1996:**1**: 83-91.
66. Barrett, SF., MR. Jerath, HG. Rylander, and A. J. Welch. "Automated Lesion Placement in the Rabbit Eye." *Lasers in Surgery and Medicine*. 1995:**17**:172-177,
67. Barrett,SF., MR. Jerath, HG. Rylander, and AJ. Welch. "Digital Tracking and Control of Retinal Images." Optical Engineering. 33:1:150 - 159.
68. Wright, CHG. , RD. Ferguson, HG. Rylander III, AJ. Welch, SF. Barrett. "A Hybrid Approach to Retinal Tracking and Laser Aiming for Photocoagulation." Journal of Biomedical Optics.} 2:2:195-203.
69. Wright, CHG. , SF. Barrett, RD. Ferguson, HG. Rylander III, and AJ. Welch. "Initial In Vivo Results of a Hybrid Retinal Photocoagulation System." *Journal of Biomedical Optics*. 5:1:56-61.

Chapter 4

LASER CARDIOLOGY
Part -A: Laser Therapy and Diagnosis*

Shmuel Einav,[1] Masayoshi Okada[2]
[1]Department of Biomedical Engineering, Tel-Aviv University, ISRAEL
[2]School of Medicine, Kobe University, Kobe, JAPAN

4.1   LASER THERAPY

4.1.1   Laser Angioplasty

Angioplasty is a method used to open coronary arteries blocked by obstructing plaques. This can be done usually using balloon angioplasty (see Figure 1). However, balloon angioplasty can be used only if there is an adequate opening that allows passages of the balloon inside the plaque. The laser catheter has been used to solve this problem.

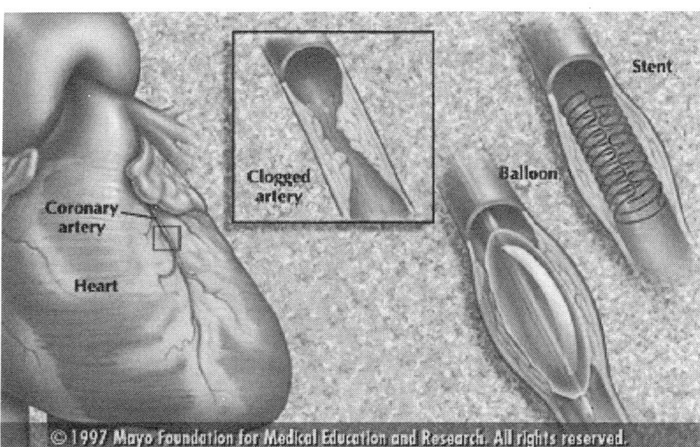

Figure 1. Balloon angioplasty with stent [1]

---

* Part-A (Sections 4.1 and 4.2) is authored by S. Einav. Part-B (Sections 4.3 to 4.5) is authored by M. Okada

When a plaque has totally blocked an artery, laser angioplasty can be used to drill a hole in the plaque to open a space for inserting the balloon catheter, so the balloon angioplasty can be successfully performed (see Figures 2 and 3).

This procedure is similar to the balloon angioplasty. A thin flexible tube, known as a catheter, is inserted through an artery in the groin and passed

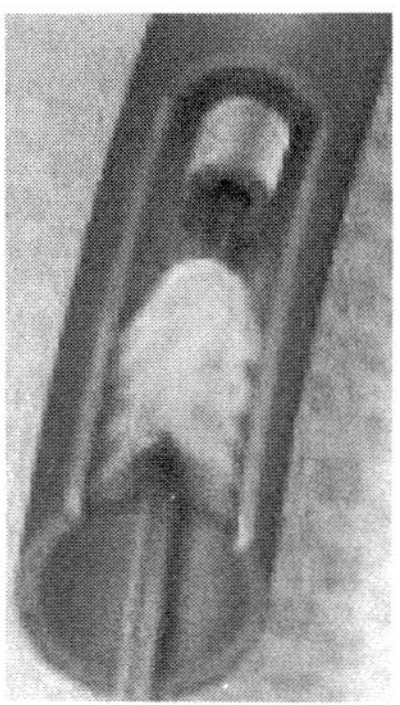

Figure 2. Laser angioplasty [2].

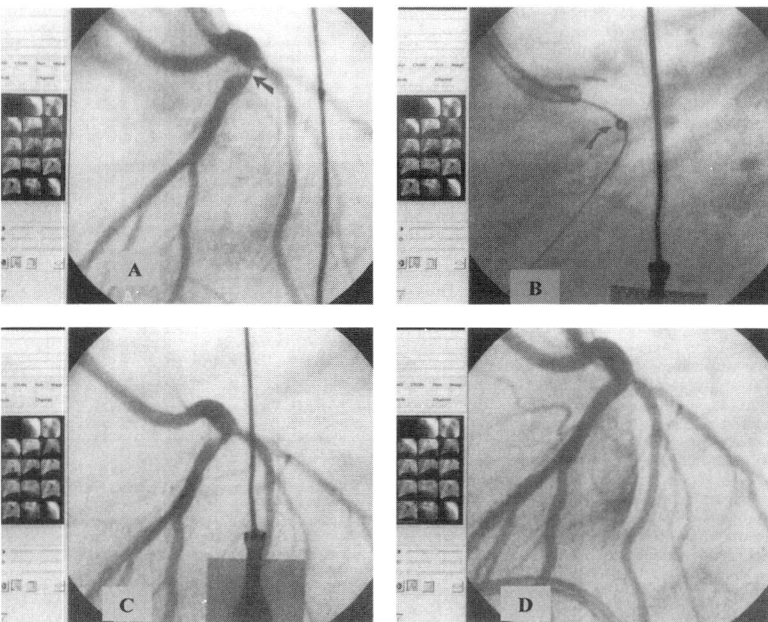

Figure 3. A) Ostial LAD stenosis (arrow). B) A 1.7-mm excimer laser catheter debulking the target stenosis. C) Immediate postlasing angiography. D) Final angiography after adjunct stenting [3].

through to the coronary arteries. A tiny laser is introduced through the catheter into the coronary artery where it vaporizes the plaque that is causing a blockage. The laser catheter contains a bundle of optical fibers, which transmit the laser light. When the laser is moved into position, it is activated to send bursts of ultraviolet (cool) laser light through the catheter and against the blockage. It is expected that the plaque is selectively vaporized using laser ablation without causing thermal damage to the blood vessel wall and without leaving debris. This procedure is often followed by a balloon angioplasty, to smooth out the artery walls, as well as the placement of a stent. The laser can vaporize a portion of the plaque and the larger balloon will follow to open up the rest of the artery. By removing a portion of the plaque with the laser, then following with the balloon, there is less chance of damage to the arterial walls and reduces the risk of restenosis.

In addition, laser angioplasty can also be used to remove in-stent restenosis (see Figure 4) or in peripheral arteries (Laser Angioplasty for Critical Ischemia), to open the smaller arteries of the lower leg. These vessels are more difficult to work on, especially in the case of diabetics [4].

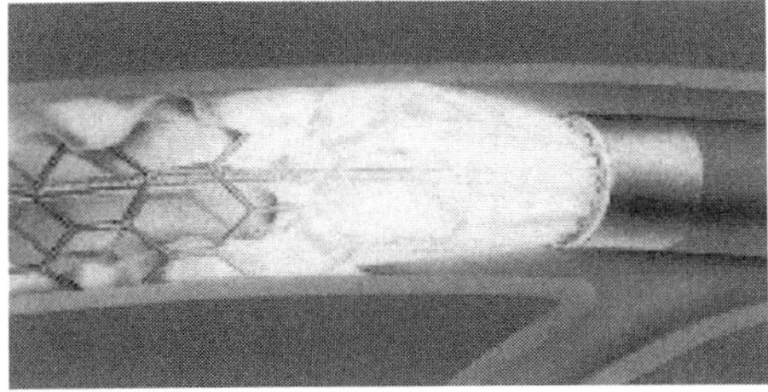

Figure 4. Excimer Laser Coronary Angioplasty (ELCA) treatment of restenosed stent [5].

There are three different methods of laser angioplasty: thermal, photothermal, and photoablative. In *thermal laser angioplasty*, an argon, or Nd:YAG laser is used to heat a biocompatible metal ally tip attached to a fiberoptic waveguide. The highest temperature is 400C, which is the temperature of the very tip of the probe. The surgeon guides the probe through the obstruction causing a small lumen for the blood to flow through. This method is not very useful since it can cause thermal damage of the tissues and carbonization and necrosis of the vessel walls. *Photothermal laser angioplasty* involves a contact of a Nd:YAG laser probe that rapidly heats the plaque to the point of vaporization using a photo-optical effect. This method is more productive and safer than the thermal method, but still can cause damage to vessel walls. The third method is *photoablative laser angioplasty* that involves the usage of excimer laser [1]. The excimer laser uses either two noble gas atoms or a noble gas atom in conjunction with a halogen atom to lase at different wavelengths, mostly Ultraviolet.

One example of laser angioplasty is Smooth Excimer Laser Coronary Angioplasty (SELCA), which uses a XeCl laser with the following properties: The excimer laser generates less heat than thermal and photothermal lasers. This reduces the carbonization and thermal damage of the blood vessels. While safer, excimer laser method still raises some safety concerns. The gases that are used for this method are typically very toxic and even fatal. No leakage of these gases can, therefore, be allowed. The UV radiation generated by the excimer laser can also cause genetic mutations of the DNA by breaking the hydrogen bonds between the two strands. Overall, laser angioplasty is also associated with many potential problems including reocclusion, vascular spasm, perforation, cardiac arrhythmias, and intimal dissection.

Up to day, the laser angioplasty is the only cardiovascular application of laser technology that has received FDA approval in the United States [7]. From 1988 to 1998, approximately, 14,000 patients were treated with excimer laser angioplasty [8]. The data underline the workability and safety of this procedure. Many works report of the significant success of excimer laser angioplasty for in-stent restenosis [9-11]. Laser angioplasty has become a safe and a cheap alternative for expensive, bypass, open-heart surgery.

However, Clinical studies have also shown that excimer laser angioplasty does not reduce the incidence of restenosis. Moreover - today it is well accepted that restenoses are extremely pronounced following excimer laser angioplasty. Their occurrence can be attributed to an enhanced proliferation of smooth muscle cells [12]. Most of these cells are undergoing DNA synthesis during two weeks after laser treatment, resulting in intimal thickening. Therefore, excimer laser angioplasty is generally being rejected today. Laser balloon angioplasty, however, is still being investigated to realize its full potential [7].

4.1.2 Laser Thrombolysis

The disadvantages of current techniques to rapidly clear large thrombus burden in occluded arteries led to the search for an alternative method that did not endanger the vessel wall. Laser thrombolysis allows selectively ablate thrombus without causing any histologic injury to the blood vessels.

The principal chromophore of thrombus in the visible waveband is hemoglobin present in the red blood cells. Since higher absorption coefficients require less energy per unit area to achieve ablation, the ablation threshold for artery is higher than that for clot. Figure 5 demonstrates the increase in absorption of nearly two orders of magnitude between clot and artery due to the presence of hemoglobin.

Pulsed-dye laser system emitting ultraviolet and visible regions waveband (400-600nm) at radiant exposures (1-2µs) can selectively remove clot [13].

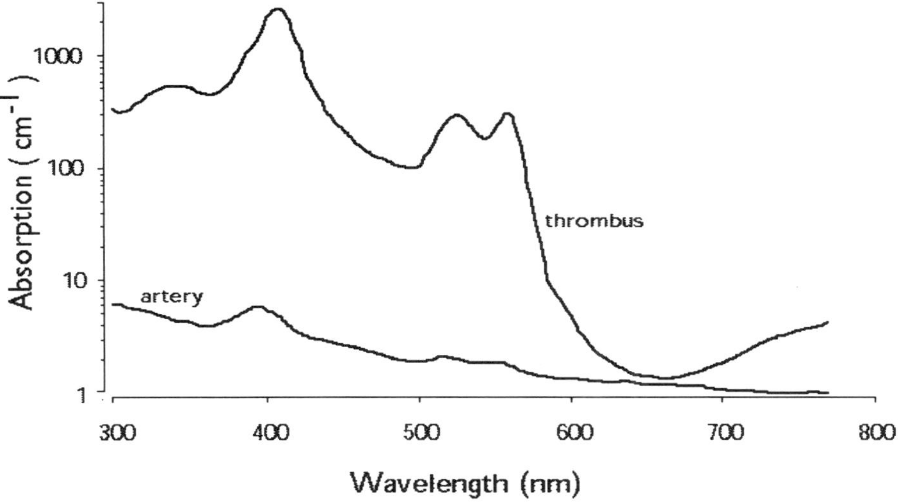

Figure 5. Absorption spectra of human thrombus and vessel wall [13].

Viator and Prahl [14] concluded from their study that ablation threshold and efficiency are independent of laser pulse duration. This result allows using Nd:YAG lasers with longer pulse (10msec) that better suites for coupling into small fibers and reduce mechanical damage to the tissue.

Figure 6 demonstrates a microsecond ablation of porcine clot in a 3mm silicon tube. The tube simulates the cylindrical geometry of a blood vessel. Light is delivered by a fluid-core catheter. The clot absorbs the light and a portion is vaporized. A vapor bubble is formed that expands and collapses causing the clot to be further disrupted. A Schematic representation of the fluid-core catheter used to deliver microsecond laser pulses to the clot during laser thrombolysis is shown in Figure 7. The laser energy is launched from the laser into an optical fiber contained in a catheter. The fiber in turn launches the light into an optically clear liquid that transmits the light to the target by total internal reflection. The distal tip of the catheter is open-ended so that the fluid can flow out of the catheter and wash away the blood in front of the clot. A clear path for direct laser delivery to the clot is thus established.

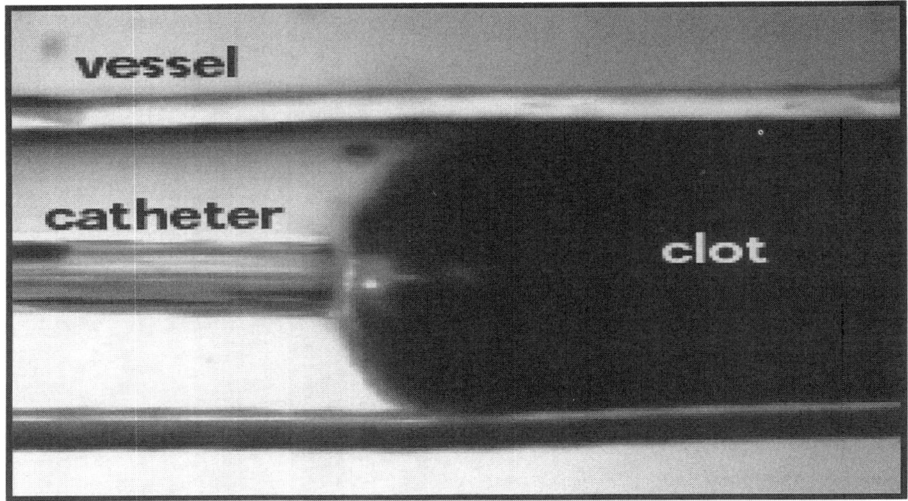

Figure 6. Microsecond ablation of porcine clot in a 3mm silicon tube. The tube simulates the cylindrical geometry of a blood vessel. Light is delivered by a fluid-core catheter. The clot absorbs the light and a portion is vaporized. A vapor bubble is formed that expands and collapses causing the clot to be further disrupted [13].

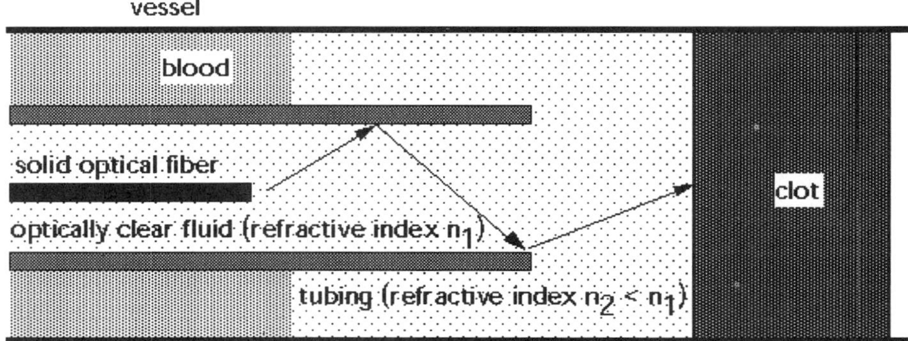

Figure 7. The fluid-core catheter [13].

Based on favorable animal studies of laser thrombolysis and approval from the FDA, a pilot study of laser thrombolysis in acute myocardial infarction in humans was performed at St. Vincent Hospital, Portland, Oregon and at St. Joseph's Hospital, Atlanta, Georgia. Effective thrombus removal was demonstrated in 16 of 18 patients [15]. A similar experiment was maid by Topaz *et al.* [16] on 6 patients, using pulse holmium laser system. Both experiments proved that laser thrombolysis could successfully remove thrombi, decrease the mean coronary artery stenosis dramatically, and therefore improve the coronary flow. The absence of any perforations or acute vessel closures supported the concept of selective thrombolysis without damage to the arterial wall. These small clinical evidences suggest that laser thrombolysis with a pulsed dye or holmium laser may offer an alternative treatment for patients with acute myocardial infraction [7]. However, current techniques for laser thrombolysis are limited because they cannot completely clear thrombotic occlusions in arteries, typically leaving residual thrombus on the walls of the artery. Shangguan *et al.* [17] suggested the possibility of using photomechanical drug delivery to enhance laser thrombolysis by delivering drugs into mural thrombus during laser thrombolysis.

4.1.3 Laser Photo-Chemotherapy

The concept of Photodynamic therapy (PDT) is the use of laser radiation to activate photosensitizers and generate free radicals. PDT has been studied and applied to various disease processes. The potential of PDT for selective destruction of target tissues is especially appealing in cardiovascular disease, in which other existing interventional tools are somewhat nonselective and carry substantial risk of damage to the normal arterial wall. Photoactivated drugs for example may inhibit smooth muscle cell proliferation and intimal hyperplasia.

Intimal hyperplasia (IH) induced by segmental injury of vessels after balloon angioplasty and is a dominant trigger for restenosis. PDT shows promise in the treatment of IH, by completely eradicating cells in the vessel wall. It results in complete vascular wall cell eradication with subsequent adventitia but minimal media repopulation. Overhaus *et al.* [18] claims that PDT alters the vascular wall matrix thereby inhibiting invasive cell migration, and as such, provides an important barrier mechanism to favorably alter the vascular injury response.

LaMuraglia *et al.* [19] argued that vascular PDT induces apoptosis as a mechanism of rapid, complete, and precise cell eradication in the artery wall. The drug is injected into the blood stream or directly injected into the diseased area with a catheter or an ultrathin endoscope. The drug is than triggered using a suitable laser wavelength and destroys the host plaque [20].

Figure 8 demonstrates for example Antrin localization in atheromatous plaque. The left picture shows a rabbit aorta, sliced longitudinally, ladened with atheromatous plaque. After receiving an Antrin injection, fluorescence analysis revealed select localization of the photosensitizer, at 750 nm, within the plaque, with little detected in the normal aortic wall [21].

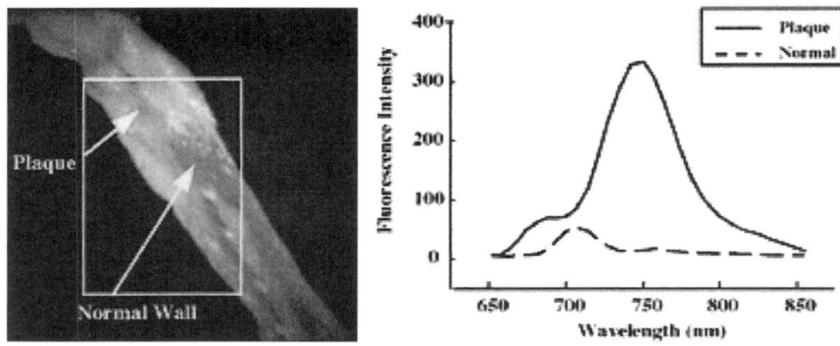

Figure 8. Antrin localization in atheromatous plaque [21]

Jenkins *et al.* [22] investigated the effect of adjuvant PDT following femoral percutaneous transluminal angioplasty (PTA) in a clinical study (7 patients). They suggested that endovascular PDT is safe and may reduce restenosis following angioplasty. Jenkins *et al.* also [23] reported of favorable influences of PDT on the arterial response to balloon injury in both the coronary and peripheral circulations in 13 juvenile pigs. Statius-van-Eps [24] suggested that inclusion of the whole injured artery or a section of an uninjured margin in the treatment field is essential for effective PDT prevention of IH.

PDT has four significant attributes of light-activated therapy: the putative selectivity and safety of photoangioplasty, the potential for atraumatic and effective debulking of atheromatous plaque through a biological mechanism, the postulated capability to reduce or inhibit restenosis, and the potential to treat long segments of abnormal vessel by simply using fibers with longer light-emitting regions [25]. The approach of systemic (or local) administration and local photoactivation of cytotoxic drugs is feasible and offers a potential powerful therapy for restenosis and atherosclerosis [7]. The available experience, coupled with the observations in human peripheral athero-sclerosis, suggest a promising future for photoangioplasty in the treatment of primary atherosclerosis and prevention of restenosis.

4.1.4   Laser Treatment of Arrhythmias

Cardiac arrhythmias have traditionally been treated with medications. However, over the years, there has come to be an appreciation for the failures and significant side effects of medical therapy because of the significant risk of side effects and adversities. Thus, more definitive methods for treatment of cardiac arrhythmias were sought such as catheter ablation. Catheter ablation of arrhythmias involves directing a catheter tip via a peripheral venous or arterial access to the site in the heart, which is critical to the maintenance of the arrhythmia circuit. Energy can then be delivered to the tip of the catheter and result in a discrete localized injury or ablative lesion. The most frequently used is catheter ablation using radiofrequency energy [26].

Lately, laser ablative approaches has been investigated for treatment of ventricular and supraventricular arrhythmias. In this approach, laser ablation is used to achieve superficial vaporization of endocardial tissue responsible for ventricular tachycardia. This can be done by ablation of ventricular foci responsible for arrhythmias and ablation of supraventricular tachyarrythmia pathways [7].

These investigations were based on the potential advantages of laser photocoagulation as compared to conventional surgical approaches or radiofrequency ablation [27]. These benefits include the fact that the treated tissues are left intact preserving structural integrity of the myocardium. Areas that are out of the reach of endocardial resection can be treated with improved access, and laser photocoagulation can be used in the absence of discrete areas of endocardial fibrosis. Laser photocoagulation can be preformed on the normothermic beating heart during ventricular tachycardia at the time of surgery. The preliminary clinical experience [28] has proven some success in this approach.

4.1.5   Laser Myocardial Ablation

The major advantage of this approach introduced with the new developed catheter that was designed to orient an optical fiber against the septum (see Figure 9). This powerful laser procedure offers the ability to perform percutaneously what otherwise would require a thoracotomy and open-heart surgery [7].

Percutaneous transluminal septal myocardial ablation (PTSMA) is a new, investigational, catheter-based treatment for severely symptomatic, medically refractory hypertrophic obstructive cardiomyopathy. Compared with surgical myectomy, PTSMA has the advantage of being minimally invasive, easily repeated, and with relatively low major morbidity/mortality risk for patients with comorbid conditions [29].

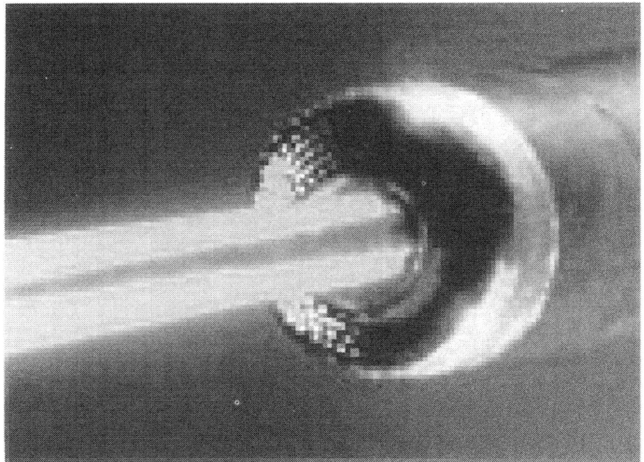

Figure 9. Laser catheter used for myocardial ablation

Laser radiation may also be effectively used for the ablation of myocardial tissue for the treatment of various cardiovascular disorders. For example performing a myotomy-myectomy by ablation of the abnormally thickened septum in idiopathic hypertropic subaortic stenosis using laser radiation.

In vitro and animal in vivo experience demonstrated that argon radiation could cut and vaporize the mayocardium producing a myotomy-myectomy morphologically similar to that produced by the conventional blade technique [30]. Moreover, this technique allowed improved visualization and cleaner resection of the septum compared to scalpel resection.

4.1.6 Transmyocardial Laser Revascularization (TMR)

Transmyocardial laser revascularization (TMR) is a new procedure for patients that suffer from severe narrowing throughout the length of their coronary arteries (angina). In this procedure, high power laser energy is used to create channels in ischemic ventricular myocardium to improve local perfusion [7,31].

Angina occurs when the heart muscle doesn't receive enough oxygen-rich blood. Most often, this reduced blood flow, called ischemia, results from cholesterol-laden plaque narrowing the coronary arteries. This situation cannot be improved or corrected by a bypass or an angioplasty. In Addition, there are many patients who because of small size vessels or diffuse disease are not good candidates for percutaneous interventions or bypass surgery. For some time now, the only option for such patients whose symptoms cannot be controlled with medications was a heart transplant [31,32].

TMR represents the rebirth of an approach ("myocardial acupuncture") abandoned in the 1960s but now being preformed with laser radiation [7]. It has been referred to as the "snake heart" procedure, because the original idea for the surgery was based on the physiology of reptile hearts, which don't really have coronary arteries but supply blood to their heart muscle through channels that extend from the cavity of the main pumping chamber of their heart.

In TMR procedure, the surgeon makes a small incision on the left side of the chest between the ribs (see Figure 10), exposing the surface of the heart and locates a viable ischemic area that is in need of improved blood flow.

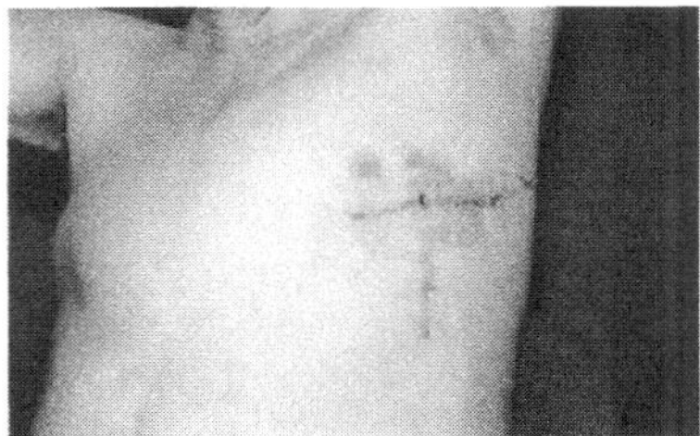

Figure 10. Incision on left side of chest for TMR surgery [33].

A computer-controlled laser is inserted into the chest opening. The computer synchronizes the laser's pulses to fire between heartbeats, hitting the left ventricle when it is filled with blood, to make very small passages through the LV (see Figure 11). The blood that has filled the ventricle protects the surrounding heart tissue from injury by the laser (Figure 12). The surgeon makes between 10 to 40 channels, about a millimeter in diameter (Figure 13), allow blood to flow into the channels, bringing oxygen to the tissues. The procedure takes about 2 hours. The holes on the heart's surface seal shut with

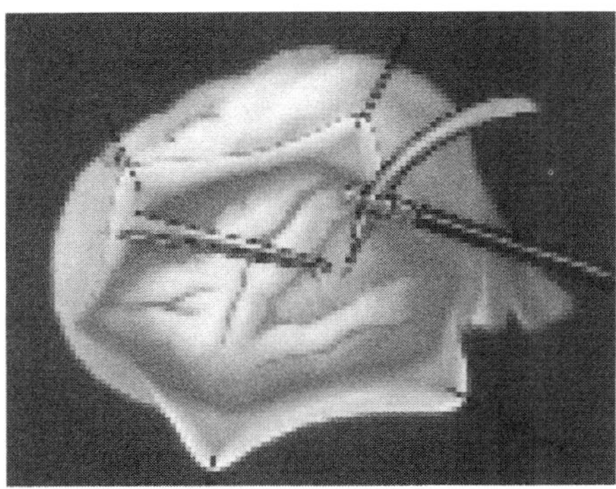

Figure 11. TMR pulse laser catheter creates channels through LV myocardium [33].

clotted blood in minutes and heal within days, but researchers speculate that the interior channels remain open so that oxygen-rich blood continues to flow into the heart's muscular wall with each contraction. The channels will eventually heal and close, but angiogenesis, the growth of capillaries, may occur in the area, sustaining improved blood flow [31,33].

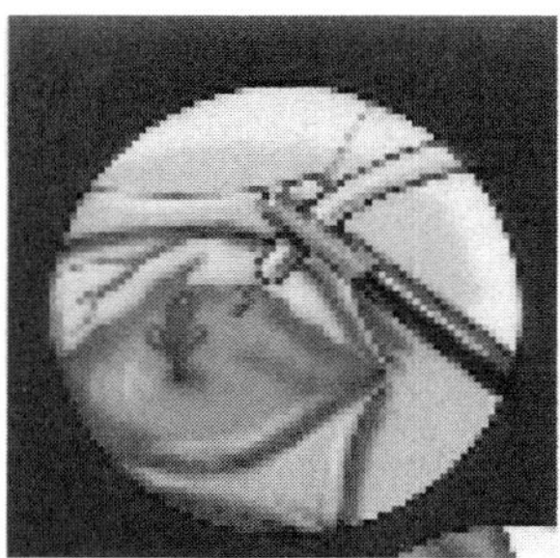

Figure 12. Blood flow through the channel, protecting the surrounding tissue [33].

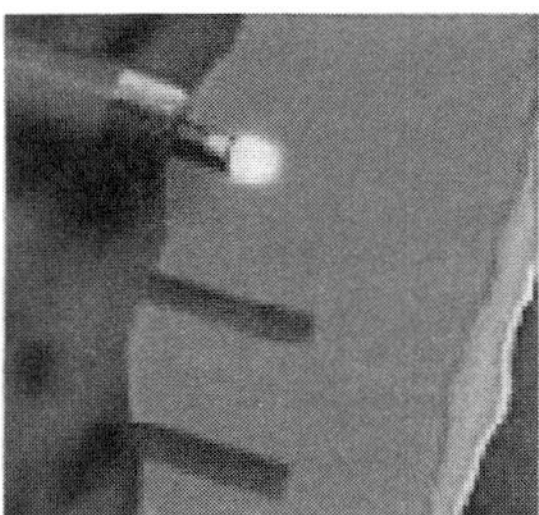

Figure 13. Illustration of channels drilled through heart myocardium using PTMR catheter [32].

TMR offers several advantages over conventional treatments. Unlike bypass surgery, which requires stopping the heart and relying on a heart-lung machine to pump the patient's blood during the procedure, TMR is performed with the heart still beating. In addition, in TMR, surgeons reach the heart through a four-inch incision between the patient's ribs, rather than by open-heart procedures. This means that recovery time is quicker, and the surgery costs about a third as much as bypass.

The results of preliminary clinical trials with TMR in terms of angina relief are impressive compared to medication [34-37] and it has shown symptomatic benefit and improvement in the exercise tolerance of patients [36]. At one-year follow-up studies, a significant improvement in the angina class, and treadmill testing (TMT) effort tolerance were observed; but without any significant change in the left ventricular ejection fraction.

For now, no one knows exactly why TMR works, and it is still considered investigational by FDA. A possible explanation is that, even though most of the laser-drilled channels are closed soon after surgery, the short-lived flow of blood through the channels, or perhaps the laser energy itself, may stimulate the growth of tiny new blood vessels, capable of carrying oxygen-rich blood to the deficient areas of the heart. In fact, several recent studies have demonstrated that blood flow to the heart does improve after TMR, despite closure of the laser-induced channels [34]. Whittaker *et al.* [38] suggests that the best results obtained when the channels connected to the LV cavity and adjacent myocardium and is surrounded by a small amount of scar in which collagen fibers are aligned parallel to the channel (see Figure 14a). If the fibers are perpendicular to the channel, the channel is closed (Figure 14b).

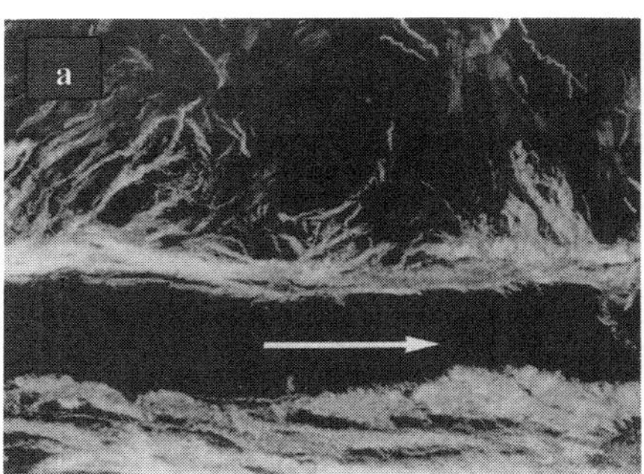
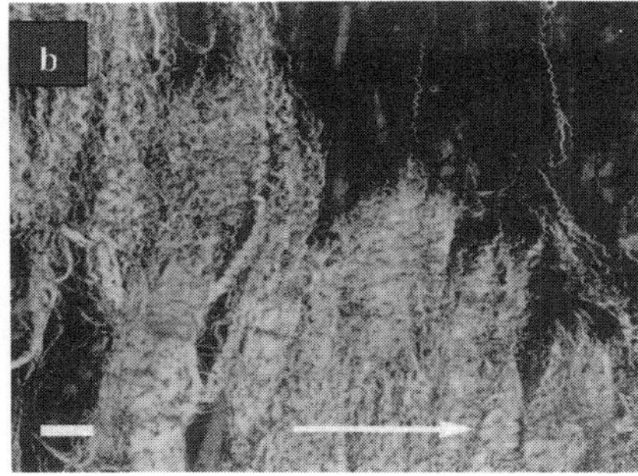

Figure 14. Sections stained with picrosirius red and viewed with polarized light of (a) open channel and (b) closed channel [38].

However, TMR procedure resulted with 10-19% perioperative mortality, in patients with unstable angina or reduced left ventricular function [36,37]. Furthermore, little information is available concerning the effect of this procedure on life expectancy [31]. The high early mortality can be brought down with careful patient selection and perioperative management [36,37].

A new, less invasive method places a catheter into the heart through an artery and creates the channels from inside the chamber of the heart into the LV muscles. This is known as percutaneous TMR (PTMR) and avoids the need to open the chest. Clinical trials using this approach were successful, and it is now in stage II of FDA approval [32].

4.1.7 Erythrocytes Protection by Low-Power He-Ne Laser

Extracorporeal circulation (ECC) systems using artificial heart-lung machines cause relatively high damage to blood erythrocytes because of the direct contact of blood with foreign bodies and the high shear stress under vacuum aspiration.

A new method for reducing the hemolysis produced by ECC circulation without administering drugs is being recently investigated [38], base on reports on protective effect of the low power helium-neon (He-Ne) laser against the damage of human erythrocytes in whole blood.

In *in-vitro* experiments [39], low power He-Ne laser beam (at 632.8 nm wavelength, 8.5 mW output power, and 1.96 eV quantum energy) was irradiated on the blood flow from distance of 22 mm. As a result, the erythrocyte deformability and erythrocyte ATP levels decreased significantly with time (comparing to a control group), and the free hemoglobin levels increased with time. There were less echinocytes (abnormal spinous erythrocytes) and more discocytes (morphologically normal cells) in the laser group when compared to the control group.

Low power lasers have been used in clinical practice although its mechanism is not fully understood. Activation of cellular function by laser exposure is considered to be a possible mechanism. Currently, no literature is available which clearly demonstrates the definite mechanism of the protective effect.

These results suggested that the irradiation of low-powered He-Ne lasers improved cytoskeletal protein activities in damaged erythrocytes. Clinical application is expected after determination of the optimal energy level [40].

4.1.8 Endothelization

Numerous reports suggest that low-power laser irradiation (LPLI) is capable of affecting cellular processes in the absence of significant thermal effect. Kipshidze *et al.* [41] demonstrated that LPLI significantly increased production of vascular endothelial growth factor (VEGF) secretion by smooth muscle cells (SMC), fibroblasts, and cardiac myocytes (see Figure 15) and stimulates human endothelial cells (EC) growth in culture. These data may have significant importance leading to the establishment of new methods for endoluminal postangioplasty vascular repair and myocardial photoangio-genesis.

4.1.9 Extraction of Pacemakers and ICD Leads

Cardiac pacemakers and Implantable Cardiac Defibrillators (ICD's) are used to control arrhythmia, or irregular beating of the heart. Once a cardiac pacemaker is implanted, a number of clinical situations may occur which require its removal, including infection, product recall or product failure. Approximately 70,000 people may face lead removal each year. Non-functional leads can cause such medical problems as reduced blood flow or thrombosis (blood clotting), migration of broken leads in the vascular system, the unavailability of veins for replacement leads, and possible electrical interactions with new leads. In addition, they are a potential source of infection [2].

VEGF SECRETION IN CELL CULTURE

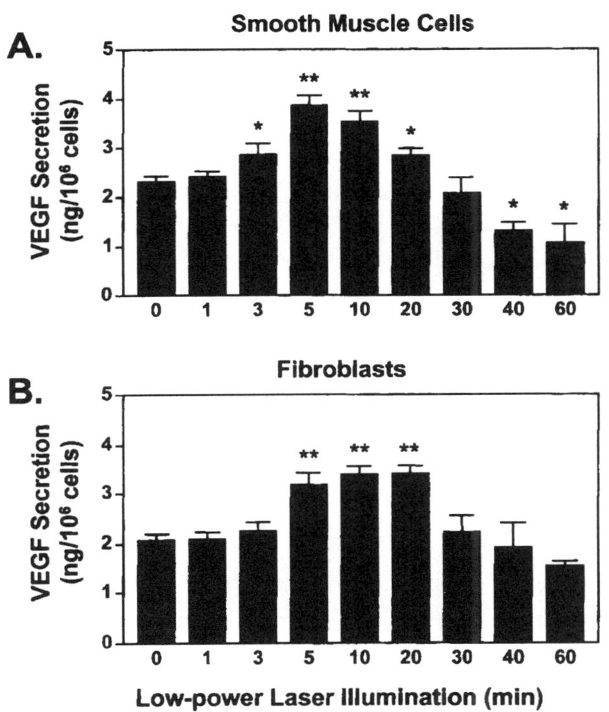

Figure 15. Laser treatment results in vascular endothelial growth factor (VEGF) secretion. Smooth muscles (A) and fibroblasts (B) [41].

Until recently, the only options for the removal of permanent pacemaker leads were surgical and traction. All of these methods can become complicated, because scar tissue will often form around the lead, binding it to the lining of the heart and blood vessels. In order to be removed, the scar tissue must be separated from the lead. Before laser extraction, physicians cut the leads from the tissue. Often, while cutting away the scar tissue, healthy tissue could be damaged [42,43].

Laser extraction is a safe and effective way to remove implanted pacemaker and defibrillator leads, because it decreases the risk of patient morbidity to practically zero by reducing the physical force required to tear the lead away from scar tissue that has accumulated over time.

Laser extraction uses cool cutting (50 degrees C) ultraviolet Excimer Laser with an absorption depth of 0.06 mm to vaporize scar tissue surrounding the lead. The laser energy is emitted from the tip of flexible 12, 14 or 16 French (Fr) probes. A new developed laser sheath (see Figure 16) is advanced over the pacemaker or defibrillator lead to cover it; when scar tissue is encountered, the laser is activated and the scar tissue at the catheter tip is vaporized. When the wire is cleared, it is pulled out through the protective sheath. The fibrotic sheaths usually surrounding leads can be cut without damaging the endothelial wall or the insulation of other leads [44].

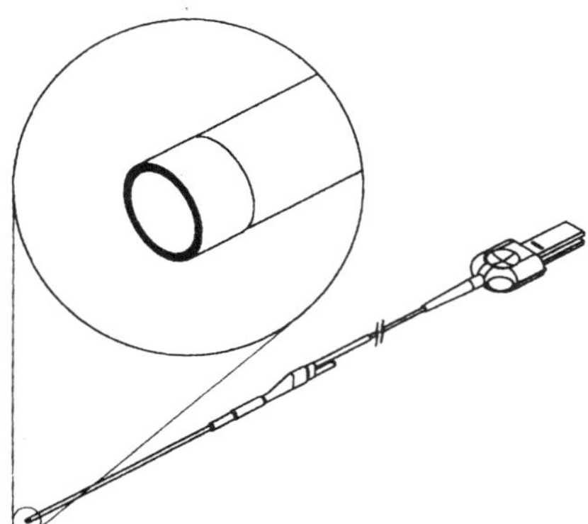

Figure 16. Laser sheath for lead removal [45].

Initial results are very encouraging [44-47]. Kennergren. [44] reviews the European multi-center experience from August 1996 to August 1998: 179 leads (104 atrial, 57 ventricular, one SVC, 17 ICD) in 149 patients were extracted in 11 centers using Excimer laser with success rate of 89%. The Plexes trial [47] randomized 301 patients to the laser sheath vs. mechanical system with success rates of 94% vs. 65%, respectively. Additionally, the success rate for lead extraction with laser after failing with the mechanical system was 88% [43,47]. In addition, the inability to pass the scar tissue binding site and lead breakage occurred less frequently in the laser-treated group. The procedure was less time consuming and therefore less traumatic to the patient [43].

Since Laser assisted lead extraction was found to be a safe and efficacious procedure, these initial results may allow broader use of the procedure to include the extraction of many non-functional leads, previously abandoned [44].

4.2   LASER DIAGNOSIS

4.2.1 Laser Doppler Anemometry, Imaging and Fluxmetry

Laser Doppler Anemometry (LDA) is a non-invasive technique that can be applied to determine the distribution of red blood cell (RBC) velocity in the blood vessels of microcirculation, such as the low-speed flows associated with nutritional blood flow in capillaries close to the skin surface and flow in the underlying arterioles and venules involved in regulation of skin temperature. The tissue thickness sampled is typically 1mm, the capillary diameters 10 microns and the velocity spectrum measurement typically 0.01 to 10mm/s [48].

The high resolution of the laser beam and its extremely narrow band ensure that sufficient illumination can be achieved with low intensity laser. In addition, the size of the focused beam can be varied to accommodate the many different blood vessels in the microcirculation. Its uniqe advantages are that it has high spatial resolution, is an absolute method, and is under operator and computer control [49,50].

Based on the heterodyning of two laser beams, the LDA offers a fast signal processing system and a means for rapidly determining flow. Basically, the LDA technique measures the velocity of suspended particles (such as RBC) in a moving fluid by detecting the Doppler shift of the laser light scattered from the moving particles [49]. Einav and Lee [51] suggested that two groups of different-sized scattering particles suspended in a fluid, which are moving with different velocities, would produce separate Doppler signals in the frequency domain, distinctly different in both amplitude and frequency.

The Doppler shift in the frequency can be derived from two distinct approaches:

1. The heterodynamic beam mode, or coherent detection at a photomultiplier tube (PMT). Incident (unshifted) laser light is heterodyned (beat or mixed) on the cathode surface of the tube, together with the frequency-shifted laser light. The tube detects only the difference between the Doppler-shifted and original frequencies. The resultant difference in the frequency is measured by frequency to voltage conversion, spectrum analysis, auto-correlation, or other equivalent data processing system. Bluestein and Einav [52] suggested to use "direct Fourier transform of short blocks of data" to reduce the variability inherent to the spectral estimation of LDA signals. The hetrodyne system makes stringent demands for the coherence and equal path length of the incident and the scattered beam.

2. The fringe beam mode. In this case, two equally intense laser beams sharing a common wave front are caused to intersect at their waist. At the intersecion, known as the measuring or sensing volume, the two beams form an interfacepattern, the fringes of which are parallel and easily seen. Particles passing through the fringes scatter light; the light has a period defined by the fixed-fringe spacing and particle velocity, and provides flow data for quantitative analysis [50].

Laser light can be directed to the tissue surface either via an optic fiber or as a light beam. For 'fiber optic' monitors (*LDF* instruments) the optic fiber terminates in an optic probe which can be attached to the tissue surface. One or more light collecting fibers also terminate in the probe head and these fibers transmit a proportion of the scattered light to a photodetector and the signal processing electronics. Normal fiber separations in the probe head are a few tenths of a mm so consequently blood flow is measured in a tissue volume of typically 1mm3 or smaller. When a larger volume of tissue is stimulated to vasodilate or vasoconstrict, or where for example a healing process results in increased blood flow, the measured blood flow changes in the small tissue volume are generally taken to be representative of the larger volume [48,53].

In a Laser Doppler blood flow Imager (*LDI*) the low intensity laser beam is scanned across a tissue surface in a raster fashion using a moving mirror. There is no direct contact with the tissue being assessed. Both large areas (a full torso) and small areas (part of a finger) can be scanned enabling the blood flow to be mapped and color coded images of the blood flow displayed. Regions of interest can be defined and statistical data calculated and recorded. Single point measurements give a high temporal resolution (40Hz data rates are typical) enabling rapid blood flow changes to be recorded, whereas the laser Doppler imager can provide spatial information and has the ability to average blood flow measurements over large areas.

Fiber optic systems can measure at tissue sites not easily accessible to a laser beam. For example measurements in brain tissue, mouth, gut, colon, muscle and bone [48,53]. Laser Doppler Imager (LDI) can be used to show heart tissue blood flow during and after coronary artery bypass graft (CABG) surgery to identify areas of poor perfusion [54].

De Graaff *et al.* [55] suggest that laser Doppler fluxmetry (LDF) may be also useful for the diagnosis of deep venous thrombosis in asymptomatic patients, as it can measure the peripheral vasoconstriction response upon an increase in venous pressure, which is hypothetically preactivated upon venous damming by a thrombus. Moreover, Ray *et al.* [56] suggest that post-occlusive Laser Doppler fluxmetry (LDF) curves may identify the distribution of arterial disease and may be useful in the non-invasive management of peripheral ischaemia.

Laser Doppler Capillary Anemometers can be positioned onto the apex of any capillary that is visible, or barely visible through the skin surface and measure capillary blood cell velocity (from 0.1 mm/s to 14 mm/s), continuously, in real time (allowing cardiac and vasomotion responses to be followed) and non-invasively [57]. An in-built CCD camera allows continuous monitoring of the capillary position either on a separate monitor or optionally on the computer screen.

4.2.2 Fluorescence Spectroscopy

Fluorescence methodology uses fluorophores, which are fluorescent organic complexes or dyes. When stimulated by light at a known wavelength, each fluorophore emits a unique fluorescence with distinguishing characteristics, particularly wavelength and intensity. This fluorescence acts as a fingerprint. The fluorophore has an affinity for the analyte of interest and attaches itself to the analyte. Wavelength and intensity are dependent upon the concentration of the analyte and this permits an analysis of the components of interest. The intensity of a fluorescence signal is a linear function of the amount of fluorophore present [58]. Several studies tried to develop laser-based spectroscopic techniques using fibre optical probes transluminally or peroperatively to identify tissue changes caused by cardiovascular diseases, and thereby potentially allow improved therapy for patients suffering from those diseases [59]. There are several different kinds of optical spectroscopic techniques to be used as laser-based minimally-invasive diagnostic techniques to identify diseased regions in the cardiac muscle and occlusions in vessels., among them: infrared spectroscopy, Raman spectroscopy, fluorescence spectroscopy and remission spectroscopy in the visible and NIR wavelength region. This diagnostic tool enables accurate detection of the presence of atherosclerotic vessel wall and the detection of early atherosclerotic changes. In order to deal with plaque blockage inside the arteries, the atherosclerotic plaque must be identified during endoscopic imaging. The Collagen to elastin ratio varies dramatically from 0.5 in normal arterial wall to 7.3 in atherosclerotic plaques, and this difference is highly reflected in fluorescence difference between normal and atherosclerotic tissue [20]. In this diagnostic approach, low–power laser radiation induces tissue fluorescence without tissue damage and can be used for diagnostic fluorescence spectroscopy. Since normal and atherosclerotic tissue have different fluorescence spectra, it may be possible to construct images of the arterial surface using fluorescence imaging.

Based on this concept, some models have been proposed to determine the chemical composition of atherosclerotic plaque based on fluorescence characteristics. These models offer not only the ability to distinguish between normal aorta and three different atherosclerotic histologic types, but also the ability to differentiate thin yellow fatty plaque from thick white atheromatous or fibrous plaque. Moreover, some models offer detection of the presence of calcification in atherosclerotic coronary artery segments or degenerative aortic valve leaflets [7].

4.2.3 NADH Fluorimetry

In normal functioning living cells that use oxygen, the ratio between nicotinamide adenine dinucleotide (NAD) and reduced nicotinamide adenine dinucleotide (NADH) varies over a large range. Under extreme conditions, however, such as lack of oxygen (anoxia) or lack of blood supply (ischemia), there is 100% reduction of NAD to NADH. Clinically, if 100% reduction of NADH can be detected at an early stage, the physician may have a chance to restore the cell viability before irreversible changes take place. If possible, the continuous monitoring of tissue NADH levels is an important means of monitoring tissue metabolism in terms of ischemia and viability [20].

Studies have shown that there is a difference in fluorescence property of NAD and NADH: The luminescence intensity is linear proportional to the number of NADH excited molecules. Using fluorescence measurements, one may determine the intracellular concentration of NADH [7,60-63].

Development of laser fluorimeter designed for measurements of NADH levels in blood-perfused organs may offer NADH fluorescence marker of the transient ischemia and/or anoxia [7] NADH fluorescence measurements, therefore, may supply information about alternations in cardiac cell metabolism and for detecting heart disease. This measurement, carried out through optical fibers, is called fiberoptic fluorimetry and may be a promising method of assessing and continuously monitoring regional myocardial ischemia andhypoxia in a clinical setting.

Using NADH laser fluorimetry, cardiologists monitored dead heart tissue (myocardial necrosis) after a heart attack (myocardial infraction) to determine the extent of damage. Laser-fiberoptic fluorimetry may become a powerful diagnostic tool, which supplies vital information to surgeons in real time during vascular surgery, bypass heart surgery, or neurosergury [20].

4.2.4 Fluorescence in Blood-flow Measurement

The fluorescence measurement of blood flow is another diagnostic method based on laser technology. This is an optical method equivalent to thermodilution, measuring blood flow, and is based on introducing a luminescent dye or radioactively labeled microspheres into the heart and measuring the rate at which it becomes diluted in the circulation using

44. Kennergren C., "Excimer Laser Assisted Extraction of Permanent Pacemaker and ICD Leads:Present Experiences of a European Multi-Center Study",*Eur J Cardiothorac Surg.*, 1999; 15(6): 856-860.

45. Reiser C., Taylor K.D. and Lippincott R.A., "Large Laser Sheath for Pacing and Defiblli- rator Lead Removal", *Lasers Surg. Med.*, 1998; 22(1): 42-45.

46. Korley V.J., Hallet N., Daoust M., Epstein L.M., "A Novel Indication for Transvenous Lead Extraction: Upgrading Implantable Cardioverter Defibrillator Systems", *J Interv Card Electrophysiol.* 2000; 4(3): 523-528.

47. Byrd C, Wilkhoff B, Love C, *et al.* "Clinical Study of the Laser Sheath: Results of the PLEXES Trial", (abstract). *Pacing Clin Electrophysiol.* 1997;20(2):1053.

48. Shepherd A.P. and P.Å. Oberg, 'Laser-Doppler Blood Flowmetry', Kluwer Academic Publishers, 1990.

49. Einav S., Berman H.J. and Dean H.C., "Fringe Mode Reflectance Laser Doppler Micro- scope system", *J. of Biomedical Engineering*, 11(1), 57-62, 1989.

50. Einav S. and Berman H.J., "Fringe Mode Transmittance Laser Doppler Microscope Ane- mometer – Its Adaptation for Measurements in the Microcirculation" *J. of Biomedical Engineering*, 10(5), 393-399, 1988.

51. Einav S. and Lee S.L., "Migration in an Oscillatory Flow of a Laminar Suspension Measured by Laser Anemometry", *Experiments in Fluids*, 6, 273-279, 1988.

52. Bluestein, D. and Einav, S. "Spectral Estimation and Analysis of LDA Data in Pulsatile Flow Through Heart Valves", *Experiments in Fluids*, 15,341-353, 1993.

53. Belcaro G.V., U. Hoffmann, A. Bollinger and A.N. Nicolaides, 'Laser Doppler', Med- Orion Publishing Co., 1994.

54. Hajivassiliou C A, Greer K, Fisher A, Finlay I G., "Non-Invasive Measurement of Colonic Blood Flow Distribution using Laser Doppler Imaging", *British J. of Surgery*, 1998; 85:52-55.

55. De Graaff J.C., Ubbink D.Th., Buller H.R. and Jacobs M.J., "The Diagnosis of Deep Venous Thrombosis Using Laser Doppler Skin Perfusion Measurements", *Microvascular Research*, 61(1): 49-55, 2001.

56. Ray S.A, Buckenham T.M., Belli A.M., Taylor R.S. and Dormandy J.A., "The Associa- tion Between Laser Doppler Reactive Hyperaemia Curves and the Distribution of Peri- pheral Arterial Disease", *Eur. J. Vasc. Endovasc. Surg.*, 17(3): 245-8, 1999.

57. http://www.bridleways.uklinux.net/cam1.html

58. http://www.fluorrx.com/white1.htm

59. http://www.mlc.lu.se/Laic/FirstReport.htm

60. http://www.elet2.sote.hu/eke/ISOTT98/Abs/A143_Coremans.html

61. http://www.evergreen.edu/user/serv_res/research/bsi/papers/NADPH.htm

62. http://mcnichols.tca.net/~roger/thesis/opening.html

63. http://www.originlab.com/www/resources/case_studies/Loyola1.asp

64. http://www.probes.com/handbook/sections/0008.html

Part-B: Some Case Studies*

4.3 TRANSMYOCARDIAL LASER REVASCULARIZATION (TMLR)

4.3.1 Introduction

Lasers have been recently used in the field of cardiovascular disease [1]. Coronary artery bypass grafting (CABG) for coronary artery disease has been widely performed in Japan as well as USA and European countries. CABG has been performed as a popular surgical therapy. Among these patients there are a few cases for whom CABG can not be carried out, because of diffuse stenosis or the small-caliber of the coronary arteries [2-4]. First of all an alternative method of transmyocardial revascularization by high energy CO_2 laser was experimentally performed to save severely ill patients with terminal stage due to ischemic heart disease [5-7]. The purpose of this study was to clarify the availability of transmyocardial revascularization from the left ventricular cavity through channels created newly by laser irradiation.

By this procedure many intramyocardial connections could be created between the coronary arteries and their veins or myocardial sinusoids in the myocardium as illustrated in Figure 17.

4.3.2 Materials and Methods

Adult mongrel dogs were used in this study. Their chests were opened through the left fifth intercostal space under general anesthesia. Acute myocardial infarction was produced by multiple ligations of the coronary arteries. At the same time, transmyocardial channels (3 to 4 per cm^2) were newly created by high energy CO_2 laser in the area of the infarcted myocardium with the heart beating or in temporary ventricular fibrillation [6].

Bleeding from the left ventricular cavity was stopped by compression with gauze for about 10 min, after which further channels could be done. Optimal condition was 60-100 W in output, and irradiation time 0.12-0.25 sec to make transmyocardial laser channels. Transmyocardial channels of 0.2mm in diameter and 10mm in depth could be safely created by high energy CO_2 laser, provided care was taken to keep to the area being lasered, since the CO_2 laser emission was remarkably absorbed by water and blood.

**Part B has been authored by M. Okada.*

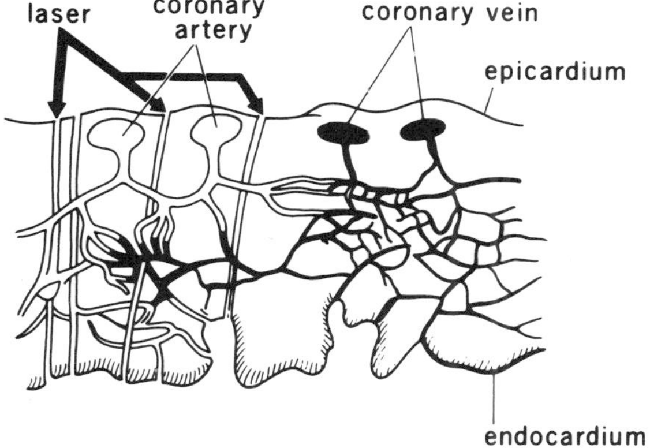

a)   Microcirculation in the myocardium

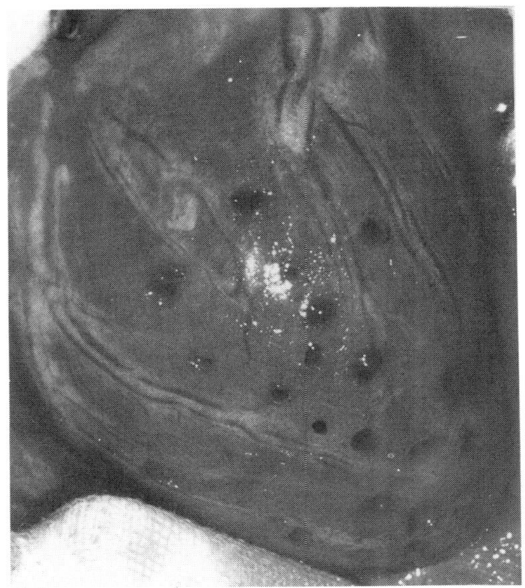

b) After completion of TMLR

Figure. 17 Mechanism of TMLR.

4.3.3   Myocardial Blood Flow and Changes of CK-MB Levels after TMLR

Myocardial blood flow was measured by laser Doppler flowmetry at the 30 minutes and 60 minutes after ligation of the coronary artery (acute myocardial infarction, AMI). Consequently, an increase of 60% in myocardial blood flow could be confirmed through TMLR between these periods. On the contrary, a decrease, more than 20% in the myocardial blood flow, was clearly observed in AMI group. There was a marked significance between two groups.

On the other hand, CK-MB activity in the blood was also evaluated between AMI TLMR group. Subsequently, the peak value of CK-MB activity was revealed at 12 hours in the TMLR group and 24 hours in AMI group after the ligations of the coronary arteries. Thus, rapid microcirculation in the myocordium was recognized through TMLR (Figure 18).

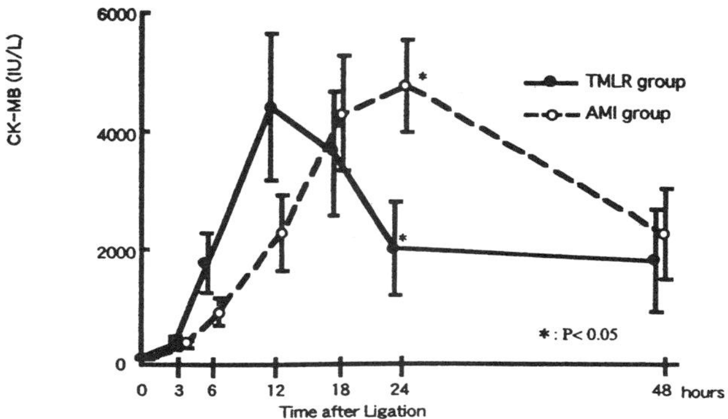

Figure 18. Changes of CK-MB levels

4.3.4 Hemodynamic Investigation

Pressure in the septal performing artery as representive of the intramyocardial pressure and the left ventricular pressure were simultaneously measured. Consequently, mean value of intramyocardial pressure was 40/30mmHg and of the left ventricular cavity 95/0mmHg. The mean pressure gradient between intramyocardial pressure and the left ventricular pressure was 55mmHg. Therefore, blood flowed from the left ventricular cavity into the ischemic myocardium during systole. On the other hand, blood flowed from the myocardium into the ventricular cavity as result of 30mmHg pressure gradient during diastole (Figure 19) [8,9].

4.3.5 Macroscopic Study

After completion of TMLR, hemodynamic and ventriculographic studies were carried out. Consequently, newly created laser channels were clearly confirmed on ventriculogram (Figure 20).

On the other hand, macroscopic findings with or without TMLR in the chronic stage after AMI were compared to each other. Subsequently, the left ventricular wall showed almost normal findings in the case with TMLR.On the contrary, a thin and infarcted area in the left ventricular wall was observed in the case without TMLR (Figure 21). Thus, TMLR revealed excellent microcirculation in the ischemic myocardium.

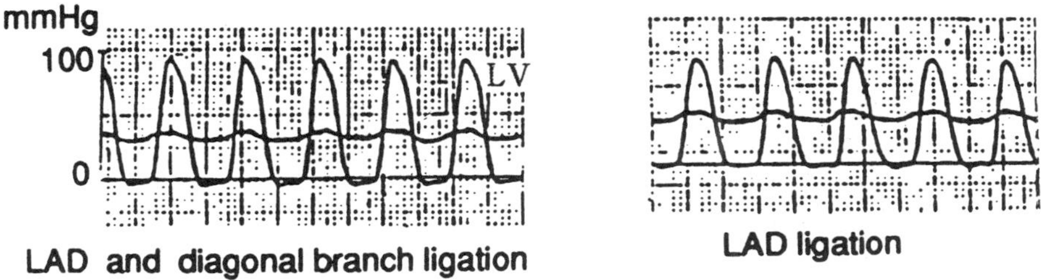

Figure 19. Hemodynamic study of myocardial pressure and left entricular pressure

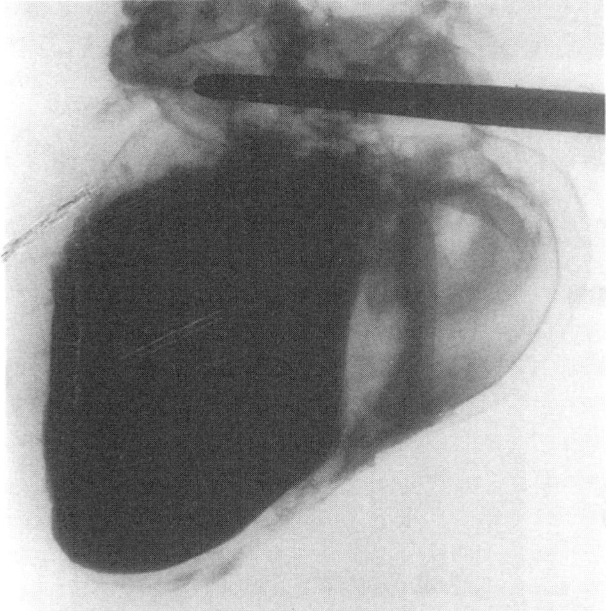

Figure 20. Left ventriculogram after TMLR

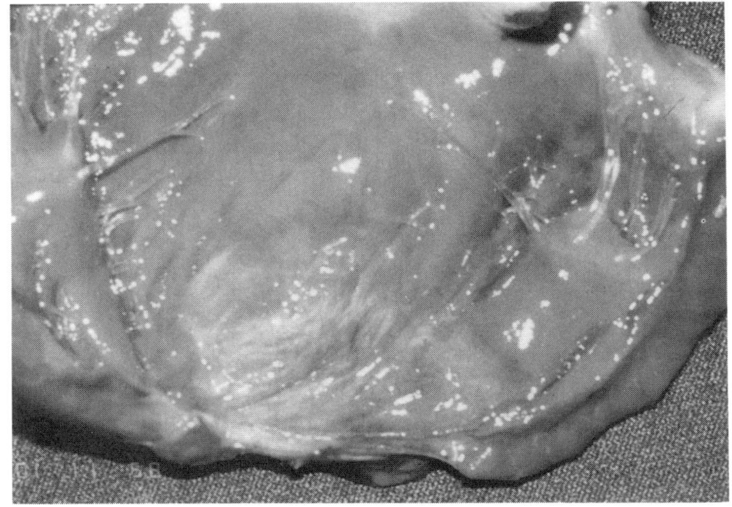

a) AMI group

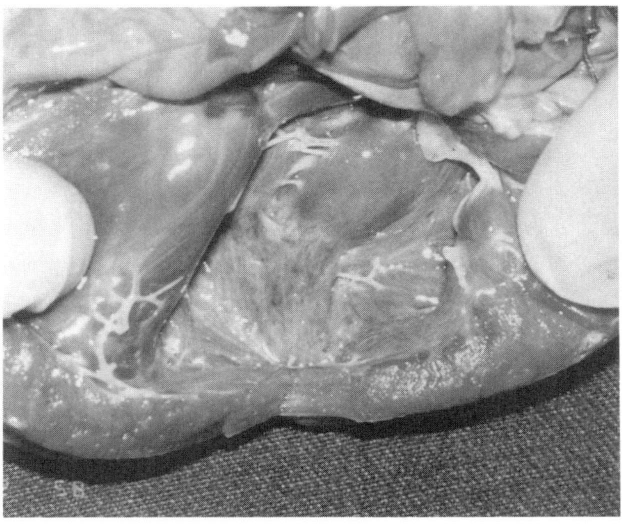

b) TMLR group

Figurer 21. Macroscopic findings of the left ventricular wall.

4.3.6 Histological Examination

Histological findings of newly created transmyocardial channels were as follows. Carbonization of the myocardium was observed in the first layer and coagulation necrosis was also recognized in the second layer of the created laser channels. Histological findings soon after creation of the myocardial channels are shown in Figure 22. In histological findings one week after TMLR, tissue reaction to laser had disappeared. Patency of the transmyocardial laser channels 3 years after TMLR could be clearly confirmed microscopically (Figure 23). These findings disclosed the feasibility of the long-term patency of the newly created channels and of clinical application [6].

4.3.7 Clinical Experience

Based on the satisfactory esperimental results the alternative laser method was applied for a 55 years-old male patient with severe anginal attack who had undergone pericardiectomy 7 years before. The patient was admitted to our Kobe University Hospital because of severe angina pectoris. A marked stenosis (90%) of the left anterior descending artery (LAD) was recognized on the coronary angiogram. An operation was planned to perform coronary artery bypass grafting to the LAD on 12 November 1985. However, the LAD could hardly be exposed, because of severe adhesion of the epicardium due to pericardiectomy. Therefore, six transmyocardial channels were created by laser (85W, 0.2sec) in the anterior wall of the left ventricle of the beating heart (Figure 24).

Postoperative course of this patient was uneventful, except for initiation of an intraaortic balloon pumping for 3 days. No abnormal changes were confirmed on ventriculogram postoperatively (Figure 25) [6]. The patient is still alive 15 years after TMLR. This patient was the first successful case with TMLR alone, in the world.

4.3.8 Discussion

A new method of transmyocardial revascularization was carried out by CO_2 laser experimentally and clinically. The principle of this procedure is to supply additional arterial blood from the left ventricular cavity into the ischemic area of the myocardium. A minimal tissue reaction was microscopically recognized in the newly created laser channels.

In the experimental study, it could be apparently confirmed that laser channels in the myocardium were patent even 3 years after TMLR. Besides, endothelial cells surrounding insides of the laser channels were clearly

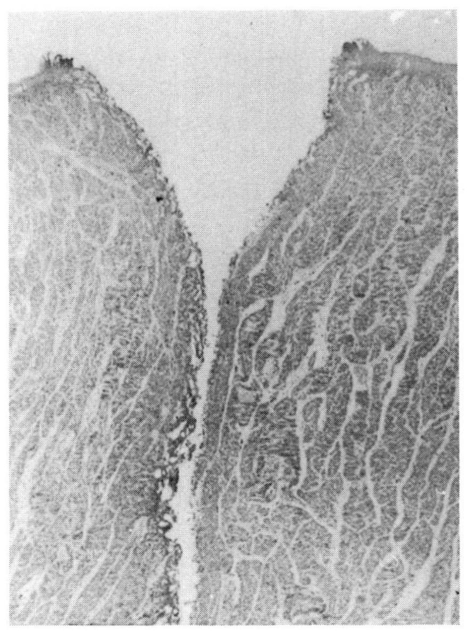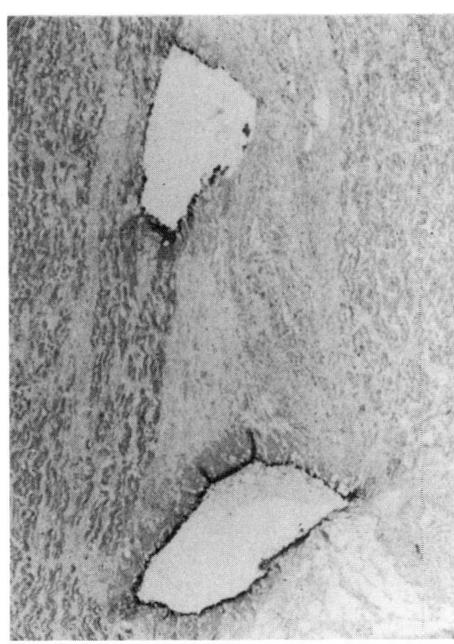

<table>
<tr><td style="text-align:center">a) Longitudinal view</td><td style="text-align:center">b) Transected view</td></tr>
</table>

Figure 22. Histological findings of laser channel.

recognized histologically [4,5]. It was considered that tissue defects of fine transmyocardial channels. From these findings the feasibility of long-term patency of laser channels and clinical applications was clearly revealed.

Until now, experimental procedure that supply arterial blood from the left ventricular cavity into the ischemic myocardium have been reported since 1965. However there were no successful results in this field [10,11].

Mirhoseini created laser channels by CO_2 in the akinetic and dyskinetic area of the left ventricle and simultaneously performed CABG in all clinical cases. Thus, myocardial revascularization by laser seems recommended for the patients for whom CABG alone is inadequate, and also where it could not be carried out at all. Our long-term experimental results and our first one patient treated so far support this statement.

In the 1990s, clinical TMLR operations have been performed in the United States as well as European countries [12-21]. Good results have been reported. These data also have been reported in some scientific papers. Thereafter, much attention has been paid to TMLR for severely ill patients with ischemic heart disease in Japan.

In 1994, Cooley has reported postoperative results of 21 cases treated by TMLR. By Canadian classification, anginal attack was decreased from 3.7±04 preoperatively 1.8±0.6 postoperatively and the blood flow ratio between the endcordium and the epicardium increased from 0.96±0.07 before, to 1.10±0.04 after. From these clinical data the availability of TMLR was insisted.

There are some excellent advantages in TMLR : 1) no requirement of extracorporeal circulation, 2) easy to operate on and short operating time, 3) shorter admission more than CABG, 4) rapid body restoration, 5) effectively low cost.

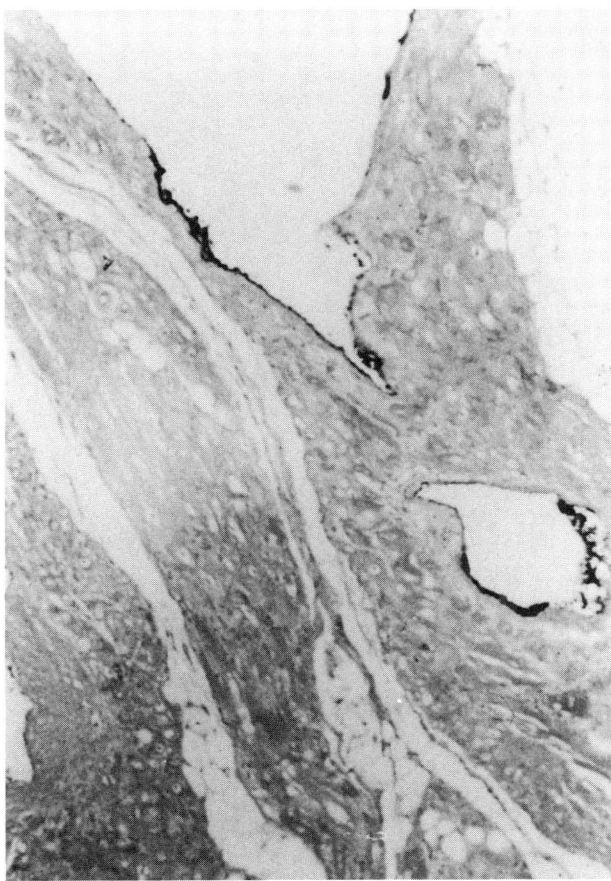

Figure 23. Microscopic findings of 3 years after TMLR.

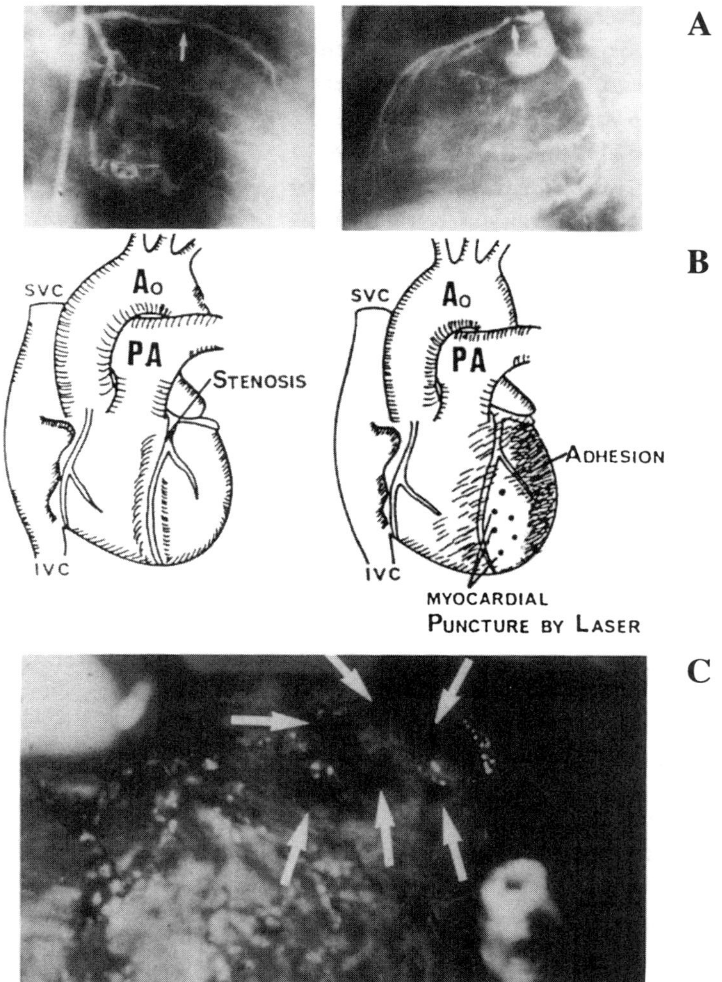

Figure 24. Clinical experience of TMLR (On 12. Nov. 1985 operated, the first successful case in the world)

By the end of 1995, 811 patients have been operated on in the world (Table 1) [15-21]. At the end of March in 1997 over 3000 patients have been treated by TMLR alone or TMLR combined CABG in the world. It is, however, very important to select the patients with end-stage coronary artery disease, for whom PTCA or CABG can not be carried out, because of diffuse stenosis and small-caliber of the coronary arteries.

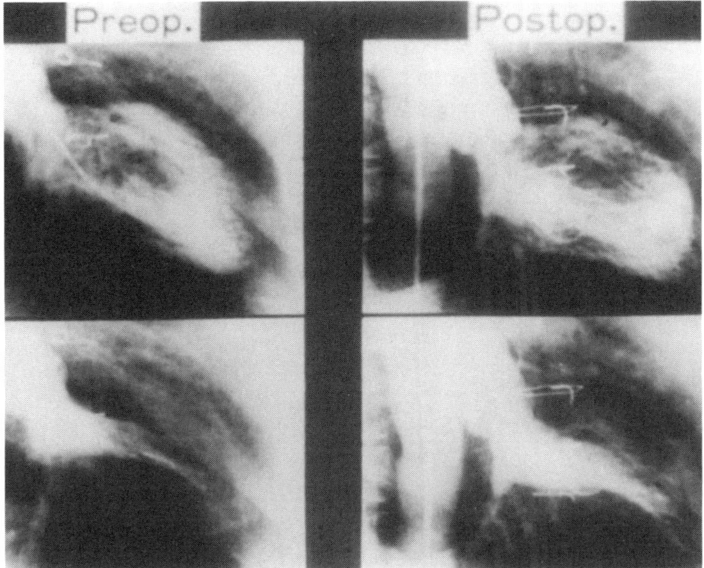

Figure 25. Pre-and postoperative left ventriculogram

4.4   LASER VASCULAR ANASTOMOSIS (LVA)

4.4.1 Procedures in Vascular Anastomosis

Lasers have been widely applied in the field of medicine and surgery, and satisfactory results have been obtained in the several medical fields [22-31]. However, laser applications are very rare in the field of cardiovascular surgery throughout the world. It has been reported for a long period that it is difficult to keep long-term patency after anastomosis of the conventional fashion with suture materials especially for small-caliber vessels. For 15 years, we have tried to perform aorto-coronary bypasses in treating patients with ischemic heart disease. There are some problems about obtaining favorable surgical results by the conventional suture method, especially in the cases with small-caliber branches of the coronary arteries. From this standpoint, a low energy CO_2 laser was used to perform coronary artery bypass grafting (CABG) [29,30].

Table 1. Clinical experience of TMLR in the world

USA (1985-1995)

Institute (Reporter)	No. of Cases
Audubon Regional Medical Center (Lansing)	77
Infinity Heart Institute (Mirhoseini)	42
Brigham & Women's Hospital (Cohn)	23
Texas Heart Institute (Cooley & Frazier)	20
Rush Prebyterian (March)	17
Seton Medical Center (Crew)	13
University of Pittsburg (Griffith)	5
Columbia Prebyterian Medical Center (Smith)	4
Total	201

(Except USA) 1985-1995

Institute (Reporter)	No. of Cases
Herz-Zentrum Bodensee (Maass)	131
The King Fahd Heart Center (Raffa)	103
Escort Heart Institute (Trehan)	90
Universität Marburg (Moosdorf)	60
Madras Medical Mission Hospital (Cherian)	52
Deutsches Herzzentrum (Hetzer)	38
Papworth Hospital (Wallwork)	30
Sheikh Zayed Hospital (Jawaid)	25
Universität Krankenhaus (Stubbe)	20
Herz und Kreislaufzentrum (Oster)	16
Cape Town City Park Hospital (Tahning)	14
Feiring Klinikken (Nordstrand)	12
Kreiskrankenhaus Völklingen (Isringhaus)	12
Klinik Im Schachen (Bertschmann)	3
Philippines Heart Hospital (Zamora)	2
Hospital Israelita Albert Einstein (Feher)	1
Kobe University (Okada)	1
Total	610

Adult mongrel dogs were used in this study. The femoral arteries and veins were gently exposed under general anesthesia. The relationship between output and irradiation time of a CO_2 laser was analyzed as well as tissue reaction to the laser in a preliminary experiment. If a laser output of 100mW continuously irradiated on the same point more than 10 seconds, swelling, disruption and vaporization of the elastic fibers of the aorta could be found in proportion to the laser output (Figure 26).

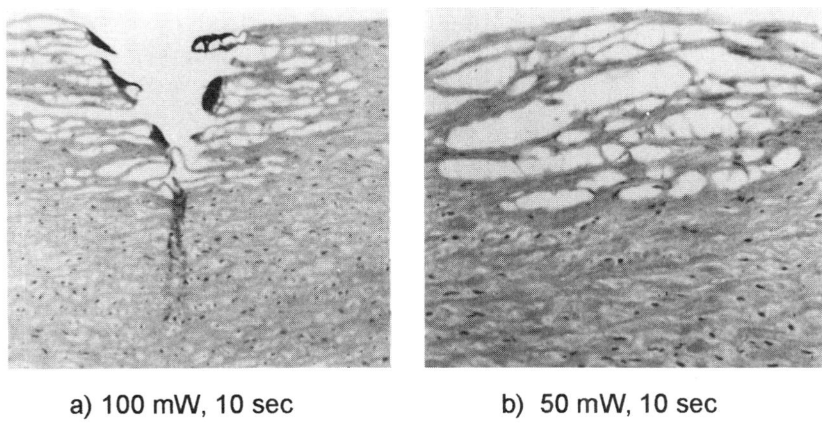

a) 100 mW, 10 sec   b) 50 mW, 10 sec

Figure 26. Laser energy and tissue reactions of the aorta

However, there were no remarkable tissue reactions to a laser output of 40mW. From these preliminary experiments it could be concluded that the optimal laser output was 20-40mW and 6-12sec/mm for vascular anastomosis of small-caliber vessels in the extremities. Side-to-side, end-to-side and end-to-end anastomosis at the site of the femoral arteries and veins or the carotid arteries and veins were carried out using a low energy CO_2 laser (Figure 27, Figure 28). Diameter of these vessels ranged from 2 to 10mm with mean of 4mm. Stay sutures of 5-0 monofilamentous suture material were anchored at the incided ends of the vessels and were located to hold tightly the rim of the vessels. The posterior wall of the femoral artery and its vein was sutured in the conventional fashion using 5-0 suture materials and sites of anastomosed were microscopically examined as a control. The anterior wall was anastomosis by low energy CO_2 (20-40mW) for 6-12sec/mm. The focused laser beam was used and moved very slowly along the anastomotic line. The distance between stay sutures was maintained at no more than 5mm.

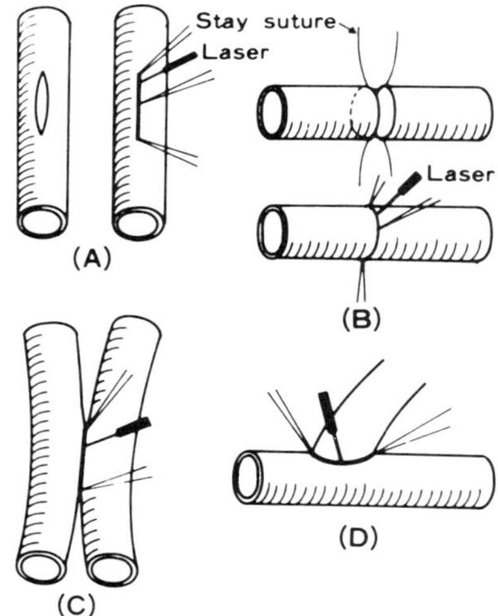

Figure 27. Schematic illustrations of laser vascular anastomosis

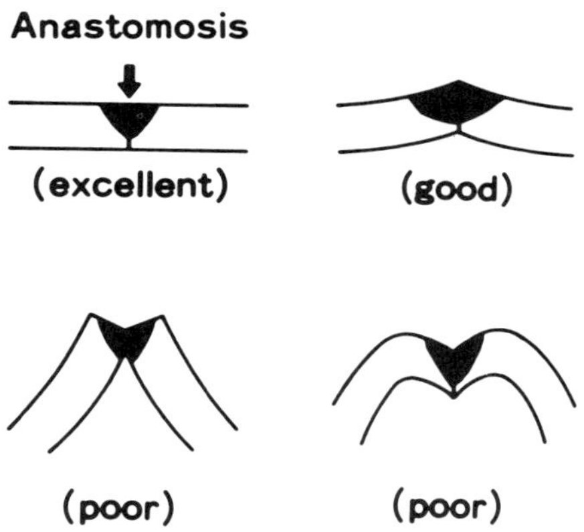

Figure 28. Important points of anastomosis

Vascular anastomosis has been routinely made by CO_2 by laser and just four stay sutures on the anastomotic line. After completion of anastomosis intravascular angioscopy was carefully carried out to observe the inside of the anastomotic portion of the vessels of which anastomotic site by laser is wide-open.

Vascular anastomosis between the left internal mammary artery and the LAD (left anterior descending artery) could also be performed by laser under the heart beating (Figure 29).

Pressure tolerance test and tensile strength test as well as histological examinations were also studied to evaluate the intensity of the laser anastomotic site of the vessels.

4.4.2   Results of LVA

The number of vascular anastomosis (end-to-end, end-to-side, side-to-side anastomosis) reached to 75 anastomoses. Bleeding from the anastomotic sites was found at only 3 points among 75 anastomotic sites.

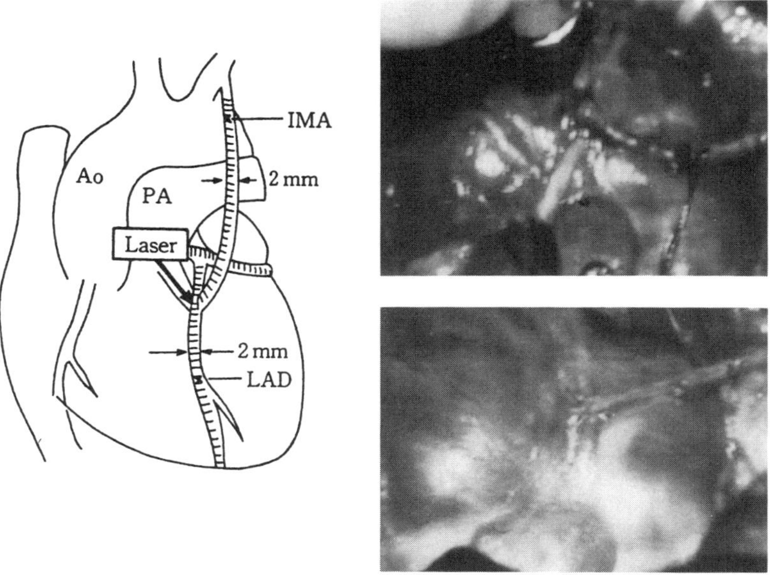

Figure 29. Laser vascular anastomosis between the left mammary artery and LAD

However, it stopped on light compression by gauze on the anastomotic line. Observation periods ranged from 6 hours to 2.5 months. There were no deaths caused by bleeding from vascular anastomosis and operative procedure. Anastomotic sites were picked out for histological examinations which were patent macroscopically at the time of exstirpation. Patency was also confirmed by angiogram and pressure tolerance test, or tensile strength test at the anastomotic sites were prudently performed after surgery.

4.4.2.1   Pressure Tolerance Test

Noradrenaline was given intravenously to maintain high pressure after completion of vascular laser anastomosis. However, there were no hemorrhages from the sites of anastomosis was effective enough for the site to tolerate high pressures without bleeding (Figure 30)

4.4.2.2   Tensile Strength Test

Intensity of the site of laser or suture vascular anastomosis was examined by weighing. Consequently, the laser anastomotic sites with only four stay sutures were separated in weights 1,034.2±103.9g. On the other hand, the sites of anastomoses sutured by 5-0 suture material were also separated into weight 1,103.7±144.8g. Thus, there were no significant differences in the intensity of the site of vascular anastomosis in each group (Figure 31).

4.4.2.3   Histological Findings

The sites of vascular anastomoses were microscopically studied after several time of intervals. A thinned fibrous membrane was observed microscopically on the adventitia of the vessels already 6 hours after laser surgery. However, thickened fibrous membrane and marked proliferation of fibroblasts were recognized at the adventitia and the media of the vessels except for the intimal layer, 1 week after laser anastomosis (Figure 32).

Furthermore, all layers of the artery and its vein were sufficiently connected by a lot of collagen fibers 2.5 months after laser anastomosis (Figure 33). Thus, good healings of sites of laser anastomoses were clearly observed histologically [32-35].

On the contrary, the suture anastomotic sites were also examined microscopically in detail. Consequently, many giant cells as well as the infiltration of several types of cells in their early stages and marked granulations in the chronic stage were clearly observed around the suture materials. The technique of laser vascular anastomosis was very easy and good results could be obtained in hemodynamic and histological findings in comparison with conventional anastomosis using suture materials. From these favorable findings it was considered that vascular anastomosis by low energy CO_2 laser might be recommended in clinical application.

4.4.2.4   Clinical Application

On the basis of excellent experiment results laser vascular anastomosis was employed in 111 patients with anginal, or chronic renal failure and peripheral vascular disorders (Table 2) [32,34].

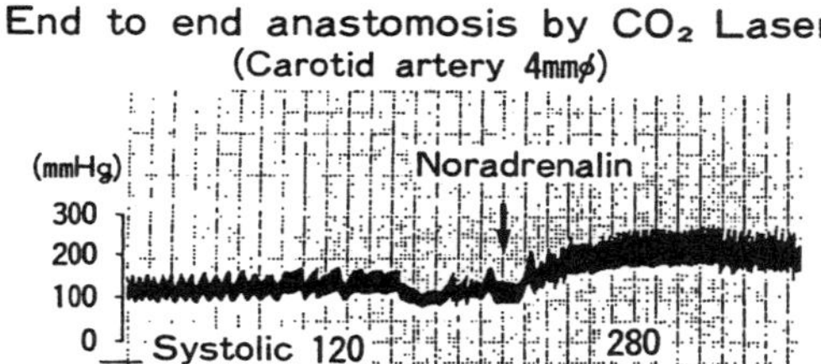

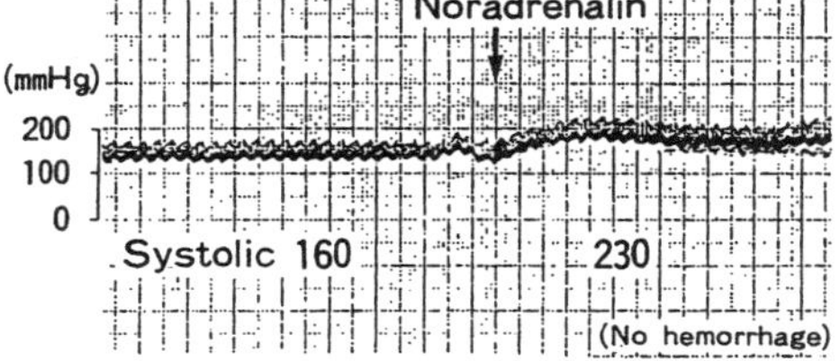

Figure 30. Pressure tolerance test

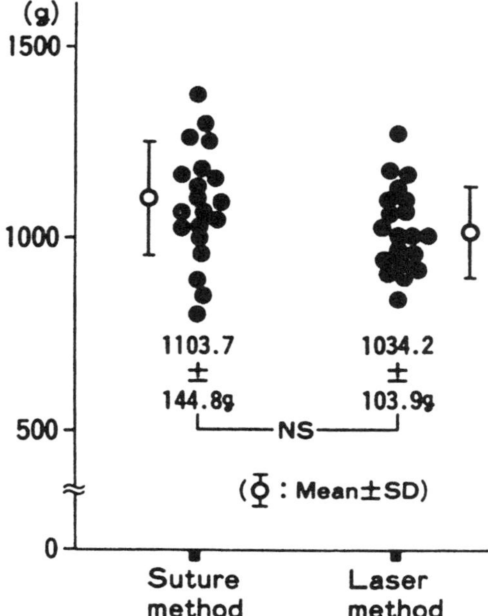

Figure 31. Tensile strength test

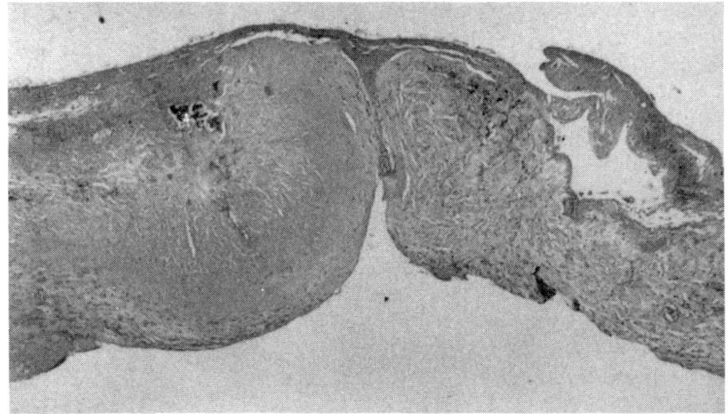

Figure 32. Histological findings of one week after laser anastomosis

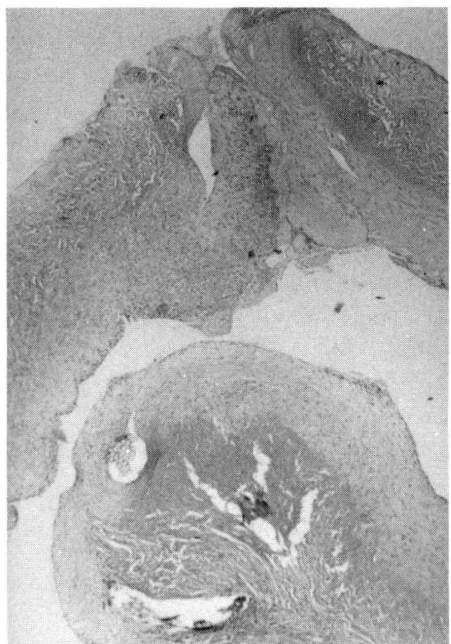

Figure 33. Histological findings of chronic stage (2.5 months) after anastomosis

A 44 year-old female patient was admitted to our Hospital, because of hypertension and uremia following renal failure (BUN 76mg/dl, Creatinine 10mg/dl, K 6.8mEq/L). A veno-arterial anastomosis at the site of the radial artery was successfully carried out using a CO_2 laser hemodialysis on February 21, 1985. The length of anastomosis was 15mm, and laser output was 30mw and irradiation time was 120sec (Figure 34). This was the first clinical successful case of vascular anastomosis by CO_2 laser in the world.

Table 2. Clinical experience of laser vascular anastomosis.

Site of Anastomosis	No. of Anastomosis
Femoral artery (EE)	69
Femoro-popliteal bypass (E-E Anaslo. By SVG)	39
Radial artery-ceph. V. (E-S)	4
Femoral vein (E-E)	3
Pop.-politeal bypass (E-E anasto. By SVG)	3
Brachial artery (E-E)	1
r-Renal artery-Ao. Bypass	1
Tibial artery (S-S, E-S)	3
SVG-LAD (E-S)	10
LIMA-LAD (E-S)	3
Total	136

E-E : End-to-end anastomosis
E-S : End-to-side
S-S : Side-to-side

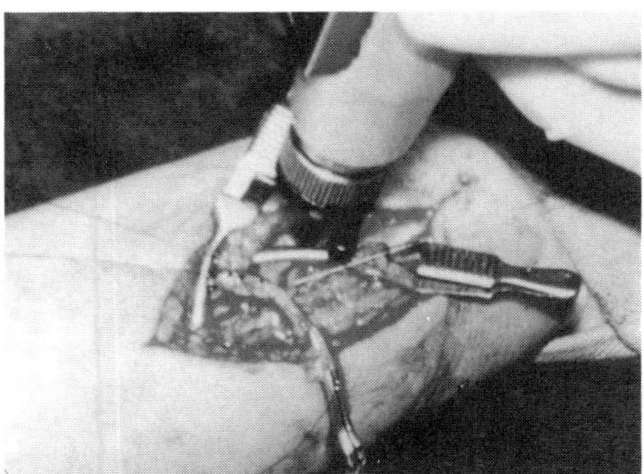
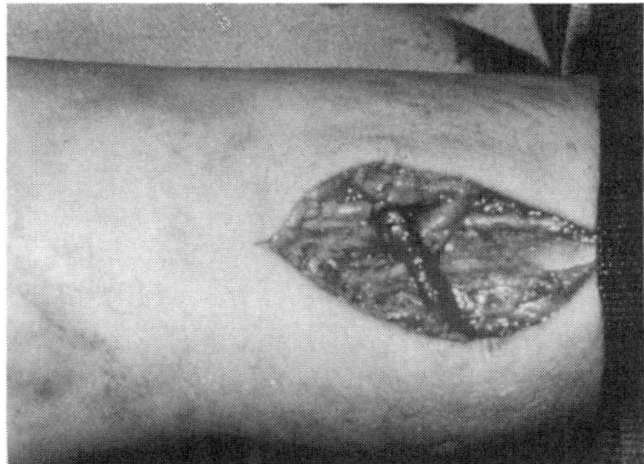

Figure 34. Clinical experience of laser vascular anastomosis

From these clinical experiences with peripheral vessels, vascular anastomosis by low energy CO_2 laser was employed in CABG for 13 patients with ischemic heart disease (Figure 35).

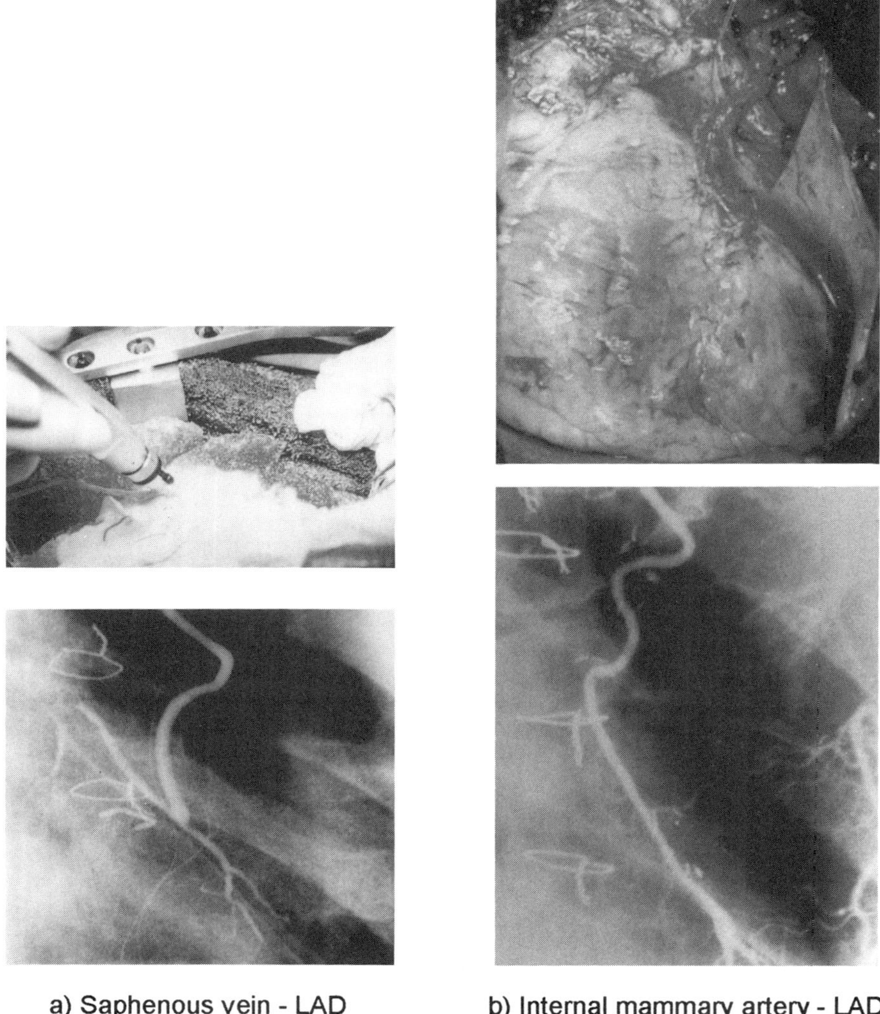

a) Saphenous vein - LAD
b) Internal mammary artery - LAD

Figure 35. Laser anastomosis in the coronary artery bypass grafting

4.4.3 Discussion of LVA Results

4.4.3.1 Tissue Reaction of Low Energy CO_2 Laser

The diameters of arteries and veins in the extremities were no more than 10 mm and the wall thickness was very thin less than 1mm. In vascular anastomosis of these vessels optimal laser output was 20-40mW and irradiation time was 6-12sec/mm. Laser beams did not reach the intimal layer in these conditions. If the output was over 50mW, a marked tissue reaction could be found such as swelling, carbonization and vaporization proportional to the irradiation time. Focused beam was convenient for making fine anastomosis on small-caliber vessels [32-34].

4.4.3.2 Important Factors in Laser Vascular Anastomosis

There were two important points in carrying out vascular anastomosis. One of them was to close the rim of the vessels tight with some fine stay sutures. The distance between stay sutures must be less than 5mm. Another one was to focus the beam on the anastomotic line. At this time the beam should be moved very slowly and repeated. Irradiation should be continued until the color along the anastomotic line changes to dark gray, or dark brown.

4.4.3.3 Intensity of the Site of Anastomosis

There is a long-term history of safety in performing vascular anastomosis with sutures. For anastomosis using many suture materials, especially for small-caliber vessels, there are some problems in their patency over the long-term period. From these standpoints a low energy CO_2 laser was employed for vascular anastomosis. Pressure tolerance was carefully tested to evaluate intensity at the site of laser anastomosis. However, no hemmorhage was observed even at the high pressure of 300mmHg. On the contrary, laser anastomotic sites were also tested for tensile strength test. However, there were no significant differences between conventional suture method and laser anastomosis. Thus, no intensity problems could be found with laser anastomosis.

4.4.3.4 Mechanism of Laser Vascular Anastomosis

Based on histological examinations, fibrous membrane, proliferation of fibroblasts and collagen fibers on the anastomotic line were observed by laser, as the time went on. Good healings were obviously recognized microscopically [32]. The reason for the healing of the anastomotic site is not now clearly recognized. It is supposed that collagen fiber as well as protein components of the tissues may be changed from a gel to a sol like a paste by laser thermal energy.

4.5 LASER ANGIOPLASTY FOR CARDIOVASCULAR DISEASE

4.5.1 Procedures for Cardiovascular Angioplasty

In recent years, endovascular intervention such as balloon angioplasty, laser angioplasty, atherectomy and the stenting method have been clinically applied for patients with atheromatous plaques of the peripheral and the coronary arteries. Among them, restenosis after endovascular intervention has been obviously confirmed in 30-40% of the patients who underwent percutaneous transluminal coronary angioplasty (PTCA) [36-41]. However, there are some problems in maintaining long-term patency by means of endovascular techniques such as balloon techniques, laser, atherectomy. For these problems, the effects of an Argon laser on vaporization of the atheromatous plaques were experimentally investigated. On the basis of our excellent experimental studies, a laser was utilized for patients with intermittent claudication, angina pectoris, and ischemic ulcer of the lower extremity. Consequently, the feasibility of laser angioplasty could be confirmed in the field of cardiovascular surgery [36].

In cardiovascular surgery, Argon, Nd:YAG, Ho:YAG, and Excimer lasers have been widely employed all over the world. An Argon laser (Trimedyne/ Laser Ionics, Model 5567, and HGM, Endocoagulator Model 20S, USA) was utilized for the vaporizing of atherosclerotic plaques in this study [36]. Animal care was in compliance with the "Principles of Laboratory Animal Care" and the "Guide for Care and Use of Laboratory Animals" (NIH Publication No.80-23, revised 1985)

First of all, the relationship between laser energy and reactions of the aortic walls to the laser was experimentally evaluated using adult mongrel dogs. A metal tip probe (Laser probe PLR-Flex, or Laser probe PLR-Plus, Trimedyne inc. CA, USA) was mainly used. Subsequently, it could be confirmed that optimal conditions for laser angioplasty were 6W in output and 3sec in irradiation time for each shot. On the other hand, a metal tip probe with thermal feedback control system (HGM, Endocoagulator, Model 20S, and Laser probe, PLAC, HGM, Salt Lake City, UT, USA) was used, for which the adequate tip temperature for vaporizing the atheromatous plaques was 200°C and the irradiation time was 5sec for each shot. These conditions were almost the same laser energy for adequacy, that is, in the case with 6W and 3sec using the MTP, the intimal layer was vaporized, and 8W and 3sec the crater reached the media.

Then, with 8W and 3sec using the bare-ended probe, arterial perforation occurred immediately. On the other hand, in the case with thermal feedback control system the arterial crater was deepened by an increase in the temperature of the MTP. In the case with 100-150°C in the temperature of the MTP, the intimal surface was slightly vaporized, with 200-300°C the crater reached deeper intimal layer. In the case with more than 300°C, the media was also vaporized. Subsequently, it was considered that suitable temperature of the MTP was 200°C.

At the time of laser angioplasty, the use of an angioscope was inevitable for observing the inside of the arteries before and after laser irradiation. At present, laser angioplasty has been performed for 125 patients with atherosclerotic changes of the peripheral and coronary arteries.

This includes 107 men and 18 women, ranging in age from 39 to 88 years-old with an average of 63. These patients consisted of 109 cases with intermittent claudication, 4 cases with rest pain and 2 cases with a refractory ulcer in the leg, including 10 cases with angina pectoris.

Angiography for the patients with peripheral and coronary arterial disease was undertaken in all patients and their operative indications were apparently decided by clinical symptoms and angiographic findings with severe stenosis of more than 75% of the internal diameter and total occlusion of the arteries. The length of occlusive and stenotic lesions in the peripheral arteries ranged from 0.5cm to 45cm with a mean of 3.2±5.0cm in stenotic lesions and 9.8±8.8cm in the occlusive lesions.

As a method of laser angioplasty, a sheath catheter was percutaneously inserted proximally for the iliac lesions and distally for the femoral and popliteal lesions under local anesthesia in the inguinal region. After this procedure, an angioscope (0.75mm in diameter) was inserted through the sheath catheter and the surface of the atherosclerotic plaques in the artery was observed. At this time, it is very important to wash out the blood with saline for clean observation. Through this procedure, the inside of the artery could be precisely observed. There are several sizes of angioscope, such as 0.75mm, or 0.45mm in diameter.

From the standpoint of image clarification, an angioscope of 0.75mm in diameter was the most useful instrument. Thereafter, laser irradiation was carefully initiated to make a laser hole for the occlusive lesion under angioscopic guidance using a bare-ended laser fiber and metal tip probe. In the case with a calcified occlusion at the site of the femoral artery, this artery first exposed and a sheath catheter was directly inserted to the atheromatous plaques under direct vision.

A guide-wire was then passed through a laser hole which was previously created using a metal tip probe (2.0-2.5mm in diameter) inserted over the guide-wire. In this study, 6W in output and 3sec in irradiation time, or 200°C and 5sec using a metal tip probe with thermal feedback control system were utilized as optimal conditions for each laser ablation. Laser ablations were continued to eliminate atheromatous plaques under angioscopoic and fluoroscopic guidances, until recanalization and a wide opening of the vessel lumen could be observed. Moving the metal tip probe slowly in the artery, it is very important to prevent vasoconstriction and fragmentation of the atheromatous plaques during laser ablation. Then, in cases where dilatation was inadequate by lasing, percutaneous transluminal angioplasty (PTA) was additionally undertaken {39].

All clinical results were expressed as the mean standard deviation. The unpaired t-test was used to test for differences in variables between the two measurements, and a P-value less than 0.05 was accepted as statistically significant.

4.5.2 Results of Cardiovascular Angioplasty

4.5.2.1 Laser Angioplasty for Peripheral Arterial Disease

At present, 115 patients (141 lesions) have been treated by laser angioplasty. This includes 98 men and 17 women who had intermittent claudication, rest pain, and refractory limb ulcers. They consisted of 114 patients with arteriosclerosis obliterans and only one thromboangitis obliterans.

Seventy-one among 141 lesions were in the iliac region, and 66 lesions existed in the femoro-popliteal region. The remaining 4 lesions were thrombogenic stenoses of implanted vascular grafts and the anastomotic site of the saphenous vein after CABG. Seventy-five lesions revealed stenotic changes, and 66 lesions showed obstructive findings (Table 3).

The criteria of clinical success were evaluated as follows: a) relief of symptom, b) improvement of arterial pulsation, c) increase of ankle pressure index of less than 0.2, and d) residual stenosis of less than 30% in the internal diameter of the lased arteries. On the basis of these examinations, all cases were strictly evaluated. Consequently, a success rate of 93% could be found in the cases with stenotic lesions. On the contrary, the success rate was 74% in the cases with occlusive lesions. Further, from the length of the lesion, a clinical success rate of 98% was observed even in the cases with femoro-popliteal lesions within 10cm in length (Figure 36). However, in the cases with lesions of more than 10cm in length, the rate decreased to 71% (Table 4).

Table 3 Patients characteristics of laser angioplasty.

Case	115 (131 legs, 141 lesions)
Gender	Male 98 Female 17
Age	43 ~ 88 (67.2 ± 9.5)
Disease	ASO 114 TAO 1
Symptom	Claudication 109 Rest pain 4 Ischemic ulcer 2
Site of Lesion	Iliac 77 Femoropopliteal artery 66 Graf stenosis 4
Type of lesion	Stenosis 75 (53%) Occlusion 66 (47%)
Lesion length (mean ± SD)	Stenosis 3.2 ± 5.0 cm Occlusion 9.8 ± 8.8 cm

Table 4. Clinical success rate in the relationship between the location and the length of the stenotic changes.

Lesion length	mean length(cm)	N	Clinical success
Femoropopliteal lesions			
< 10cm	3.2±2.5	45	44 (98%) ⎤ ※
≧ 10cm	21.3±8.7	21	15 (71%) ⎦
Total	9.0±9.9	66	59 (89%)
Iliac lesions			
< 5cm	2.2±1.0	53	48 (91%) ⎤ ※
≧ 5cm	9.7±4.4	18	8 (44%) ⎦
Total	4.1±4.0	71	56 (79%)

Clinical success : increase (> 0.2) of ankle pressure index
relief of patient's symptom   ※ $p < 0.01$

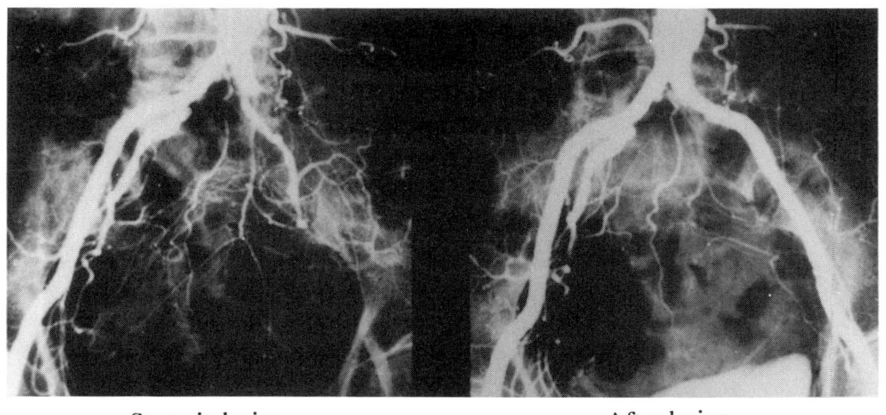

(a)

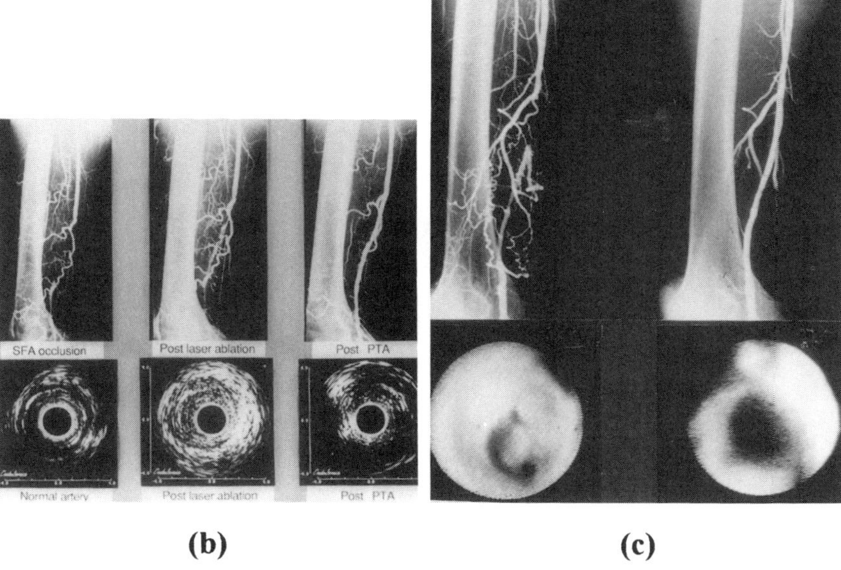

(b)   **(c)**

Figure 36. Clinical experience of laser angioplasty. a) For the occlusion of the common iliac artery, b) For the occlusion of the popliteal artery under intravascular ultrasound, c) For the occlusion of the popliteal artery under angioscopic guide.

On the other hand, a clinical success rate of 91% was obtained in the cases with iliac lesions of less than 5cm in length. Thus, there were significant differences in comparison with the success rate and the length of the lesion between both groups. The tortuorsity and severe calcification in these regions were considered to be the reason for this significance.

A long-term follow-up study of 120 months was performed on 99 limbs with clinical success by angiography, measurement of ankle pressure index and clinical symptoms except for angioscopy. Subsequently, the cumulative patency rate in the follow-up of 120 months was 85% for the stenotic lesions and 75% for the occlusive lesions (Figure 37).

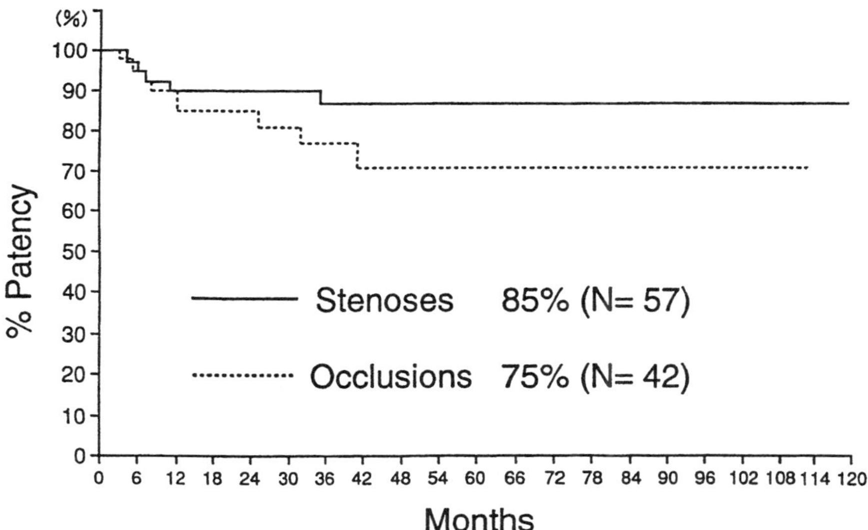

Figure 37. Cumulative patency rate after laser angioplasty for the peripheral occlusive diseases.

4.5.2.2 Laser Angioplasty for Coronary Arterial Diseases

Laser coronary angioplasty was intraoperatively performed for 10 patients with multiple stenoses in a coronary artery (Table 5).

This included 9 men and one woman, ranging in age from 39 to 67 years old with a mean of 58. A metal tip probe (1.5-2.0mm in diameter) was used with angioscopic guidance, by which laser angioplasty could be safely carried out in all cases (Figure 38).

First of all, a coronary incision was made longitudinally and the angioscope was inserted prior to the stenotic lesion. Then, the metal tip probe was passed to the lesion to vaporize the plaques under chilled heart protection. In the case of laser coronary angioplasty, the optimal conditions were 4-5W in output and 2sec in irradiation time for each shot. In addition to this, the diameter ratio between the metal tip probe and the coronary artery was an important factor for the prevention of coronary vasospasm during laser irradiation. That is, a small size metal tip probe, less than 30% of the diameter of the coronary artery, should be applied. The patients are doing well without severe complications throughout the therapy.

Table 5 Clinical experience of laser angioplasty for coronary artery disease

Case	Age	Gender	Symptom	CAG findings			CABG	Laser irradiation
1) K.N.	59	M	UAP	LMT	(5)	90%	LAD	
				LAD	(7)	75%	DI	LAD
					(9)	90%	RCA	(6W, 3sec, 3times)
				RCA	(3)	50%		
2) I.K.	41	M	PIA	LAD	(6)	90%		
					(7)	75%	LAD	LAD
				Cx	(11)	99%		(6w, 2sec, 3times)
				RCA	(1)	100%		
3) S.K.	61	F	PIA	LAD	(6)	90%		
					(9)	90%	LAD	RCA
				Cx	(13)	100%	RCA	(6w, 3sec, 7times)
				RCA	(1)	100%		
4) T.Y.	56	M	UAP	LAD	(6)	75%	LAD	
				Cx	(13)	100%	Cx	RCA
				RCA	(2)	90%	RCA	(6w, 3sec, 5times)
					(3)	75%		
5) T.Y.	39	M	PIA	LAD	(7、8)	75%	LAD	LAD
				Cx	(13)	90%	Cx	(6w, 3sec, 3times)
				RCA	(2)	90%	RCA	
6) M.N.	67	M	UAP	LAD	(6)	100%	LAD	RCA
				Cx	(14)	90%	Cx	(5w, 2sec, 2times)
				RCA	(1)	75%	RCA	(6w, 3sec, 3times)
7) T.A.	65	M	PIA	LAD	(6)	100%	LAD	LAD
				Cx	(13)	99%	Cx	(6w, 3sec, 3times)
				RCA	(1)	100%	RCA	
8) M.M.	65	M	UAP	LAD	(6)	100%	LAD	
				Cx	(11)	75%	Cx	LAD
					(12)	90%	RCA	(4w, 2sec, 4times)
				RCA	(3)	100%		
9) Y.N.	61	M	OMI	LAD	(6)	100%	LAD	RCA
				RCA	(2)	90%	RCA	(2w, 2sec, 10times)
10) A.U.	65	M	UAP	LMT	(5)	75%	LAD	LAD
				Cx	(14)	90%	Cx	(200℃,5sec,12times)
				RCA	(2)	75%	RCA	

UAP : Unstable angina pectoris   LMT : Left main trunk lesion
PIA : Post infarctim angina   LAD : Left anterior descending artery
OMI : Old myocardial infarction   Cx : Circumflex artery
CAG : Coronary arteriogram   RCA : Right Coronary artery
CABG : Coronary artery bypass grafting

Subsequently, laser coronary angioplasty was a useful procedure for multiple stenoses in a coronary artery, saving time in the operation and maintaining the long-term patency rate of CABG, because of minimized invasiveness.

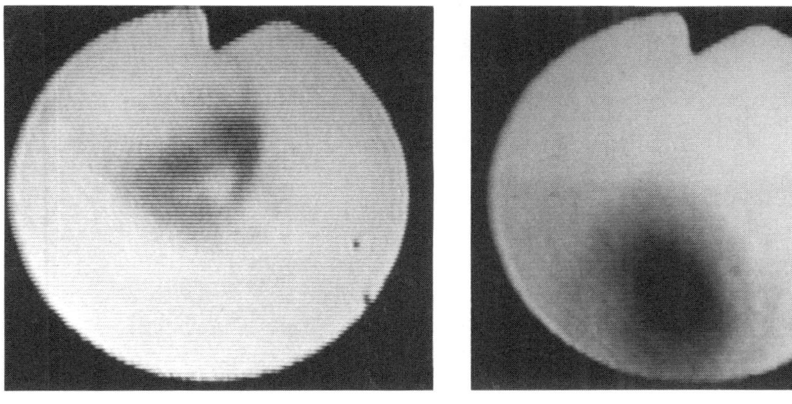

<table>
<tr><td align="center">a)   Stenotic lesion</td><td align="center">b) After lasing</td></tr>
</table>

Figure 38. Laser angioplasty for coronary artery disease.

4.5.2.3 Discussion

Recently, Argon, Nd:YAG, Ho:YAG, and Excimer lasers have been widely utilized for laser angioplasty [34-56]. The optimal conditions for laser angioplasty by Argon laser were 6W in output and 3sec in irradiation time, 200°C in output and 5sec in irradiation time in our serial studies [39,49].

On the other hand, several laser conditions (6-12W in output, 3-10sec in irradiation time) have been reported according to the kinds of laser system and laser fibers. At the time of laser angioplasty, angioscopic and intravascular ultrasound guidance were necessary to evaluate the characteristics of the atheromatous plaques and the arterial wall before and after the laser ablation. And sometimes, it was angioscopically recognized that the proximal-and the distal portions were composed of tight atheromatous plaques and the middle portion was not occluded or filled with fresh thrombus.

On the basis of our clinical experience, laser angioplasty should be recommended to eliminate, or reduce the stenotic, or occlusive changes of short segments within 10cm in length for a peripheral artery, and within 2cm in length for a coronary artery.

In recent years, laser angioplasty has been widely employed in United States and European countries. The initial success rate by laser angioplasty has been reported to be 65-95% in comparison with 70-85% for percutaneous transluminal angioplasty. In our clinical series, the clinical success rate was 91% in the cases of stenotic lesions in comparison with 71% for occlusive lesions. Thus, satisfactory results by laser angioplasty were clearly confirmed [49].

On the other hand, the clinical success rate was 98% in cases with femoro-popliteal lesions of less than 10cm in length. Thus, there were slight differences in the laser effects between stenotic and occlusive lesions as well as in the relationship between initial success and clinical success in the long-term period. Cumberland has reported that 50 of 56 totally occluded arteries were recanalized by laser and that the ankle pressure index increased from 0.53 before to 0.84 after laser irradiation [34]. In addition to this, technical success was 88% and clinical success was 77%. In Japan, similar results have been reported in recent years.

In general, complications in laser angioplasty include hematomas in the inguinal region, the subintimal pathway of the laser fiber, and dissective change of the artery by additional PTA. We have also experienced 11 dissections and 3 subintimal pathway of the arteries by additional PTA, and 4 intimal injuries of laser probe and guide-wire. However, there was no urgent surgical intervention for them.

Thus, there are some differences in the clinical success due to indication, techniques and antithrombogenic management after laser angioplasty in several hospitals. On the other hand, intraoperative coronary laser angioplasty was a safe and effective procedure under direct vision [49,50]. However, Litvack and Sanborn have reported a high incidence of complications after percutaneous transluminal laser coronary angioplasty [51,52]. All cases treated by laser methods should be follow-up even in the long-term period.

In conclusion, laser angioplasty was effective to significantly open the lumen of occlusive and stenotic lesions of the peripheral artery. At present, excellent results have been revealed within 10cm in length for femoro-popliteal lesions. On the contrary, satisfactory results were obtained with 5cm in length for iliac lesions. In the case of coronary arteries are good indications, stenotic lesions within 2cm in length. However, the indication for laser angioplasty will change in the long-term period.

REFERENCES (Part B)

1.   Okada M, Ikuta H, Shimizu K, Horii H, Nakamura K: An alternative procedure of myocardial revascularization by CO_2 laser. Jpn J Laser & Med 1984; 4:201-202

2. Mirhoseini M, Shelgikar S, Cayton MM: New concepts in revascularization of the myocardium; Ann Thorac. Surg., 985; 45:415-420

3. Okada M, Ikuta H, Shimizu K, Horii H, Nakamura K: Myocardial revascularization by CO_2 laser. Rev Eur Technol Boimed 1985; 7:100-103

4. Okada M, Ikuta H, Shimizu K, Horii H, Nakamura K: Alternative method of myocardial revascularization by laser. Experimental and clinical study. Kobe J Med Sci 1986; 32:151-161

5. Okada M, Ikuta H, Shimizu K, Horii H, Nakamura K: A new myocardial revascularization by high energy laser. Surg & Med Laser 1988; 1:61-64

6. Okada M, Ikuta H, Shimizu K, Horii H, Nakamura K: A new method of myocardial revascularization. Thorac Cardiovasc Surgeon 1991; 39:1-4

7. Beck CS: The development of new blood supply to the heart by operation. Ann Surg 1935; 102:801-813

8. Goldman L, Rockwell RJ: Laser action at the cellar level. JAMA 1966; 198:641-644

9. Pifarre R, Jaca ML, Lynch RD, Neville WE: Myocardial revascularization by transmyocardial acupuncture. J Thorac Cardiovasc Surg. 1969; 58:424-431

10. Sen PK, Udwadia TE, Kinare SG, Parulkar GB: Transmyocardial acupuncture. J Thorac Cardivasc Surg 1965; 50:181-189

11. Vineberg AM: Development of an anastomosis between the coronary vessels and transplanted internal mammary artery. Can Med Assoc J 1946; 55:117-119

12. Crew JR, Transmyocardial revascularization by CO_2 laser. Surgical Technol International 1991; 1:236-238

13. Horvath KA, Smith WJ, Jaurence RG, Schoen FJ, Appleyard RF, Cohn LH: Recovery and viability of an acute myocardial infarct after transmyocardial laser revascularization. J Am Coll Cardiol 1995; 25:258-263

14. Cooley DA, Frazier OH, Kadipasaoglu KA, Lindenmeir MH, Rehlivanoglus S, Kolff JW et al: Transmyocardial revascularization: Clinical experience with twelve month follow-up. J Thorac Cardiovasc Surg 1996; 111:791-799

15. Okada M: Transmyocardial laser revascularization: Indication, Technique, Results. J Jpn Surg Soc 1996; 97:234-239

16. Okada M: Transmyocardial laser revascularization (TMLR): A long way to the first successful clinical application in the world. Ann Thorac Cardiovasc Surg 1998; 4:119-124

17. Landolfo CK, Landolfo KP, Hughes GC, Coleman ER, Coleman RB, Lowe JF: Intermediate-term clinical outcome following transmyocardial laser revascularization in patients with refractory angina pectoris. Circulation 100(19 Suppl): II, 128-133

18. Lee LY, O'Hara MF, Finnin EB, Hachamovitch R, Szulc M, Kligfield PD, Okin PM, Isom OW, Rosengart TK: Transmyocardial laser revascularization with excimer; Clinical results at 1 year. Ann Thorac Surg 200; 70:498-503

19. De-Oliveira SA, Dallan LA, Lisboa LA, Chavantes MC, Cesar LA, Pardi MJ, Jatene AD: Transmyocardial laser revascularization: Early clinical experience. Arq Bras Cardiol 1999; 72:441-450

20. Allen KB, Dowling RD, Delrossi AJ, Realyvasques F, Lefrak EA, Pfetter TA, Fudge TL, Mostovych M, Schu D, Szentpetery S, Shaar CJ: Transmyocardial laser revascularization combined with coronary artery bypass grafting: A multicencer, blined, prospective, randomized, controlled trial. J Thorac Cardiovasc Surg 2000; 119:540-547

21. Lutter G, Sarai K, Nitsche E, Saurbier B, Frey M, Hoegerie S, Martin J, Zipfel M, Spillner G, Beyersdorf F: Evaliation of transmyocardial laser revascularization by following objective parameters of perfusion and ventricular function. Thorac Cardiovasc Surgeon 2000; 48:79-85

22. Ascher PW: Vorteile und Moglichkeit des CO_2 Laser in der Neurochirurgie. Wien Med Wochenschr 1977; 128:260-262

23. Baggish MS: In: Bellina, J.H.,ed.,Gynecologic Laser Surgery, CO_2 laser surgery for benign and malignat lesion of the vagina., Plenum Press, New York, 1981

24. McNally KM, Sorg BS, Welch AJ, Dawes JM, Owen ER: Photothermal effects of laser tissue soldering. Phys Med Biol 1999; 44:983-1002

25. Gorisch W, Boergenm KP, McCord, RC, Weinberg W, Heillenkamp F: Temperature measurements of isolated mesenteric blood vessels of the rabbit during laser irradiation. In: Kaplan,I.,ed.,Laser Surgery II Jarusalem Academic Press Jerusalem,1978

26. Jain KK, Gorisch W: Repair of small blood vessels with the Neodymium-YAG: A preliminary report. Surgery 1979; 85:684-688

27. Jainm, KK: Sutureless microvascular anastomosis using a Neodymium-YAG laser. J Microsurg 1980; 1:436-439

28. Stewart RB, Benbrahim A, LaMuraglia GM, Rosenberg M, Litalien GJ, Abbott WM, Kung RTV: Laser assisted vascular welding with real time temperature control. Laser Surg Med 1996; 19:9-16

29. Klein SL, Chen H, IsraelGraff J: A comparison by burst testing of three types of vascular anastomosis. Microsurg 1998; 18:29-32

30. Demaria RG, Lhote FM, Dauzat MM, Oliva-Lanraire MC, Juan JM, Vernnhet H, Aymard T, Chaptal PA, Godlewski G: Arterial wall compliance after diode laser assisted microanastomosis: A comparative study with conventional manual microanastomosis on the rabbit femoral artery. Laser Med Sci 2000; 15:207-213

31. Maitz PKM, Trickett RI, Dekkey P, Tos P, Dawes JM, Piper JA, Lanzetta M, Owen ER: Sutureless microvascular anastomosis by a biodegradable laser-activated solid protein solder. Plastic Reconstr Surg 1999; 104:1726-1731

32. Okada M, Ikuta H, Horii H, Nakamura K: A new method of vascular anastomosis by low power CO_2 laser. J Jpn Soc Laser Med 1985; 5:209-214

33. Okada M, Nakamura K: Current problems and managements in aortocoronary bypass. Operation 1985; 39:101-109

34. Okada M, Yoshida M, Tsuji Y: Klinische Erfahrungen der Laseranwendung in der Cardiovascularen Chirurgie. Langenbeck Arch Chir (Suppl), 1994;717-719

35. Phillips AB, Ginsburg BY, Shin SJ, Soslow R, Ko W, Poppas DP: Laser welding for vascular anastomosis using albumin solder: An approach for MID-CAB. Laser Surg Med 1999; 24:264-268

36. Okada M, Yoshida M, Tsuji Y, Nakamura K: Laser angioplasty with vascular endoscope in the field of the peripheral and the coronary artery. Surg Med Lasers 1988; 1:53-60

37. Vlestra RE: Percutaneous transluminal coronary angioplasty: Initial clinic experience. Mayo Clin Proc 1981; 56:287-291

38. Gruentzig A: Results from coronary angioplasty and implication for the future. Am Heart J 1982; 103:779-783

39. Okada M, Tsuji Y, Yoshida M, Nakamura K: Clinical and experimental studied on laser application for coronary and the peripheral arterial disease. Revue Euro Technol Biomed 1990; 12:27-31

40. Ginsburg R, Kim DS, Guthaner D, Mitchell RS: Salvage of an ischemic limb by laser angioplasty: Description of a new technique. Clin Cardiol 1984; 7:54-58

41. Diethrich EB, Timbadia E, Bahadir I, Colurn K, Lenzen S: Argon laser assisted peripheral angioplasty. Vasc Surg 1988; 22:77-87

42. Cumberland DC, Sanborn TA, Taylar DI, Moore DJ, Welsh CL, Greenfield AJ, Gulber JK, Ryan TJ: Initial clinical results with a laser probe in total peripheral artery occlusion. Lancet 1986; 1:1457-1459

43. Sanborn TA, Cumberland DC, Greenfield AJ: Percutaneous laser thermal angioplasty: Initial results and 1 year follow-up in 129 femoropopliteal lesions. Radiology 1988; 168:121-124

44. Bittl JA, Excimer laser angioloplasty for saphenous vein graft lesions. Saphen Vein Bypass Dis 1998; 33:231-243
45. Strebel RT, Utzinger U, Peltola M, Schneider J, Niedere PF, Hess OM: Excimer laser spectroscopy: Influence of tissue ablation on vessel wall fluorescence. J Laser Applic 1998; 10:34-40
46. Topaz O, Mclvor M, Stone GW, Krucoff MW, Perin EC, Fosch AE, Sutton J, Nair R, deMarchena E: Acute results, complications, effect of lesion characteristics on outcome with the solid-state, pulsed-wave, mid-infared laser angioplasty system: Final multicenter registry report. Lasers Surg Med 1998; 22:228-239
47. Nazzal M, Kaidi A, Thanh P: A safe procedure in peripheral vascular surgery. J Cardiovasc Surg 1998; 39:131-135
48. Dahm JB, Kuon E: High enrgy eccentric excimer laser angioplasty for debulking diffuse restenosis leads to better acute and 6 month follow-up results. J Invasive Cardiol 2000; 12:335-342
49. Okada M, Yoshida M, Tsuji Y, Nakamura K: Laser angioplasty for the peripheral and the coronary artery disease. Angeiologie 1990; 42:121-127
50. Diethrich EB, Hanafy HM, Santiago OJ: Intraoperative coronary excimer laser angioplasty: Preliminary clinical experience. Angiology 1990; 41:777-779
51. Litvack F, Grundfest W, Hickey A, Jakubowski A: Percutaneous coronary angioplasty: Results of the first 110 procedures. J Am Coll Cardiol 1990; 15:25A
52. Sanborn TA, Faxon DP, Kellett MA, Ryan TJ: Percutaneous coronary excimer laser assisted balloon angioplasty: Initial multicenter experience. J Am Coll Cardiol 1990; 12:25A
53. Liu ML, Chow WH, Kwok OH, Jim MH, Yip A, Fan K, Chan E: Treatment of in-stent coronary restenosis with excimer laser angioplasty. Chinese Med J 2000; 113:14-17
54. Haase J, Storge H, Hofman M, Schwarz F: Excimer laser angioplasty with adjunctive balloon dilatation versus balloon dilatation alone for the treatment of in-stent restenosis: Results of a randomized single center study. J International Cardiol 1999; 12:513-517
55. Koster R, Kahler J, Terres W, Reimers J, Baldus S, Hartig D, Berger J, Meinetz T, Hamm CW: Six month clinical and angiographic outcome after successful excimer laser angioplasty for in-stent restenosis. J Am Coll Cardio 2000; 36:69-74
56. Topaz O, Janin Y, Bernardo N, Bailey NT, Mohanty PK: Coronary revascularization in heart transplant recipients by excimer laser angioplasty. Laser Surg Med 2000; 26:425-431

Chapter 5

LASER TOMOGRAPHY

Dmitry A. Zimnyakov and Valery V. Tuchin
Saratov State University, Russian Federation

5.1   INTRODUCTION

Comparative analysis of the modern optical technologies based on the use of laser light for tissue structure diagnostics and imaging is given in this chapter. A great interest to the development and medical applications of optical imaging methods that has appeared in the last two decades, was stimulated by such undoubted advantages of these techniques as safety, potentiality to obtain high spatial resolution on the cellular and even subcellular level in combination with relatively large penetration depths of the probe laser light in the visible and near-infrared regions, possibility to provide the multifunctional diagnostics and imaging of tissues and organs, etc. It is necessary to note that various aspects of laser diagnostics and imaging in biology and medicine were discussed in a series of special issues and books of selected papers [1-6]. Here we will discuss the basic physical principles, potentialities, limitations and instrumentation design for such laser tomography methods as various diffusing light technologies, laser confocal microscopy, optical coherence tomography and speckle imaging techniques. Also, the most important examples of clinical and laboratory applications of laser imaging for structure and functional diagnostics of tissues and organs will be presented.

5.2   DIFFUSING LIGHT TECHNOLOGIES

Most of the modern diagnostical and imaging technologies with use of laser light scattering by probed tissue can be determined as the "diffusing light technologies" and are based on the analysis of spatial distributions of certain parameters of scattered light in the dependence on mutual positions of light source (laser), probed object (tissue), and detector (or set of detectors). All these approaches can be classified in several groups depending on the applied principles of the optical signal processing and, correspondingly, the parameters of the scattered optical field used to reconstruct the image of the probed tissue structure. In general, these are:

continuos-wave (CW) imaging techniques in the transmission and back-reflection mode;

modulation techniques widely known as frequency-domain and time-domain techniques and based on the application of the harmonically modulated laser radiation (with ultra-high modulation frequency) or ultra-short pulses of laser light for tissue structure imaging; if only phase measurements are provided such technique is named as "phase method";

diffusing-wave imaging techniques used in general to identify into the tissue volume the site of the localized dynamic inhomogeneity with blood perfusion level differing from that for background tissue (such as, e.g., early breast or brain tumor or a small amount of bleeding in tissue volume).

Definition "diffusing light technologies" shows that the central point in the background theory for these techniques and, correspondingly, analytical approaches to the inverse problem solution during the tissue image reconstruction is the application of diffusion approximation to describe the laser light propagation in the probed tissue. Of course, this approximation is not always valid and is limited by the certain restrictions for scattering geometry and optical parameters of the probed media (large scattering and small absorption coefficients, large distances between light source and detector in the scattering media which at least in several times exceed the inverse value of the reduced scattering coefficient [7], observation of scattered laser light pulses at large times corresponding to "tails" of temporal distributions of the photon density) but it is mathematically simple and has been shown experimentally to be a reasonably good approximation in most of the dense weakly ordered media, particularly human tissue.

Diffusion equation used to describe the light transport in dense scattering media is usually written [8] as:

$$\nabla D \nabla U(\bar{r},t) - v\mu_a U(\bar{r},t) - \partial U(\bar{r},t)/\partial t = S(\bar{r},t) \qquad (1)$$

where $U(\bar{r},t)$ is the light energy density also interpreted as the photon density; v is the speed of light in the scattering medium; $S(\bar{r},t)$ is the source term; $D = v\left[3\left(\mu_s' + \mu_a\right)\right]^{-1}$ is the light diffusion coefficient in the medium, μ_s' is the scattering factor, or the reduced scattering coefficient of the medium, and μ_a is the absorption coefficient of the medium. For such scattering media as human tissues the scattering factor is typically significantly (in many times) large than μ_a for visible and NIR light; for instance, typical values of μ_s' and μ_a for human brain are equal to 17.5 cm^{-1} and 0.04 cm^{-1}, respectively (probe light wavelength is 820 nm). For human breast these values are equal to 15 cm^{-1} and 0.035 cm^{-1}, respectively (at 780 nm) [9,10].

Thus, spatial-temporal distributions of the scattered light energy, or dynamic intensity patterns carry the information about the inner structure of the scattering media and analysis of these patterns can provide the tomographic reconstruction. In this case, contrast of reconstructed images can result from changes in tissue blood volume and blood oxygenation. Similar changes cause the spatially distributed variations of the wavelength-dependent absorption into the tissue volume. Also, such variations can be induced by the administration of the special chemicals that preferably accumulate in the region of the disease location. Another factor influencing the contrast of the reconstructed images is the spatial variations of the scattering coefficient, which can be connected with the presence of the fat, water and perhaps even with glucose concentration in tissue [10]. One of the promising areas of the further development of the light diffusion technologies is the brain studies due to that the light in near-infrared penetrates the skull much more effectively, then does, for example, ultrasound. In addition, the nature of medical optical imaging favors the widespread use of diffusing light probes because these instruments are compact, portable and inexpensive and rely only upon electro-optical components that are small and efficient, such as laser diodes and miniature photomultiplier tubes [10]. In accordance with the above introduced classification the basic light diffusion imaging technologies will be sequentially considered.

5.2.1 CW Imaging Techniques

One is the simplest approaches to the reconstruction of images of inner structure of dense media masking the hidden inhomogeneities with differing optical parameters is to use the continuos-wave laser source with the simultaneous analysis of patterns of the scattered light intensity in the transillumination or back-reflection mode. Early works dedicated to application of the light technologies for diagnostical purposes in medicine showed that significant information can be obtained by the analysis of the diffusing light field induced by CW laser sources in transillumination mode [10]. Measurements of the spatial distributions of CW light intensity at the object surface in combination with a conventional back-projection image reconstruction were reported by Jarry *et al.* [11], Jackson *et al.* [12], Tamura *et al* [13], Oda *et al.* [14] and very many other researches. It seems intuitively that CW intensity distributions contain the less useful information for image reconstruction in comparison with analysis of dynamic intensity patterns carried out by use of time-resolved detection of the diffusing light. Indeed, results from both simulated and experimentally measured data indicate that the presence of absorbing centers in a scattering object is rather noticeable being determined by use of the light path statistical analysis from the time-resolved measurements than by use of the light intensity distributions at the object surface (Arridge *et al.* [15,16], Fishkin *et al.*[17], Berndt and Lakowicz [18]. But it should be noted that in tissue, when the background absorption coefficient is large (for instance, greater than 1.0 cm^{-1}), image of absorptive heterogeneities are not significantly improved by use of high-frequency modulated probe light (with the modulation frequency of the order of 1 GHz) and corresponding time-resolved detection technique [10].

Generally, quality of the reconstructed image can be improved by use of the modulation technique only in the case if the modulation frequencies exceed the photon absorption rate ($v\mu_a$) for the probed scattering medium. CW and low-frequency modulation techniques can give the additional opportunities in case of regional functional imaging of tissues with relatively low resolution, where it is necessary. A simple example is the early localization of a head injury that causes brain bleeding or hematomas. Here CW light imaging devices can detect minor bleeding in the brain [10] that is at the limit of detection of X-ray computed tomography.

5.2.2 Frequency-domain Techniques

In case of the turbid media probing by laser light with intensity harmonically modulated at angular frequency ω its value within the probed medium can be written as the composition of time-independent and time-dependent parts:

$$U(\bar{r},t) = U_{dc}(\bar{r}) + U_{ac}(\bar{r})\,exp(\,-j\omega\,t) \qquad (2)$$

Time-dependent part of the scattered light intensity (the second term in the right-hand side of equation 2) can be obtained as the partial solution of the light diffusion equation 1. Considering the harmonically oscillating point-like source at the origin, equation 1 is reduced to the well-known form of the Helmholtz equation for coordinate-dependent amplitude:

$$\left(\nabla^2 + K^2\right)U_{ac}(\bar{r}) = \delta(\bar{r})A/D \qquad (3)$$

with $K^2 = \left(-v\mu_a + j\omega\right)D$. Here A represents the product of the source modulation and strength, and the medium is assumed to be homogeneous. In case of an infinite scattering medium the solution of the Helmholtz equation describes the highly damped spherical wave propagating outward from the source and inducing the regular spatial-temporal oscillations of the photon density into the scattering medium. Such kind of oscillations is usually considered as a diffuse photon density wave. In typical imaging system based on the detection of the photon density waves the intensity-modulated laser light is delivered into a probed sample (e.g., by use of the fiber-optics cable); laser diode or more complex laser system is used as an illumination source).

Diffusing light is detected by the single movable detector or by the system of spatially distributed detectors; harmonically modulated component of the detected photoelectric signal is processed by standard phase-sensitive technique. As it follows from equation 2, photon density waves demonstrate the common features typical for any form of classical waves: i.e., in case of interaction with any obstacle embedded into the scattering medium the diffraction of the photon-density wave will take place [19]. Being passed through the interface between two scattering media with different optical properties such wave exhibits the property of refraction [20]. Also, intensity "interference patterns" will be formed in case of interaction of photon density waves propagating from two or more oscillating light source [21]. Finally, the dispersion of these waves was mentioned Tromberg *et al.* [22]. One of the prospective directions in further development of the laser imaging techniques for biomedical applications can be the modulated optical systems that employ several well-chosen, discrete modulation frequencies or that use continuous frequency variation and provide the essential information being at the same time relatively simple and inexpensive.

One of the typical phase imaging systems for *in vivo* studies was designed in the University of Illinois at Urbana-Champaign [23]. The optical signal at 760 nm from the mode-locked Titanium Sapphire laser (Mira 900, Coherent) was modulated at 160 MHz. The heterodyne mixing at the dynode chain of the PMT produces a cross correlation signal (1.25 kHz), carrying the same phase and amplitude information, as the original signal. The imaging system provides a sub-second data integration times per pixel (10^4 total pixels, 8×8 cm^2 grid in a gradation of 101 steps of 0.8 mm each) resulting in a total measurement time of about 10 min. To partially compensate for limits on the detector's dynamic range and reducing the influence of the boundary effects the human hand under investigation was immersed in a highly scattering aqueous solution of Liposyn III (20%) (an intravenous fat emulsion) which scattering and absorption properties were approximately matched to those of the hand, by diluting the emulsion with water and serial additions of black indian ink.

Another example of frequency-domain imaging system is that has been designed by University of Pennsylvania and NIM Inc. for regional imaging of brain tissue [24]. The system can operate at selectable RF ranging from 50 to 400 MHz. Dual wavelength light source (two laser diodes at 779 and 834 nm), avalanche photodiode detection (APD), and single side band (SSB) modulation/demodulation electronics are the main features of the imager. It was successfully used for a preliminary clinical study, i.e., the positions of the shunt components were defined on the basis of reconstructed images (at a depth of 1.2 cm) of brain tissue of a patient with hydrocephalus (abnormal increase in the amount of cerebrospinal fluid) who was undergoing surgery to have a shunt replaced.

Very stable and fast scanning imaging system uses the diffraction of diffuse photon density waves [25]. The system consists of a RF modulated (100 MHz), low-power (about 3 mW) diode laser (786 nm). The source light is fiber guided to the tissue. A detection fiber couples the detected diffuse wave to a fast APD. The SSB IQ demodulation electronics were used. The dynamic range of the system is about 2500. The source position was fixed, a single detection fiber was scanned over a square region 9.3×9.3 cm^2, the amplitude and phase of the photon density wave were recorded at each position for a total of 1024 points. To obtain projection images of hidden macro-inhomogeneities in a highly scattering tissue imaging algorithms based on K-space spectral and Fast Fourier Transform (FFT) analysis were recently developed and tested clinically [26]. The FFT approach has yielded clinical projection images with processing times much smaller than current collection times. It was shown that boundary effects present important problems. Matching substances might be used to reduce the boundary effects, nevertheless, the boundary effects may be incorporated in the reconstruction algorithm.

A schematic diagram of the F/D optical mammography apparatus (LIMA), developed at Carl Zeiss is shown in Figure 1 [27]. It uses two diode lasers at 690 and 810 nm. Lasers' intensities are sinusoidally modulated at 110.0010 and 110.008 MHz, respectively. The average power is about 10 mW. Both laser beams (2 mm in diameter) are collimated, made collinear, and directed to the object. An optical fiber (5 mm in diameter) located on the opposite side of the breast delivers light to the detector. A PMT with modulated gain at 110 MHz is used as a detector. The differences frequencies of light and gain modulation are $\Delta f_1 = 1$kHz (relative to the signal at 690 nm)

and $\Delta f_2 = 0.8$ kHz (relative to the signal at 810 nm), and called cross-correlation frequencies. An appropriate electronic filtering allows for separation of signals at these frequencies, i.e., at the two wavelengths.

The breast is slightly compressed between two parallel glass plates. The dual-wavelength laser beam and the detector fiber are scanned in tandem along the upper and lower plane, respectively, so that source-detection separation is fixed. The entire compression assembly with the two glass plates can be rotated by 90^0 to allow for data acquisition in craniocaudal and mediolateral projections. The extension of the scanning step (the image pixel size) can be set by software, but it is generally defined by needed spatial resolution, the total acquisition time and signal-to-noise ratio. For this system the scanning step of 1.5 mm in both directions gives about 3 min the total acquisition time for whole mammogram and noise of about 0.2^0 for phase and 0.1% for amplitude measurements. The boundary effects were overcome using an appropriate algorithm [$N(x, y)$ function] based on the idea to explore the phase information in a given pixel (x, y) to obtain an estimate of the breast thickness in that pixel. As a second step, the dependence of the amplitude signal with tissue thickness is modeled using the empirically determined dependence on thickness in the optically homogeneous case. LIMA system was clinically tested on 15 patients affected by breast cancer.

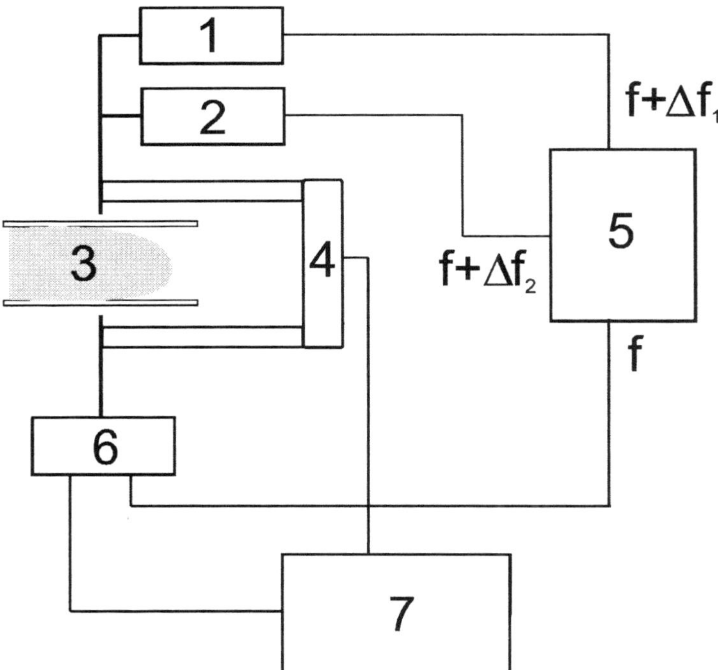

Figure 1. Frequency-domain optical mammography apparatus [27]; 1,2 – laser diodes; 3 – sample (breast) under study; 4 – XYZ translation stage; 5 – oscillator; 6 – detector; 7 – data processing and control unit.

A comparison of X-ray and optical mammograms illustrates that developed optical technique has a good contrast and tumor detectability, rather than high spatial resolution, which is intrinsically limited by the diffusive nature of light propagation in tissue. The promise of optical imaging methods lies in high contrast, detectability, and specificity, that allow for diagnostic capabilities. Further enhancement in contrast can be achieved by introducing additional light sources, wavelengths, modulation frequencies, and/or multiple detectors (see above discussion). In addition to contrast enhancement, frequency-domain and time-domain methods have the potential to provide an *in situ* optical biopsy by measuring localized optical properties [28, 29].

5.2.3 Phased Array Technique

In the NIR the wavelengths of diffusive photon-density waves in tissues are equal to 5 – 14 cm for modulation frequencies from 500 to 100 MHz. That means low resolution of imaging with the usual source and detection combination in spite of providing the high accuracy of phase and amplitude measurements. The so-called photon-density waves interference method (phase and amplitude cancellation method or phased array method), described for the first time in 1993 [30], is very promising for the improvement of a spatial resolution of the modulation technique [31-33].

The idea of this method is based on the usage of either duplicate sources and a single detector or duplicate detectors and a single source so that the amplitude and phase characteristics can be nulled and the system becomes a differential. If equal amplitude at 0^0 and 180^0 phases are used as sources, an appropriate positioning of the detector can lead null in the amplitude signal and a crossover between 0^0 and 180^0 phase shift, i.e., 90^0:

$$A\sin(\omega t + 0^0) + A\sin(\omega t + 180^0) = 2A\cos(90^0)\sin(\omega t + 90^0) \qquad (4)$$

where ω is the light modulation frequency.

In a heterogeneous medium the apparent amplitude's null and phase's crossover may be displaced from the geometric midline. This method is extremely sensitive to perturbation by an absorber or scatterer. The spatial resolution of about 1mm for the inspection of an absorbing inhomogeneity was achieved, the same resolution is expected for the scattering inhomogeneity. Another good feature of the technique is that at the null condition, measuring system is relatively insensitive to amplitude fluctuations common to both light sources. But from the other hand, inhomogeneities, which affect a large tissue volume common to the two optical paths, can not be detected. The amplitude signal is less useful in imaging since the indication of position is ambiguous. Although this can be accounted by further encoding, the phase signal is robust and the phase noise less than a 0.1^0 (signal-to-noise ratio more than 400) for a 1 Hz bandwidth can be provided [31].

The phase modulation system requires, for optimal results, SSB measuring technology [(see Figure 2)]. For instance, the nine source and four detectors are used in 50 MHz single wavelength (780 nm) phase array imaging system [34]. The number of sources and detectors can readily be increased, furthermore, multiplicity of source/detector combinations can be increased simply by moving the source detector pad in two dimensions with respect to its original position by half the minimal distance between source and detector, equal to 2.5 cm. The image pad dimensions are 9×4 cm.

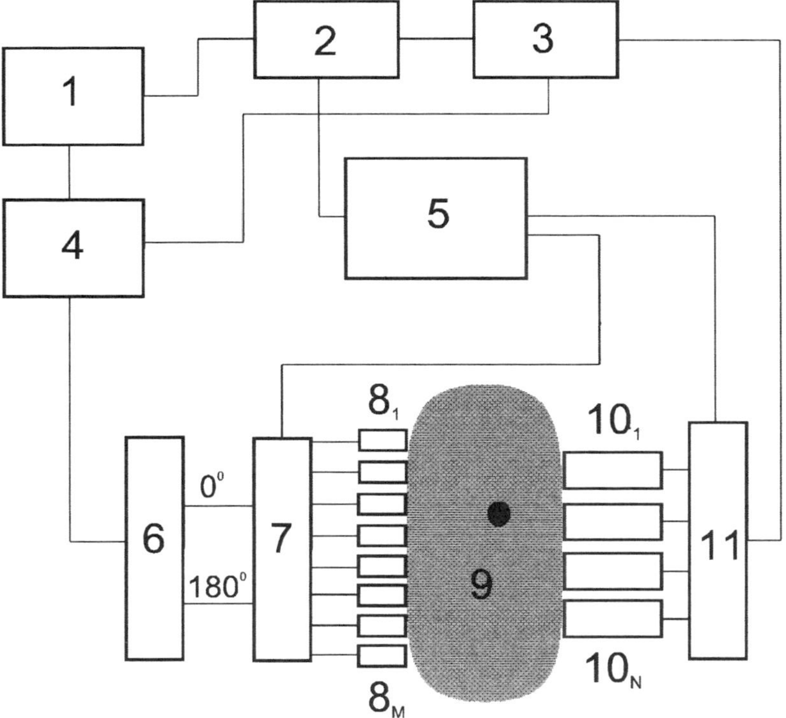

Figure 2. Schematic of multiple-channel frequency domain imaging system; 1 – local oscillator; 2 – phase detector; 3 – SSB receiver; 4 – SSB transmitter; 5 – PC-control and image output; 6 –splitter; 7, 11 – switches; $8_1,\ldots,8_M$ – laser diodes; 9 – object with inhomogeneity; $10_1,\ldots,10_N$ –photomultiplier tubes.

A local oscillator at 1 kHz modulates a 50 MHz SSB transmitter, the RF output of which is connected to a $0^0/180^0$ phase splitter/inverter and then to nine switches appropriate to the nine light sources which are sequenced at 0^0

and 180^0 phase by 1 Hz switches. The four PMTs are sequentially connected to the 50 MHz SSB receiver (0.5 mV sensitivity), and hence the audio output at 1 kHz is coupled to a zero crossing phase detector to give the phase signals in sequence. The phase detector is coupled via controlling computer to a computer for image computation and display (not shown). The transmitter and receiver are phased locked by RF coupling. The phase noise of the system is less than 0.1^0 (1 Hz bandwidth). A complete set of data from 16 source/detector combinations is obtained every 16 s.

More universal and comprehensive phased array imaging system, that can be used for testing neonates brain function, has been described [35]. Each of single wavelength laser diode light sources was replaced by a set of two laser diodes (750 and 830 nm, totally 18 lasers) with a 20 mW source power. The wavelength of 780 nm was shifted to 750 nm because at 750 nm the signal gain is more than twice due to the respective extinction coefficients. Detection of the optical signals was provided by four PMT (TO8 Hamamatsu). Two independent phasemeters and 2 SSB radio transmitters/receivers were used with 50 and 52 MHz frequencies. The size of the optical probe is slightly larger (10×5 cm), because two lasers are located in a point, but a source-detection separation was the same, 2.5 cm.

A dual wavelength phased array imaging system can be used for testing neonates brain function, and its relationship with some neurological disorders by means of metabolic activity indicated by oxygen concentration or glucose intake to the brain cells.

Another dual wavelength imaging system (750 and 830 nm) that uses a simple amplitude cancellation technique was applied for the human breast imaging [36]. The optical probe of the imager consists of nine laser diode light sources and 21 silicon photodetectors. Imager sequences through all sources and detectors in a millisecond and gives high quality breast tumor images every 8 second. Detection limit in localizing of macroinhomo-geneities, hidden in a highly scattering tissue, using phased array imaging systems has been discussed by Papaioannou *et al.* [37].

5.2.4 Time-domain Techniques

Another approach is based on the application of the sequences of ultra-short laser pulses for tissue imaging and diagnostics. Two versions of this technique are possible; one of them supposes the detection of only non-scattered, or "ballistic" photons by use of time-gating, or time-of-flight techniques with further reconstruction of the tissue image similarly to that it takes place in X-ray tomography. Another method deals with multiply scattered components that form the broadened light pulse traversing the medium. In this case, the peak time delay of such broadened pulse depends on the scattering coefficient of the probed sample as well as terminal slope depends on the sample absorption coefficient. The close relation between two modulation techniques should be mentioned: in particular, transport of light pulses in the scattering media can be considered in terms of a superposition of diffuse photon density waves at the equidistantly disposed frequencies; each such wave as the spectral component of the time sequence of pulses scatters independently on each other.

It is necessary to note that it is very difficult to provide measurements of the absolute concentrations of absorbers and absolute values of the scattering coefficients for the optical tomograpy purposes (although this is desirable), but this allows to provide the high-performance image-reconstruction procedures. Generally, the imaging is aimed at detection of pathology or at localization of lesions. The detection of a lesion is achieved by recording a 2-D image with sufficient contrast, while localization needs optical slicing and tomographic reconstruction to obtain the 3-D images, by which the size, shape and position of the hidden object can be determined [38].

The imaging systems usually use 2-D or 3-D scanning of a narrow laser beam or translation optical stage with the attached object. Nonscanning systems are more robust and correspondingly fit much better to medical applications. Such nonscanning systems use multichannel fiber-optical arrangement with fixed positions of light sources and detectors, or low-noise, high sensitive and fast CCD cameras with microchannel plate optical amplification. In any case the measurement procedure is completed by sampling the intensity of each pixel as a function of time, to obtain a time-space intensity mapping. The image is numerically reconstructed by attributing to each pixel the intensity measured over the selected integration time [38].

A multi-channel NIR imager-spectrometer based on the time-correlated single photon counting technique was designed for breast imaging in clinics (see Figure 3) [35, pp.284-288]. The instrument uses two NIR wavelengths 780 and 830 nm, the average power of each laser diode is about 40 μ W, they pulsing at 5 MHz with a pulse width of about 50 ps. A high-sensitive R5600U-50 GaAs photomultiplier (PMT) has been chosen for the breast examination. For enhancement of carcinoma images contrast, an intravenous administration of Infracyanine®25 (IC25), an NIR contrast agent, was used. Optical absorption changes was calculated using the following relation:

$$\Delta\mu_a = -\frac{2}{c\Delta t^2} \int_{t_1}^{t_2} \ln\frac{J_2(r,t)}{J_1(r,t)} dt \tag{5}$$

where c is the speed of light in the medium; Δt is the time resolution of the pulse-height analysis (PHA, Hamamatsu Inc.) of the multi-channel analyzer

(MCA, Hamamatsu Inc); J_1, J_2 is the photon current measurement pre- and post-IC25 injection respectively and t_1, t_2 is the width of the J_1 time resolved curve. Equation 5 gives accurate values of $\Delta\mu_a$ for small absorption changes.

The relative displacement of the light sources and detectors, the positions of the projection plane and pathology (carcinoma, black sphere) are shown in Figure 4.

The calculations of absorption coefficient differences along the straight lines connecting those source-detector pairs in space that have comparable separations allows for estimation of IC25 distribution in tissue. Tests with patients were done simultaneously with the standard MR imaging examination protocol.

One of the examples of a potential of time-resolved diffusion imaging for mammography applications is presented [35]. In this case, the possibilities of a time-resolved optical diffusion mammography were compared with MR image study. Measurements were done for the patient (70 years old Caucasian) was diagnosed with an Infiltrating Ductal Carcinoma approximately 10 mm in diameter. For light diffusion imaging, 6 sources and 8 detectors were employed. A good correspondence between the MR and the NIR images was demonstrated. In the 780 nm light image there are two objects resolved, either due to measurement noise or due to actual physiology of the tissue. Due to more absorption (12%) of IC25 at 780 nm compared to the 830 nm, there is actually expected differences to be enhanced more.

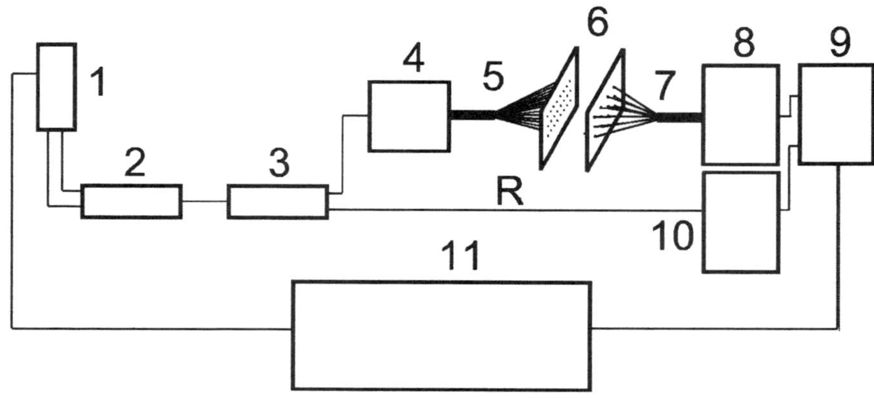

Figure 3. Typical scheme of the multi-channel time-correlation NIR imager-spectrometer for mammography; 1 – laser diode assembly; 2 – fiber-optical coupler; 3 – signal splitter; 4 – fiber-optical switcher; 5, 7 – bundles of optical fibers; 6 – breast soft compression plates; 8, 10 – detector units; 9 – router; 11 – data processing unit; R – reference branch.

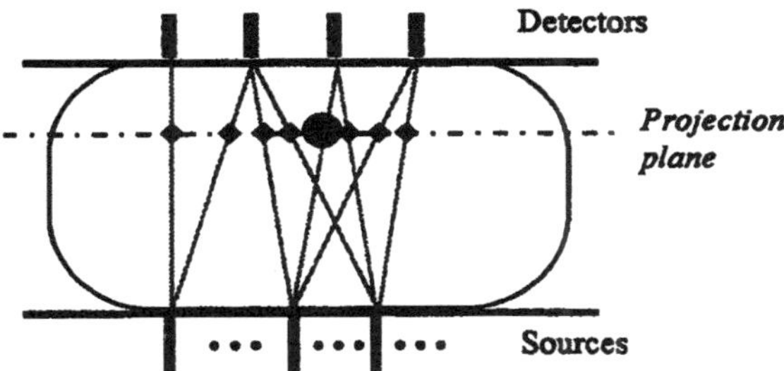

Figure 4. Geometric interpretation of the tumor localization procedure.

Much more comprehensive time-resolved optical tomography system employing 32 channels and designed for imaging of the neonatal brain and the human breast is the MONSTIR (Multi-channel Optoelectronic Near-infrared System for Time-resolved Image Reconstruction) [35, pp.120-122]. Light from a pulsed high-power picosecond laser source is switched sequentially into one of 32 fibers, which are attached to the surface of an object under study.

The detection system serves for recording the temporal distribution of light exiting the tissue at certain positions around the object with a temporal resolution about 80 ps and the rate of photon counting up to a few 100k per second per channel. This is accomplished by utilizing 32 fully simplex ultrafast photon-counting detectors. Scattered photons are collected by 32 low-dispersion, large diameter (2.5 mm) fiber bundles which are coupled to 32 stepper motor driven variable optical attenuators (VOAs).

Because of the large dynamic range of light intensities around the object, the VOAs are required to ensure that the detectors are not saturated or damaged and that the system operates within the single photon counting mode. Light transmitted via VOA is collected by a short 3.0 mm diameter single polymer fiber and than is transmitted via a visible blocking filter to the photocathodes of four ultrafast 8-anode microchannel plate-photomultiplier tube (MCP-PMT). The resulting electronic pulse is preamplified, converted into a logic pulse, and a histogram of photon flight times recorded and transfered to the control computer.

A dedicated image reconstruction software package, TOAST (Time-resolved Optical Absorption and Scattering Tomography, TOAST Website: http://www.medphys.ucl.ac.uk/toast/), is used for reconstruction of tomographic images of the absorption and scattering profiles.

5.2.5 Diffusing-wave Tomography

Differing from other above considered diffuse light technologies, this method uses the coherence property of laser light multiply scattered by the probed tissue. Partial components of the diffuse optical field, being mutually coherent and superposed, will form the random interference pattern, or *speckle pattern* inside and outside the scattering medium. Motions of the structure-forming elements into the scattering system will be manifested as the speckle pattern dynamics, whose parameters will mirror the dynamics of the scattering medium. Typically, correlation or spectral analysis of temporal fluctuations of the scattered field amplitude at the fixed detection point is applied to measure the dynamic properties of the scattering medium or to image its inner structure. Thus, diffusing-wave, or correlation spectroscopy and tomography are in general the tools for probing and imaging of dynamic inhomogeneities in tissue such as local diseases or traumas with level of the blood perfusion differing from that for the background tissue (such as, e.g., tumors).

The basic object usually used to establish the relations between dynamic and optical properties of the detected inhomogeneity as well as the background tissue and temporal fluctuations of the scattered optical field is the field correlation function $G_1(t,\tau)$ introduced as:

$$G_1(t,\tau) = \left\langle E(t+\tau)E^*(t) \right\rangle \tag{6}$$

where * denotes the complex conjugation procedure and averaging is carried out over all possible configurations of the scattering system. For stationary and ergodic scattering systems temporal correlation function of the field fluctuations depends only on the time lag value: $G_1(t,\tau) = G_1(\tau)$. Considering the formation of the fluctuating optical field due to the multiple scattering of the plane monochromatic light wave by the system of non-interacting statistically independent movable scatterers, we can obtain the following well-known relation for [39] $G_1(\tau)$:

$$G_1(\tau) \sim \int_0^\infty exp\left(-\frac{k_0^2 \left\langle \Delta \bar{r}^2(\tau) \right\rangle s}{3 l^*}\right) \rho(s) ds \tag{7}$$

where probability density function $\rho(s)$ describes the statistical properties of distribution of optical paths which characterize the propagation of partial components of scattered optical field into the scattering medium; k_0 is the wavenumber of the probe light in the scattering medium; l^* is the transport mean free path which is an inverse of the reduced scattering coefficient μ'_s; $\langle \Delta \bar{r}^2(\tau) \rangle$ is the variance of the scatterer position for the observation time, characterizing the type of scattering system dynamics. The probability density $\rho(s)$ is associated with the photon density that corresponds to the sertain value of effective optical path; in particular, for given scattering and detection conditions it can be obtained by solution of the diffusion equation. Such solution should describe the temporal dependency of the diffuse light intensity at the detection point for given boundary conditions and δ-like temporal dependence of the probe light intensity. Presence of inhomogeneities into the scattering volume will change the path statistics and thus such inclusions can be detected and localized by evaluating the decay parameters of the field correlation function $G_1(\tau)$ [40].

Actually in typical dynamic light scattering measurements the measured value is the temporal correlation function of speckle intensity fluctuations:

$$G_2(\tau) = \langle I(t+\tau)I(t) \rangle$$

if any specific optical techniques such as diffusing-wave interferometry [41] are not applied. For optically dense non-stationary random scattering systems consisting of many statistically independent scatterers the relation between normalized field and intensity correlation functions (these are $g_1(\tau) = G_1(\tau)/G_1(0)$ and $g_2(\tau) = G_2(\tau)/G_2(0)$, respectively) is given by the Siegert formula:

$$g_2(\tau) = 1 + \beta |g_1(\tau)|^2 \tag{8}$$

where the factor β is determined by the detection conditions; for ideal conditions, then the used detector aperture is much smaller than the coherence area of the detected optical field, or the speckle size, β is equal to 1.

Figure 5 illustrates typical scheme [40] of the diffusing-wave diagnostical and imaging system available for tomographical applications. The probe laser light (this may be, possibly, the radiation of Ar-ion laser, or first or second harmonics of the diode-pumped AIG:Nd laser, or radiation of the laser diode) is delivered into the scattering medium by the multimode optical fiber. The backscattered (or, possibly, the transmitted) diffuse light is collected by the single-mode fiber and detected by the photomultiplier tube operating in the photon-counting mode. Such procedure is repeated several times at different positions of the source and detector to provide enough information for tomographical reconstruction of the inhomogeneity image. Single-mode fiber as the light-collecting system is used in order to provide as much better value of β as possible. The sequence of photo-counts is processed by the digital autocorrelator to measure the temporal correlation function of the speckle intensity fluctuations $G_2(\tau)$. After this, normalized correlation function of the scattered field fluctuations is obtained by use of Siegert formula and its parameters (e.g., slope in semi-logarithmic coordinates or correlation time) are applied as the diagnostical or visualization parameters.

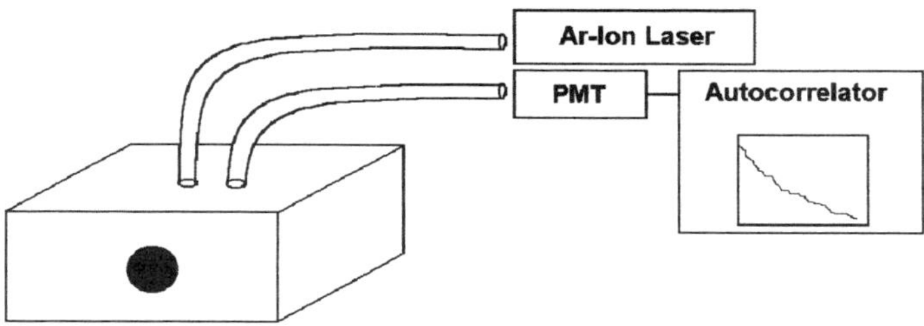

Figure 5. Typical scheme of the diffusion tomography experiment based on the photon correlation measurements.

One of the prospective approaches in the diffusing-wave tomography of the non-stationary turbid media is the analysis of correlation transport viewed as propagation of correlation "wave" outwards from sources and its scattering by macroscopic inhomogeneities associated with spatial variations of dynamical or optical properties. It should be noted that evolution of the spatial-temporal correlation function of the optical field fluctuations due to the light propagation in free space has been analyzed in works of Born and Wolf [42]; corresponding wave equation for the field correlation function has been obtained. Later, it has been shown by Ackerson *et al.* [43] that certain analogies exist between the transport of correlation in the disordered scattering media and transport of photons which can be described by the well-known radiative transport equation. The main feature of correlation transport relates with the accumulation of the decay of correlation function caused by each scattering event during the propagation of correlation wave in the scattering system. In this case, considering the "stationary correlation transport" through the scattering medium (steady state) probed by continuos-wave source, one can modify the radiative transfer equation in its usual form in order to obtain the corresponding correlation transport equation:

$$\nabla G_1(\bar{r},\widetilde{\Omega},\tau) + \mu_t G_1(\bar{r},\widetilde{\Omega},\tau) =$$
$$= \mu_s \int G_1(\bar{r},\widetilde{\Omega}',\tau) g_1^s f(\widetilde{\Omega},\widetilde{\Omega}') d\widetilde{\Omega}' + S(\bar{r},\widetilde{\Omega}) \tag{9}$$

Temporal correlation function of the scattered field fluctuations $G_1(\bar{r},\widetilde{\Omega},\tau)$ depends on the detection point position ($\bar{r}$) and direction in turbid medium ($\widetilde{\Omega}$) chosen for correlation analysis; $\mu_t = \mu_s + \mu_a$. Term $g_1'(\tau) = exp\left(-\frac{1}{6}q^2\langle\Delta\bar{r}^2(\tau)\rangle\right)$, that corresponds to single scattering, describes the accumulation of correlation decay due to sequences of scattering events; $f(\widetilde{\Omega},\widetilde{\Omega}')$ is the phase function of the scattering medium and $S(\bar{r},\widetilde{\Omega})$ is the light source distribution.

In the case of validity of standard diffusion approximation, the stationary correlation transport equation 9 can be rewritten in the following form:

$$\left(D_\gamma\nabla^2 - c\mu_a - \frac{1}{3}c\mu_s' k_0^2\langle\Delta\bar{r}^2(\tau)\rangle\right)G_1(\bar{r},\tau) = -cS(\bar{r})$$

where $D_\gamma = cl^*/3$ is the photon diffusion coefficient, c is the light speed in the scattering medium and μ_s' is the reduced scattering coefficient. It should be noted that term $\frac{1}{3}v\mu_s' k_0^2\langle\Delta\bar{r}^2(\tau)\rangle$ describes the additional losses of correlation due to the dynamic scattering in the disordered medium and can be interpreted as "correlation absorption" caused by the dynamic processes.

Presence of any kind of scattering medium dynamics is manifested as the appearance of additional "absorption" term in the correlation diffusion equation. Thus, numerical solution of this equation for given sequence of the source and detector positions with respect to probed scattering object with embedded dynamic inhomogeneity can be used as the basis for inverse problem solution (reconstruction of the inhomogeneity "image"). Similar technique has been developed by **Boas** *et al.* [44] and was verified in the experiments with phantom multiply scattering "static" object (titanium dioxide-resin cylinder) containing "dynamic" inhomogeneity (spherical space filled by water solution of Intralipid). Sample was illuminated by semiconductor laser radiation through fiber-optic light-guiding system; scattered light was collected by single-mode fiber-optic light collector and detected by photon-counting system. Scattered light intensity fluctuations as random sequences of photo-count pulses were processed by digital autocorrelator to obtain $G_2(\tau)$ for given illumination and detection conditions. Apart from geometry of the scattering system, angular scanning of the object was carried out; measurements were made every 30^0 at the surface of the cylinder with source-detector angular separations of 30^0 and 170^0. Results of the inhomogeneity image reconstruction are shown in Figure 6.

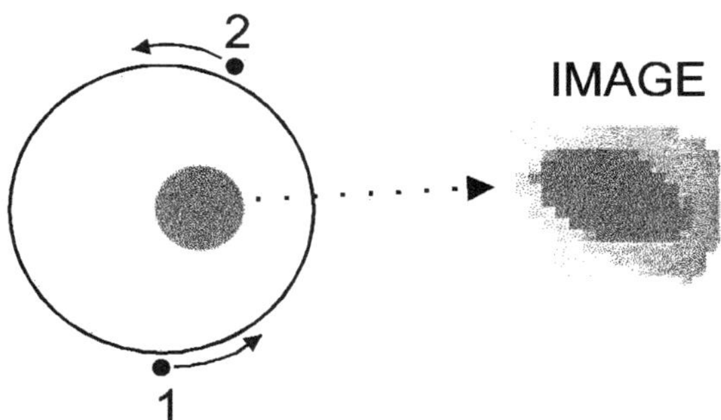

Figure 6. Imaging of the dynamic multiply scattering inhomogeneity embedded in the static scatterer, by means of the correlation diffusion analysis [44]. Light source is laser diode with fiber-optics light-delivering system. 1 – source; 2 – detector. Static scatterer is a 4.6 cm diameter cylinder with l^* = 0.25 cm and μ_a = 0.002 cm^{-1}. Dynamic scatterer is a 1.3 cm diameter spherical cavity filled with a colloid with l^* = 0.25 cm, μ_a = 0.002 cm^{-1} and D_B = 1.5×10^{-8} cm^{2}s^{-1}. A slice of image is presented in (b). The values of the reconstructed particle diffusion coefficient are imaged by using the linear gray-level scale (darkest level corresponds to D_B =1.5×10^{-8} cm^{2}s^{-1}, white level – to 0).

5.3 LASER SCANNING CONFOCAL MICROSCOPY

Laser scanning confocal microscopy is one of the most powerful tools for high-resolution imaging of cellular and subcelular structures of thin tissue sections without dissecting the tissue sample. Basic ideas and various aspects of practical applications of this imaging technique have been developed by various researchers [45-58].

Basic principles of confocal microscopy are illustrated by Figure 7. Small source of light is used to illuminate a small region within the probed tissue by use of the condenser lens. The image of this region is transferred by the objective lens onto a photodetector with a small aperture. The positions of the light source, probed volume of the tissue and detector aperture are chosen to provide the conjugation of the object and image plane and thus source, probed volume and photodetector aperture can be considered as the confocal to each other. Another condition is the optical matching of sizes of the photodetector aperture and the light source due to appropriate choice of the magnification of the image transferring optical system (condenser lens and objective lens). These conditions lead to that only portion of light from very small region optically conjugated with detector aperture will induce the photodetector signal. On the contrary, contributions to photoelectric signal induced by the portions of light from regions located before and after the optically conjugated plane will be negligibly small as it is shown in Figure 7.

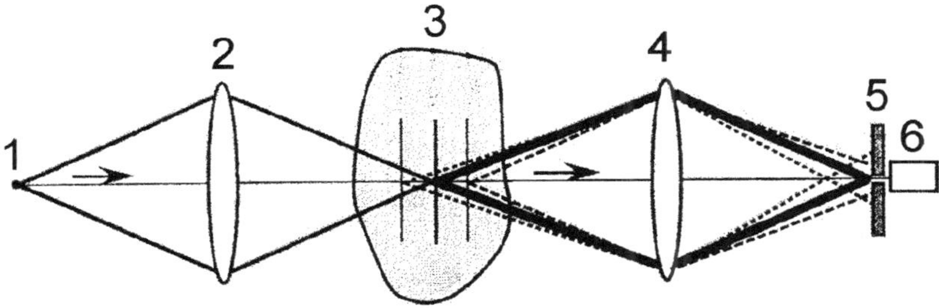

Figure 7. Optical scheme of confocal microscope; 1 –small source of light; 2 – condenser lens; 3 – sample under study; 4 – objective lens; 5 – pinhole diaphragm; 6 - detector.

Thus, such instrument allows to probe the thin slices of tissue (optical sectioning) with high optical resolution and high contrast. Such device allows only to probe a small region into the tissue volume at a time. To provide the reconstruction of the image of the whole sample it should be scanned in a desired manner: by moving the sample relative to a stationary positioned optical system (object scanning) or by moving the optics relative to the sample located at the fixed position (beam scanning). For imaging of in-vivo tissues the latter procedure (beam scanning) is definitely more convenient. In this case preferable configuration of the confocal scanning system is the reflection one, as it is shown in Figure 8.

Application of the laser as the light source in the confocal microscopic system provides the additional opportunities for reconstruction of the high-fidelity 3D tissue images due to very high levels of spatial coherence and spectral density of the laser radiation.

The portion of the detected light reaching the detector from the each element of the probed tissue depends on the incident irradiance, the velocity of the sample scanning, the numerical aperture of the illumination and light-collecting optics, the detector aperture size, the wavelength of illumination, and the scattering cross-section of the probed tissue. For in-vivo imaging, these parameters can be optimized to provide nearly diffraction-limited images of optically dense tissue such as skin to depths of 500 μm [49].

Two of the most important performance parameters for confocal systems are the numerical aperture of the illumination and light-collection lenses and illumination wavelength λ. In the case of equal values of numerical apertures of condenser and objective lenses in the object space (as it takes place for reflection configuration, Figure 8), the lateral resolution of the confocal system is proportional to the ratio λ/NA [50]:

$$\Delta x = \frac{0.46\,\lambda}{NA} \tag{10}$$

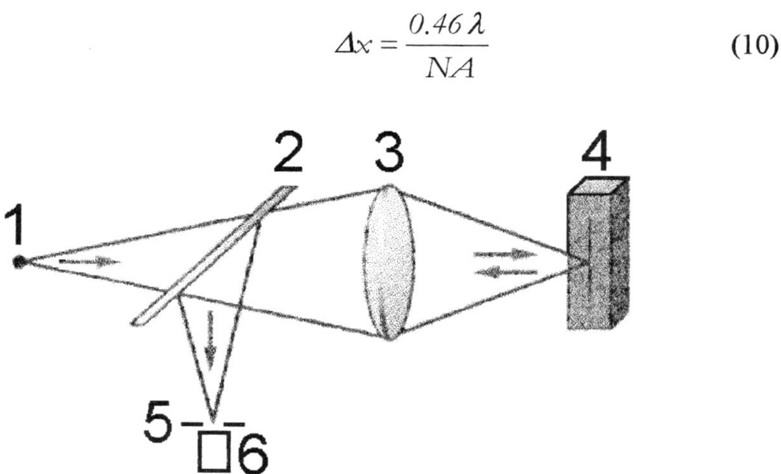

Figure 8. Confocal optical system for the backscattered light detection; 1 – point-like light source; 2 – beamsplitter; 3 – condenser and objective lens; 4 – sample under study; 5 – pinhole diaphragm; 6 - detector.

The axial resolution defining the thickness of the probed slice into the tissue volume or section thickness is evaluated by the ratio λ/NA^2 [51]:

$$\Delta z = \frac{1.4\,n\lambda}{NA^2} \tag{11}$$

where n is the refractive index of the objective lens immersion medium. For instance, application of microscope objective with a magnification of $100^\times$ and numerical aperture of 1.2 allows one to obtain the lateral resolution of about 1 μm and axial resolution of 4 μm at the illuminating wavelength of 1.06 μm.

The range of optimal values of numerical aperture for illumination at 1.06 μm is between 0.7 and 0.9, as it has been shown in experiments with the Massachusetts General Hospital-developed confocal scanning laser microscope for in-vivo human skin imaging [49]. Higher value of numerical aperture should provide the better spatial resolution and contrast of reconstructed image but actually all these advantages are accompanied by the increased off-axis aberrations, small working distance and field of view. On the other hand, numerical apertures less than 0.7 provide low contrast image reconstruction because of the too large values of the section thickness in comparison with typical thickness of the individual cell layers. For NA values less than 0.7 or larger than 0.9 reconstructed confocal images have the quality estimated in terms of contrast and spatial resolution that is similar to the quality of the conventional microscopic images.

Another parameter influencing on the performance of the confocal scanning system is the detector aperture (pinhole) diameter. A small pinhole provides the better sectioning but with the less value of the detected intensity of the backscattered light. Wilson and Carlini [52,53] and other researchers [54] have considered the axial resolution of the confocal system in case of imaging of plane mirror surface; it has been found that the axial resolution remains constant up to a normalized pinhole radius of $v_p = 2$ and then rapidly falls off for larger pinholes. The dimensionless value v_p is equal to:

$$v_p = \frac{2\pi}{\lambda} NAr_p \qquad (12)$$

where r_p is the actual pinhole radius at the object.

The important question is the appropriate choice of the wavelength of the probe light as it depends on a number of different factors. NIR spectral range (from 0.7 to 1.2 μm) which in general is typical for biomedical applications, is characterized by the maximal penetration depth due to the small absorption and scattering of the probed tissues. But reduced scattering for these wavelengths of the probe also causes the decrease of the backscattered intensity and, as a result - the reduction of the signal-to-noise ratio. In case of imaging of the human derma tissue the best choice is to use illuminating wavelengths around 800 nm; this provides a good compromise between increasing penetration and good signal sensitivity if silicon avalanche photodiode is used as the detector.

To obtain high-quality confocal images, the microscopic system should operate at high frame rates enough to reduce blur and motion artifacts in the tissue caused by living object motions or dynamic changes, such as blood microcirculation in capillary net [49]. For standard video scan rates (about 20 -30 frames per second) and pixel densities the integration time per single pixel will be of the order of 100 ns, so the efficiency of the photon detection will be about 10^{-6}.

For such low levels of the detected signal (one photon in one million) caused by the short integration time, quantum shot noise limits the signal-to-noise ratio and, correspondingly, the maximum depth of imaging. The latter one can be increased by the increase of the imaged tissue irradiance level, but it is necessary to keep in mind that used optical power should be limited in order to prevent the optical damage of in-vivo studied specimen. The critical level of the tissue irradiance strongly depends on the used wavelength; in NIR spectral range penetrating radiation causes the heat damage due to absorption. In experiments [49] with wavelengths from 800 to 1064 nm and irradiance energies from 0.2 to 0.3 J/cm^2 per each imaged pixel histology showed no damage.

Optical scheme of video-rate confocal scanning laser microscope for in-vivo imaging of human tissues [50] is shown in Figure 9. The collimated laser beam is scanned in the fast (X) direction with a rotating polygon mirror and in the slow (Y) direction with an oscillating galvanometric mirror. The scanning is at standard video rates of 15.734 kHz along X and 60 Hz along Y, so the images can be displayed in real time on a television monitor. The X and Y scanning produces a raster of laser beam spots in the back focal plane of the objective lens. The raster width (16 mm) is comparable with the typical value of diameter of aperture (18 mm) in the eyepiece of a conventional microscope.

The raster size, being demagnified by the objective lens, defines the field of view at the tissue. 20^{x}- 100^{x} objective lenses usually used in such system provide the field of view changing from 800 to 160 μm. The XY plane is a horizontal plane that is parallel to the surface of the tissue, and the Z axis (the optical axis of the confocal microscope) is perpendicular to it. The intermediate optics consist of folding mirrors and achromatic lenses. There is a telescope system between the polygon mirror and the galvanometric scanners and a single lens between the galvanometric scanner and the objective lens. Water-immersion objective lenses with high numerical apertures (NA) are usually used in this system. Water as immersion liquid provides an adequate matching of refractive index with living tissue and, consequently, leads to:

1) diminishing of spherical aberration due to refractive indices mismatch in case of imaging of deep layers into the tissue volume;

2) increase of image brightness due to reduced internal reflections of the backscattered light back into the tissue volume.

The objective lens aperture is overfilled by ~3× in order to keep resolution close to diffraction limit and to allow the lateral motions of the objective lens within ± 5 mm range.

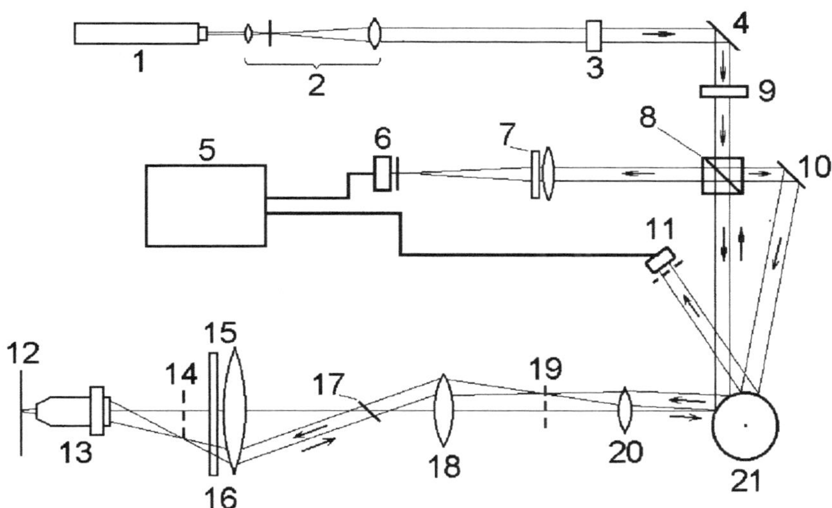

Figure 9. Optical scheme of the video-rate confocal laser scanning microscope for imaging human skin and oral mucosa *in-vivo* [50]; 1 –laser; 2 – beam expander and spatial filter; 3 – linear polarizer; 4, 10 – mirrors; 5 – signal processing unit; 6 – avalanche photodiode with pinhole; 7 – crossed polarizer; 8 – polarizing beamsplitter; 9 – neutral density filter; 11 – split diode; 12 – target surface; 13 – microscope objective lens; 14 – raster plane; 15 – f/2 lens; 16 - $\lambda/4$ retarder; 17 – galvanometric mirror; 18 – f/5.3 lens; 19 – raster line; 20 – f/2 lens; 21 – polygon mirror.

Light backscattered by tissue passes through objective lens and two scanning devices once again; in order to cut-off the background light induced by backreflections of the p-state illuminating beam crossed polarizers with a quarter-wave retarder are used. The returned light is descanned by by two scanning devices (the galvanometric mirror and the rotating polygon mirror) and then separates from the illumination path at the polarizing beam splitter. After this, the backscattered light is detected by an avalanche photodiode with the pinhole diaphragm. With used optics (100$^{\times}$, 1.2 NA objective lens) lateral resolution (Δx) and axial one, or section thickness (Δz) were estimated as 0.4 µm and 1.4 µm, correspondingly. Optimal value of the objective lens numerical aperture was obtained by the estimations of the contrast value for the images grabbed with different objective lenses and was found to be in range of 0.7-1.2. Detector aperture diameter was chosen using the above described criterion by Wilson et al. For skin examination, the optimal values of illumination power for the considered system was 20-40 mW at the skin surface. Over a field of view 160×120 μm obtained with $100^{\times}$, 1.2 NA objective lens such optical power results in an irradiance $100 - 200$ W/cm^2. For 15 min imaging there is no optical damage of the living tissue as it has been shown by histologic examination carried out in three sites. Further experiments with freshly excised, living, melanin-containing bovine epithelial cells (as a model for pigmented living human skin) have showed that, at the wavelength of 1100 nm, cell death occurs for irradiance exceeding 500 W/cm^2 following approximately 5-10 min of confocal imaging. For described system used for skin tissue imaging the level of the detected power was typically equal to $10 - 100$ nW that corresponds to $1000 - 10000$ photons per single pixel at 100 ns pixel integration time. Thus, the calculated rms value of the signal-to-noise ratio of detector output was found to be 13-40.

One of the most important questions is how to provide the stable and reliable optical contact of the confocal system with the examined in-vivo tissue sample. For the considered system [50], a mechanical arm facilitating access to any site on a human body was built; this arm pivots on the same axis as the galvanometric scanner of the confocal system. The optical elements following the galvanometric scanner were mounted upon the arm, and the microscope objective lens was enclosed in an aluminum housing. A brass ring-and-template arrangement was attached to the skin with medical adhesive. The ring forms a well for holding the immersion medium. The site to be imaged was located with a hole in the template that was 0.3 mm thick. Hole diameters ranged from 0.2 to 10 mm, permitting precise location of either small or large sites. The template was thin enough that the skin could protrude through the hole and be accessible to the objective lens, especially for lenses with short working distances of few hundred micrometers. By locking the ring-and-template assembly into the housing of the objective lens the reliable microscope-to-skin contact was achieved that effectively minimized gross skin motion to within ± 25 μm (± 2 cells) in the lateral (XY) direction. The microscope objective lens was mounted upon a three-axis micrometer stage, and by translating the objective along the objective along the axial (Z) direction relative to the template one could image confocal sections at various depths in the skin.

The ring-and template assembly was attached to a pair of surgical tweezers thus forming the clamp that could hold oral tissue. The clamp effectively kept lip or tongue tissue immobile for $3 - 4$ min necessary to grab the confocal images.

Some (but not all) possible applications of laser confocal systems in basic and clinical medical research can include [55]:
- detection of tumor margins in basal cell carcinomas;
- proliferative and inflammatory skin disorders;
- oral (lip and tongue) mucosa;
- freshly excised head and neck specimens; and
- superficial tissue layers in the bladder and organs of living rats (after removing the overlying skin and muscle).

Other investigations may include the distribution of melanin, cell-cell interactions (diapedesis, phagocytosis, melanin transfer, apoptosis), microcirculation, drug delivery and distribution, photoageing, wound healing, and artificial tissue.

5.4   OPTICAL COHERENCE TOMOGRAPHY

One of the most prospective optical imaging technologies for medical and biological applications is based on the usage of the interferometers with low-coherent light source. Such devices, with probed object as the retroreflector in the object arm of interferometer and scanning mirror in the reference arm can serve as tomographic system being provided the transverse XY-motions in the object surface plane (Z-direction is provided by reference mirror scanning). The resulting two-dimensional or three-dimensional data sets can be used for reconstruction of spatial distributions of the sample reflectance. The basic ideas and principles of this method, widely known as optical coherence tomography (OCT), were given by classical works of various workers [56-60]. During the last decade the outstanding research activity in this field has stimulated an abundance of theoretical and experimental works dedicated to various aspects of low-coherent imaging in biology and medicine.

Typical optical scheme of low-coherent imager with fiber-optics interferometer that can be used in medical diagnostics is presented in Figure 10 [61]. In this case, the light-beating signal due to the interference of the object and reference beam is detected and it will only be measured as the optical lengths of reference and object channels will differ by length not larger than the coherence length of the used light source. The typical point spread function of the low coherent interferometer defining its axial resolution is shown in Figure 10(b). This function is actually defined by the envelope of the interferometer output signal in case of approximately equal optical path lengths for both arms of interferometer and can be obtained, say, in experiments with backreflecting mirror as a sample.

A super-luminescent diode (SLD) light sources or solid state lasers generating ultra-short light pulses are usually used as the low-coherent illumination sources; SLDs have typically tunable spectral bandwidth $\Delta\lambda$ of 30-100 nm and femtosecond lasers are characterized by a higher bandwidth up to 100 nm.

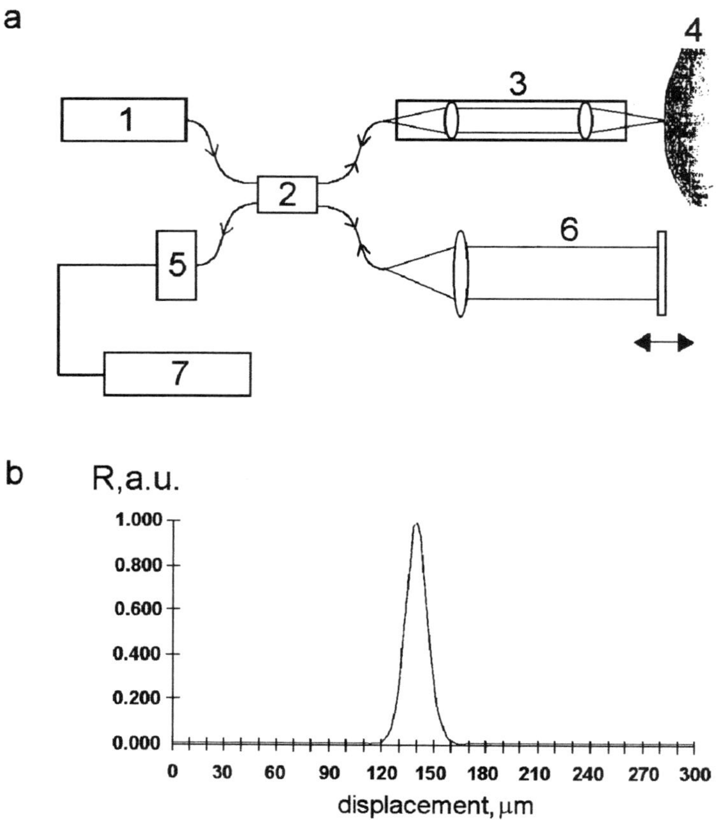

Figure 10. a - schematic sketch of OCT instrument; 1 – low coherence light source; 2 – fiber-optical interferometer; 3 – sample arm; 4 – sample; 5 – detector; 6 – reference arm; 7 – signal processing unit. b - typical form of the point spread function of OCT imager.

For given median wavelength of the probe light, λ, the axial, or depth resolution of low-coherent interferometer can be evaluated as [62]:

$$\Delta_z = \frac{2\ln 2}{\pi} \cdot \frac{\lambda^2}{\Delta\lambda} \tag{13}$$

Typically, the depth resolution changes from 20 - 30 up to several microns (in the dependence on the used light source) and it can be concluded that such technique "fills a nishe between confocal microscopy and imaging modalities such as US [ultrasound], MRI [magnetic resonance imaging], and CT [computed tomography]" [63]. Maximal imaging depth is determined by the extinction of the probe light into the imaged tissue and in the case of transparent media such as eye tissues can be very large. As for the wide variety of optically dense tissues such as, e.g., skin maximal penetration depth of the probe light for the appropriate levels of the signal-to-noise ratio is of the order of 1 mm. The results of comparative study of imaging potentialities of confocal microscope and full field OCM (optical coherence microscopy) instrument were presented by Wang *et al.* [64]. The significantly better quality of the reconstructed images was obtained in the latter case. Onion tissue was used as the imaged sample and full field OCM system, which is schematically shown in Figure 11, was examined in these experiments. The sample arm of the low-coherent interferometer consists of a high speed scanning confocal microscope with a fast scanner (a resonant scanner or a rotating polygonal mirror) and a slow scanner (a galvanometric scanning mirror); the slow scanner was positioned at the image plane of the fast scanner. To exclude the mechanical scanning of the phase delay in the reference arm, a 40 MHz acousto-optic modulator (AOM) in combination with fixed mirror is used for frequency shifting of the reference arm light due to double passage through AOM. In such a way, the reference arm length was fixed to match the optical path length of the sample arm. The same setup was modified for confocal microscopy by blocking the reference arm and detecting the DC centered signals from the sample arm.

Both sets of images with confocal microscope and OCT imaging system were recorded at 8 frames per second with polygonal mirror as a fast scanner. Each image is a single frame extracted from the video. Since the rotating polygonal mirror causes path length change in the sample arm of the interferometer during the OCM image reconstruction, additional frequency shift of operating frequency of acousto-optic modulator was introduced during the sample scanning. This shift was equal to 3 MHz from one side of the image to the other side. Thus, by moving the center frequency from 80 to 83 MHz, a full-field OCM image was captured.

Application of the fiber-optical light-delivering and light-collecting cables allows one to built the flexible low-coherent imaging system providing the possibility of endoscopic analysis of human tissues and organs. In particular, OCT system developed for endoscopic applications (high speed *in vivo* intra-arterial imaging) is described by Tearney *et al.* [65]. Solid state Cr^{+4}:Forsterite laser with Kerr lens mode locking is used as an illumination source with a median wavelength of 1280 nm and a bandwidth of 75 nm. Thus, the theoretical axial resolution of the system can be estimated as 10 μm (see equation 13); actual depth resolution measured with mirror as a standard technique for resolution evaluation gave the axial pixel size equal to 9.2 μm. The lateral resolution of this system that depends on the spot size of the used lens system on the output tip of the light delivering fiber, was equal to 30 μm with confocal parameter equal to 1.74 mm. Electronics allowed one to capture 4 frames at second for 512 transverse image pixels. The optical power incident on the imaged tissue was approximately 10 mW. Corresponding signal-to noise ratio was 106 dB. Reference-arm phase delay scanning device consists of oscillating galvanometer mirror, lens and grating.

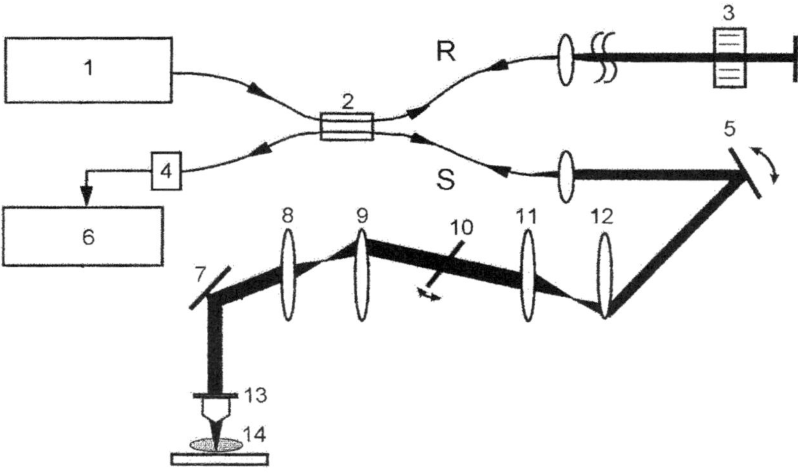

Figure 11. Optical scheme of high speed, full field optical coherence microscope [64]; 1 – low coherence light source; 2 – fiber-optical interferometer; 3 – acousto-optic modulator; 4 – detector; 5 – resonant scanner; 6 – computer-based data processing unit; 7 – mirror; 8,9,11,12 – lenses; 10 – galvanometer; 13 – microscope objective; 14 – sample under study; R – reference arm; S – sample arm. By blocking the reference arm, this system can also be used as confocal scanning microscope.

Various fiber-optical devices designed for endoscopic OCT imaging have been described [65]. One of the examples is the fiber-optical scanning catheter used for intra-arterial imaging. It consisted of an encased, rotating speedo-meter cable carrying a single mode optical fiber. Such catheter consists of an optical coupling at its proximal end, a single-mode fiber as the light-delivering channel, and focusing and beam directing elements at the distal end. Beginning at the proximal end of the device, incident light from a fixed single-mode optical fiber is coupled through a narrow air gap into a second single-mode fiber that can rotate. The drive assembly of the catheter, located at the proximal end, uses an optical fiber connector. A gear is attached to the connector and a shaft assembly consisting of the connector, the fiber in the catheter, and the distal focusing elements. A dc motor is used to drive the shaft assembly through a gear mechanism.

The beam is focused by a graded index lens and is directed by a microprism. The beam was scanned circumferentially by rotating the cable, fiber and optical assembly inside the non-movable housing. Power losses caused by suboptimal coupling and internal reflections within the catheter were 3-4 dB. For instance, *in-vivo* image of the rabbit trachea, which was obtained with the above described system, allows to differentiate various tissue structures such as the pseudostratified epithelium, mucous, and surrounding hyaline cartilage [65].

Principles of design and implementation of various fiber-optical forward-imaging instruments for optical coherence tomography were discussed Boppart *et al.* [66]. In comparison with the side-imaging devices, these instruments have such advantage as possibility to collect the backscattered light before the introducing of the light delivering system into tissue. Also, it makes possible the image-guided placement of the device in surgery and for monitoring interventional procedures such as tissue incision, resection, and laser surgery.

In one of these instruments, piezoelectric cantilever provides the translation motion of a single-mode fiber together with a gradient-index (GRIN) lens. Such design allows to assemble both a light-delivering fiber with focusing lens and a transverse scanning device in a compact small-sized unit but disadvantage is a fixed magnification of such system.

For practical applications, this instrument was constructed with a 6.4 mm × 38.1 mm lead zirconate titanate piezoelectric cantilever (Morgan Matroc, Inc.) as the transverse scanner. It provides displacement of 1 mm for 300 V driving voltage. Cantilever arm length was increased by a 38-mm extension tube in order to provide 2 mm transverse scan length. This extension tube was used as a housing for a single-mode optical fiber and a 0.7-mm-diameter, 0.25-pitch GRIN lens. This lens was placed at the distance of 0.29 mm from the fiber tip. The faces of the fiber tip and the GRIN lens were angled to reduce the intensity of backreflected light that could saturate the detector. Such construction provided a 31-μm spot with 1.2-mm confocal parameter. Working distance was equal to 3 mm.

Another design provides a variable magnification due to application of two-lens focusing system. A cleaved fiber tip scans in the focal plane of the first lens in a telescope. Two-lens system transfers the image of the fiber tip onto the imaged sample. Magnification can be varied by change of the focal length of the second lens. In this case, changing the magnification scales both the focused spot size and the transverse scan length congruently, making the ratio of the transverse pixel spacing to spot size constant.

Rigid forward-imaging device such as laparoscope provides visualization of tissue at distant (10-50 cm) internal sites while maintaining a small instrument diameter for insertion through small incisions during minimally invasive surgical procedures. A beam splitter and imaging lenses are mounted in order to provide the simultaneous low-coherent imaging and a conventional visualization of the tissue surface. White-light illumination fibers were located around the perimeter of the rod lens to provide illumination for visualization.

Potentialities of the OCT imaging technique as applied for morphological study of the human tissues are demonstrated by a great number of examples. For instance, these are the images of normal and diseased glands with pathologic morphology (inflammation) [67]. In the latter case, inflammation is depicted by a high backscattering area in the OCT image. Areas of hemorrhage, center, are noted in the OCT image as disruption of the normal mucous morphology and resultant loss of crypt structure. Another good example is the result of three-dimensional OCT image reconstruction for in-vitro sample of the ampulla of a human fallopian tube [68]. In this case, fifty cross-sections were acquired with a lateral spacing of 100 µm. Variation in the structure of the ampulla toward the infundibulum such as decrease of the mean size of folds should be noted. In the considered case, the imaging depth was limited to 2.5 mm.

Typical axial resolution of OCT imaging systems with such universally adopted broadband light sources as SLDs or mode-locked solid lasers varies from 10-15 µm (SLD) to 4-5 µm (short-pulse laser sources such as organic-dye and Ti:sapphire lasers). To provide significantly higher axial resolution (e.g., on the subcellular level) the broadband light sources covering few hundred nanometers in the visible range are required. Drexler *et al.* [69] have described such ultrahigh-resolution OCT instrument for *in-vivo* imaging. Corresponding optical scheme is presented in Figure 12. Longitudinal resolution is of the order of 1 µm that is the highest OCT resolution achieved to date, was demonstrated for such construction. A Kerr-lens mode-locked femtosecond Ti:sapphire laser is used as an illumination source; it emits sub-two-cycle pulses corresponding to bandwidths of up to 350 nm with a center wavelength at 800 nm. Such high performance is achieved with specially designed double-chirped mirrors with a high-reflectivity bandwidth and a controlled dispersion response, in a combination with low-dispersion calcium fluoride prisms for intracavity dispersion compensation. A pair of fused-silica prisms and razor blades are used to spectrally disperse the laser beam and spectrally shape the laser output. Optical scheme of the low-coherence interferometer was optimized for the ultrabroad bandwidth of the illumination source. Specially designed lenses with a 10-mm focal length and a numerical aperture of 0.30 in combination with single-mode fibers and special broadband fiber couplers were used. Polarization controllers were also used to exclude the broadening of the shape of the interference envelope due to polarization mismatch. Dispersion was matched by use of variable-thickness fused-silica and BK7 prism in order to reach a uniform group-delay dispersion. Such instrument is characterized by the halfwidth of the point spread function (see Figure 10, b) of the order of 1.5 µm [69].

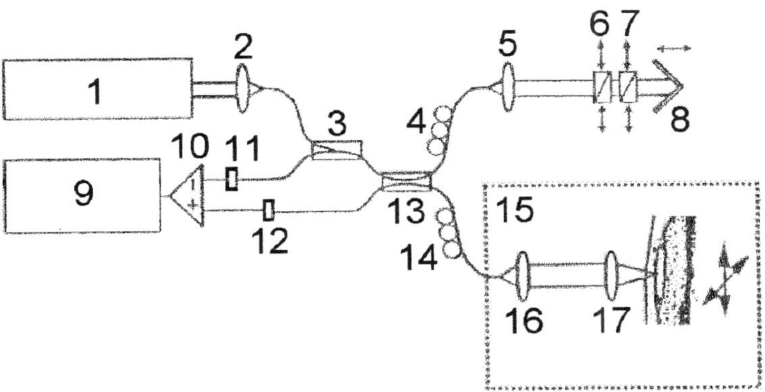

Figure 12. Ultrahigh resolution fiber OCT system with a Kerr-lens mode-locked Ti:sapphire laser [69]; 1 – KLM Ti:sapphire laser; 2,5,16,17 – specially designed lenses; 3,13 – special broadband fiber couplers; 4,14 – polarization controllers; 6,7 – dispersion-matching elements; 8 – reference mirror; 9 – computer-based data processing unit; 10,11,12 – dual balanced detector; 15 – scanning system.

The *in-vivo* subcellular level resolution (1µm × 3µm; longitudinal × transverse) tomograms of an African frog tadpole (*Xenopus laevis*) were obtained to demonstrate the potential of the above described ultrahigh-resolution OCT instrument. Obtained images clearly depict the multiple mesanchymal cells of various sizes and nuclear-to-cytoplasmatic ratios, olfactory tract and intracellular morphology, as well as mitosis of several cells. It should be noted that high lateral resolution throughout the different depths has also been achieved.

One of the promising applications of OCT imaging technology is its simultaneous application together with the laser surgery. One of the examples of such combination is the high-resolution OCT-guided laser ablation system described by Boppart *et al.* [70]. Figure 13 represents the schematic of this system; laser ablation was performed using a continuous wave argon ion laser operating at a wavelength of 514 nm with 1-3 W power output. Argon laser radiation was coupled into a fiber and focused onto the tissue surface as 0.8 mm diameter light spot. Light source used for OCT imaging was superluminescent diode with a 1.3 μm center wavelength. Axial resolution was equal to 18 μm in free space. The signal-to-noise ratio was 115 dB for 5mW power of SLD radiation falling onto the sample.

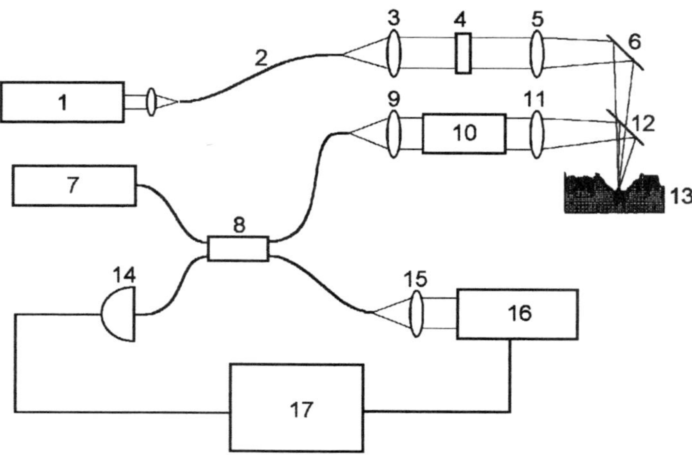

Figure 13. Schematic of OCT-guided laser ablation system [70]; 1 – Ar laser; 2 – fiber-optical light delivering system; 3,5,9,10,15 – lenses; 4 – shutter; 6 – mirror; 7 – SLD source; 8 – fiber-optical interferometer; 10 – XY-scanning system; 12 – dichroic mirror; 13 – laser treated tissue; 14 – detector; 16 – optical delay line; 17 – data processing and acquisition unit.

Possibility of monitoring of the laser ablation procedure by means of OCT imaging system was demonstrated in experiments with tissue ablation. A 10-s, 3-W argon laser exposure was used to form an ablation crater in rat rectus abdominis muscle. The specimen was then translated on a multiaxis translational stage to provide 3D-imaging of the crater with the OCT system. Sixty cross-sectional images were acquired at 100-μm intervals to reconstruct the image that provides information on the depth- and distance-dependent damages of the muscle tissue. For smaller distances from the crater center the larger damages occur, resulting in carbonization of the tissue into the crater.

Modification of the low-coherence imaging technique based on the detection of the photon horizon positions under short-pulse illumination of the probed sample was reported by Hausler *et al.* [71]. This method is based on the application of the low-coherence source (laser diode at 670 nm operating below the threshold) in combination with a Mach-Zehnder interferometer. Multiply scattering sample (solid polyester with the embedded monodispersive SiO_2 spheres; reduced scattering coefficient is 92 cm^{-1}; anisotropy parameter is 0.84) was placed in one of the arms of interferometer (Figure 14). Light scattered out of the surface of the scattering sample and the reference wave were superimposed upon the CCD sensor. The fraction of components of the scattered optical field with effective optical paths matched with the propagation path of the reference beam induces the speckle modulation in the corresponding regions of the image of the sample surface; others fractions cause the incoherent summation of intensities with the intensity of the reference beam. Image as a result of superposition of the reference and the object wave is recorded by the CCD sensor.

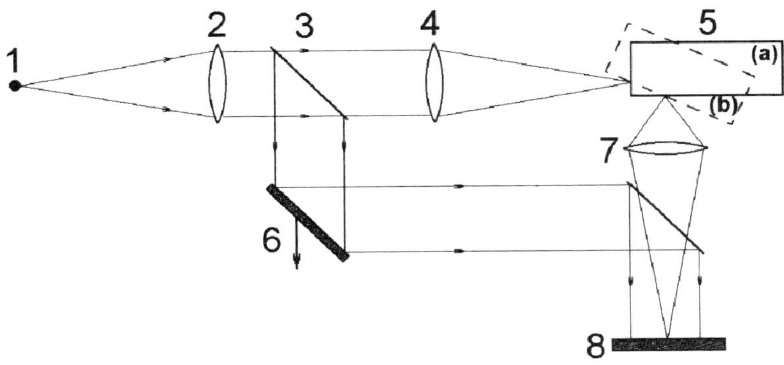

Figure 14. Imaging system with low-coherence interferometer for the study of the path distributions in multiply scattering media by means of speckle contrast analysis in the image plane [71]; 1 – low coherence light source; 2,4 – lenses; 3 – beam splitter; 5 – sample; 6 – adjustable mirror; 7 – imaging lens; 8 – CCD sensor; a – observation of the transversal cross-section; b – observation of the surface.

To improve the quality of the analyzed images the subtraction technique was used: after the exposure the reference phase is shifted by π. The incoherent fractions of the signal are the same in both exposures. Therefore the difference between these two images will contain only the coherent fraction of the signal. In the processed in such a way image dark spots, or speckle modulation of the surface image, will be caused by the partial components of the scattered field that have run the same path length but along the different individual paths. A particular feature of the recorded image is a sharply curved edge of the impulse response, the "photon horizon". This curve defines the maximum penetration depth in the analyzed scattering system for each reference path length. Thus, different penetration depths can be visualized by suitable adjustment of the reference path length. Figure 15 shows the character of these images obtained with different light sources.

The pathlength resolution for this system is determined by the coherence length l_C of the used light source and for used source with $l_C = 30$ μm the resulting time resolution is about 100 fs [71].

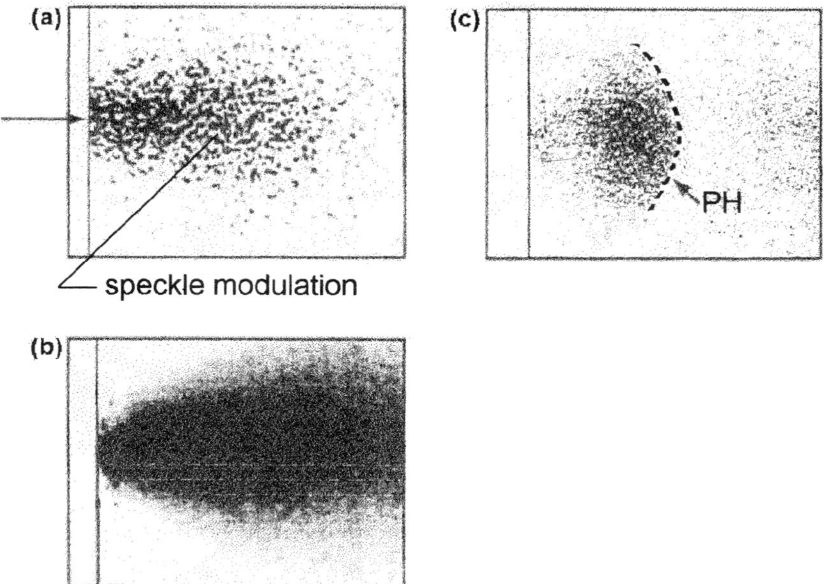

Figure 15. Images of the scattering process with different coherence lengths and different kinds of observation [71]. (a) - fully coherent illumination, direct observation; (b) - broad band illumination, direct observation; (c) - broad band illumination, extraction of the coherent part; dashed line shows the position of the photon horizon (PH).

Being applied for imaging of macroscopically inhomogeneous scattering phantoms and human skin *in-vivo*, the photon horizon detection technique demonstrated promising results [72]. In the case of human skin, the smaller exposure times are required than for motionless scattering system because of the time integration of speckle-modulated images during the exposure. Nevertheless exposure time of 40 ms is enough small to provide the adequate quality of the photon horizon images of human tissues.

On the basis of the obtained results, it can be concluded that photon horizon detection makes it possible to observe light propagation in two dimensions, at the surface of strongly scattering media with a resolution better than 10 fs and with the measuring range about 350 μm in depth. This gives the possibility to use such low-coherence imaging technique for the detection of pathological alterations of human skin (e.g. melanoma maligna).

Finally, it is necessary to note that one of the possible ways to increase the penetration depth of OCT with an appropriate level of the signal-to-noise ratio is the application of the tissue optical clearing technology. Recent researches in this field have demonstrated the high abilities of such technique for tissue structure diagnostics and imaging [73-75].

5.5 SPATIAL SPECKLE CORRELOMETRY

One of possibilities to visualize tissue scattering structures by means of the correlation analysis of dynamic speckles is the scanning of the probed object by a laser beam and the simultaneous detection of the intensity fluctuations of the scattered light; this technique can be determined as the spatial speckle-correlometry [76]. In particular, in the case of the morphological analysis of *in-vitro* tissue samples and tissue replicas, the most convenient scheme for the scanning system consists of a light source and a detector located in fixed positions, with the object under study undergoing a translation scanning movement with respect to the illuminating beam. A typical setup for such a scanning speckle correlometer designed for tissue structure analysis and visualization using transmitted light is shown in Figure 16.

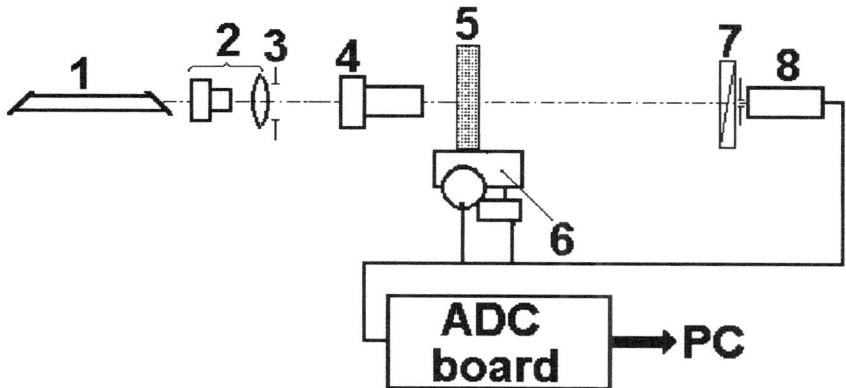

Figure 16. Typical optical scheme of a scanning speckle correlometer for the morphological analysis of *in-vitro* tissue samples and tissue replicas using transmitted light. 1 - CW laser; 2 - beam expander with spatial filter; 3 - iris diaphragm; 4 - microscope objective as focusing lens; 5 - sample under study; 6 - 2D scanning device; 7 - polarizing filter; 8 -photomultiplier tube with pinhole diaphragm.

A single-mode He-Ne laser 1 is used as the illumination source. Two modes of tissue illumination can be used in this technique: a broad collimated beam or a sharply focused beam. A telescopic system 2 is used as the collimator and beam expander. A microscope objective 4 is used as the focusing lens in the case of focused beam scanning; if the broad beam illumination is required, a collimated probe beam with adjustable diameter is used. The diameter of the collimated beam is adjusted by the iris diaphragm 3. Two-dimensional scanning of the probed sample 5 is provided by a computer-controlled XY-translation stage 6 with stepper motors. In order to provide a sufficiently uniform translation motion of the sample during the scanning process, stepper motors with high operation frequencies are used (not less than 700 - 750 Hz for the arrangement used). The speckle intensity fluctuations induced by the sample scanning are detected by a photomultiplier tube (PMT) 8 assembled in a housing with a pinhole diaphragm; the photodetector is placed in the far-field diffraction zone with respect to the characteristic size of the structural inhomogeneities of the object under study. In the case of multiple scattering systems, a polarization filter 7 is used to provide correlation analysis of linearly polarized components of the scattered field with different polarization azimuths. Also, correlation analysis of the speckle intensity fluctuations can be carried out in the image plane by placing an imaging lens between the sample and the photodetector. Typical example of the speckle intensity fluctuations detected in the diffraction plane in the case of scanning an *in-vitro* sample of optically cleared human sclera is shown in Figure 17.

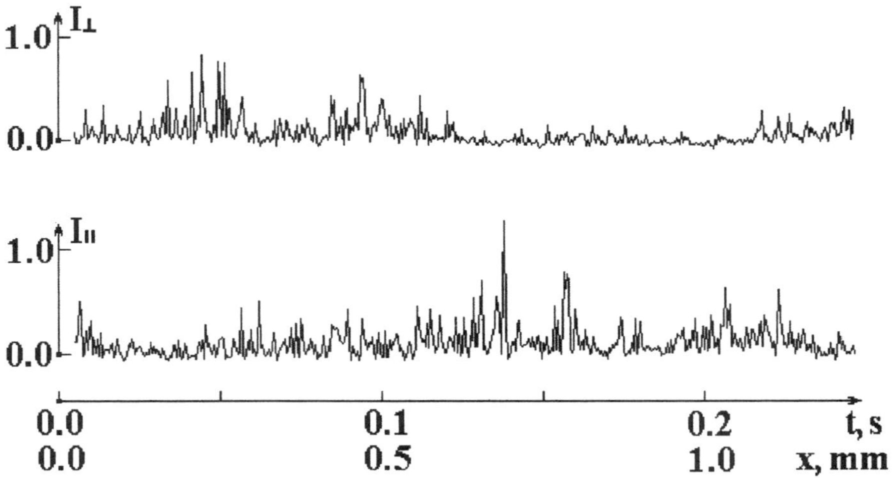

Figure 17. Typical example of the detected intensity fluctuations in the case of scanning an *in-vitro* sample of optically cleared human sclera (upper trace - polarization filter 7 is directed perpendicularly to the polarization azimuth of the illuminating beam; lower trace – parallel direction). Scanning velocity - 5 mm/s.

The spectral width of the detected intensity fluctuations depends on the scanning velocity, the characteristic scales of the structural inhomogeneities of the studied object, the type of scattering mode encountered by the probe light during its transmission through the sample (single scattering or multiple scattering) and the aperture of the illuminating beam. Single scattering or low step scattering takes place if the thickness of the sample under study is of the order of or less than the transport mean free path l^* that characterizes the scattering properties of the tissue. For the single scattering mode, if the characteristic size of the tissue structural inhomogeneities is less than the illuminating spot size and the detector is placed in the far-field diffraction zone, then the spectral width of the detected speckle intensity fluctuations is determined by the ratio of the scanning velocity to this size. At the same time, the shape of the spectrum of the detected speckle intensity fluctuations is determined by the intensity distribution across the illuminating beam aperture [77]. When the size of this aperture is reduced so that it is comparable with the characteristic size of the structural inhomogeneities, the shape of the observed spectrum of the intensity fluctuations and its width become dependent on the statistical and spectral properties of the refractive index fluctuations in the probed volume [77].

In the case of multiply scattering tissues, the second-order statistics and, correspondingly, the spectral properties of the detected light fluctuations, will be determined by the statistical properties of the distribution of the effective optical paths for the given illumination and detection conditions. In particular, the temporal correlation function of the field fluctuations of light scattered by a moving multiply scattering medium can be expressed in terms of the scalar wave approach (equation 7):

$$G_1(\tau) = \left\langle E(t)E^*(t+\tau) \right\rangle \sim \int_0^\infty exp\left(-k^2\left\langle \Delta\bar{r}^2(\tau)\right\rangle s\big/3l^*\right)\rho(s)\,ds$$

where the variance of the displacements of the scattering particles during the observation time τ can be formally expressed as $\left\langle \Delta\bar{r}^2(\tau)\right\rangle = v^2\tau^2$ (v is the scanning velocity) and the probability density function of the effective optical paths is determined by taking into account the specific illumination and detection conditions (including, e.g., the presence of free space between the probed sample and the photodetector and the finite size of the detector aperture).

It should be noted that for most typical cases of the morphological analysis and functional imaging of *in-vitro* tissue samples scanned with velocities in the range 1 - 10 mm/s, the spectral width of the detected intensity fluctuations does not exceed a few hundred kHz. This allows us to use a conventional **PC-compatible ADC** board to provide the data acquisition procedure with further correlation analysis of the detected signal.

The signal processing algorithms discussed in this section are based on the evaluations of the local values of the scale characteristics of the detected intensity fluctuations. These scale characteristics are associated with one-dimensional random processes with pre-fractal properties [78] (demonstrating the self-similarity of the local estimations of the statistical moments in the finite range of space or time scales). A typical way to analyze the scale behavior of the detected time-dependent intensity fluctuations $I(t)$ is to study the dependence of the corresponding structure function on the time lag τ. The structure function $D_I(\tau)$ is introduced as:

$$D_I(\tau) = \left\langle \{I(t+\tau) - I(t)\}^2 \right\rangle \tag{14}$$

The structure function $D_I(\tau)$ is related to the correlation function of the intensity fluctuations $G_2(\tau)$ by: $D_I(\tau) = 2G_I(0) - 2G_I(\tau)$; for fractal-like intensity fluctuations, $D_I(\tau)$ exhibits a power-law increase with increasing τ:

$$D_I(\tau) \cong L_I \tau^{v_I} \tag{15}$$

where the parameter L_I, called the topothesy, is determined by the distance between two points on the curve $I(t)$ for which the average slope of the chord is equal to 1 (in the appropriately chosen coordinate system). The exponent v_I varies between 0 and 2 and is related to the fractal dimension H of the random curve $I(t)$ by [78]:

$$v_I = 2(2 - H). \tag{16}$$

The half value of the structure function exponent, or exponential factor $v_I/2$ is usually known as the Hurst parameter [79]. Fractal-like random fluctuations exhibit a power-law decay of the spectral density in the high frequency region: $S(\omega) \sim \omega^{-\alpha}$; the corresponding spectral exponent is related to the exponential factor v_I by: $\alpha = v_I + 1$. It should be noted that, as a rule, the vast majority of real physical processes are restricted to a limited range of space or time scales spanning no more than 1 to 2 decades (so-called pre-fractal behavior).

The exponential factor of the speckle intensity fluctuations v_I demonstrates a high sensitivity to variations in the optical properties of weakly ordered scattering systems (such as, e.g., tissues) in the case of the transition from the multiple scattering mode of light transport in the system to the single scattering one. This sensitivity can be illustrated, e.g., by the experimental results obtained with optically cleared samples of human sclera [79]. Such clearance can be provided by the diffusion of special immersion agents [such as, e.g., trazograph (x-ray contrasting drug), glucose, etc.] into the tissue volume and the matching of the refractive indices of the different components of the tissue structure (collagen fibrils and ground substance in the case of sclera tissue).

The transition from multiple scattering of the probe light to the low order scattering and single scattering mode in the later stages of optical clearing is characterized by a sharp increase in the exponential factor of the intensity fluctuations. It should be noted that, if in the early stages of optical clearing the normalized correlation function of the intensity fluctuations $\tilde{g}_2(\tau) = G_2(\tau)/<I>^2 - 1$ is quasi-exponential (i.e., the corresponding value of the exponential factor is close to 1), then for the later stages the Gaussian form is more typical (the corresponding value of the exponential factor is close to 2). This is a direct manifestation of the above-mentioned peculiarities of the spectral and correlation properties of the scattered light fluctuations in the case of single scattering by a regularly moving medium with small-scale fluctuations in refractive index and detector position in the far-field diffraction zone. In this case the shape of $\tilde{g}_2(\tau)$ is determined by the intensity distribution in the illuminating beam, which is close to Gaussian.

Locally estimated values of the exponential factor ν_I of the speckle intensity fluctuations obtained during two-dimensional scanning of the probed tissue can be used for reconstruction of the two-dimensional functional images of various tissue diseases ("ν_I-maps"). These local estimations can be carried out by using a moving window to select the processed data block from the discrete time sequence of the detected intensity values. The sequence of the local values of the structure function of the speckle intensity fluctuations is calculated for given values of the time lag and then the local value of the exponential factor is evaluated for each position of the moving window as:

$$\nu_I(j) = \frac{\sum_i^N ln\{D_I(\tau_i)\} \sum_i^N ln\,\tau_i - \sum_i^N ln\{D_I(\tau_i)\}\,ln\,\tau_i}{N\sum_i^N ln^2\tau_i - \left(\sum_i^N ln\,\tau_i\right)^2} \tag{17}$$

where j indicates the current position of the moving window along the scanning trace, N is the number of τ_i used for the estimations of ν_I.

Figures 18 and 19 illustrate the application of this technique to the functional imaging of diseased human skin (psoriasis). These figures show the typical examples of v_I-maps obtained by scanning the *in-vitro* samples of epidermal layers of normal (Figure 18) and psoriatic (Figure 19) skin. Two scanning modes have been used: a sharply focused beam and a collimated beam (beam diameter was ≈ 2 mm). The probed samples have been prepared using skin stripping technology [80].

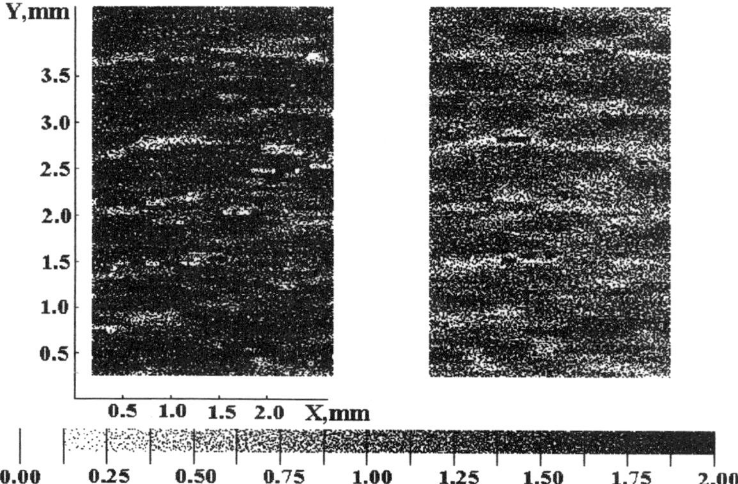

Figure 18. v_I-maps of the upper epidermal layers of healthy human skin. The left image was obtained using a focused probe beam, and the right image using a collimated probe beam.

Each v_I-map can be quantified by the first-order statistical moments of the spatial distributions of the exponential factor (average value and variance). Figure 20 shows the histograms of v_I as a function of the stage of the disease. For early and mid-stage psoriasis, $\overline{v}_I$ and $\left\langle \Delta v_I^{\,2} \right\rangle$ are less than for normal skin due to impregnation of the diseased epidermis by tissue fluids. This causes partial suppression of the volume scattering of the probe beam in the diseased region. In the later stages of psoriasis ("desquamation" stage), the volume scattering increases because of the appearance of microspaces filled by air in the tissue volume.

Scanning speckle correlometry has also been used for the quantification of skin dryness measurements and in the morphological study of various skin diseases using specially prepared skin replicas.

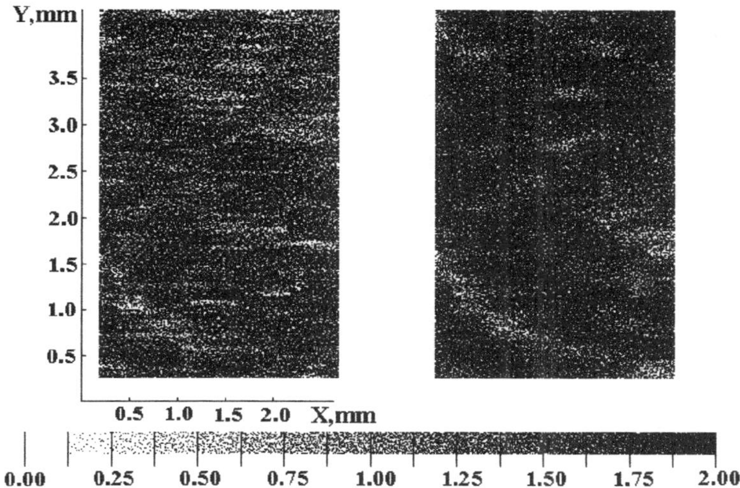

Figure 19. As in Figure 18. Later stage ("desquamation") of psoriasis.

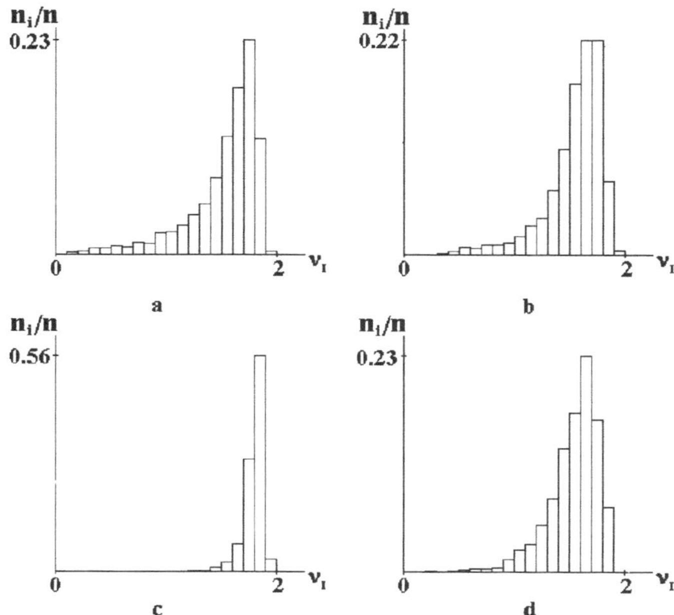

Figure 20. Histograms of V_I for the functional images of the normal (a) and diseased (b-d) *in-vitro* human skin (focused beam illumination); b – early stage of psoriasis; c – middle stage; d – later stage ("desquamation").

5.6 IMAGING TECHNIQUES BASED ON SPECKLE CONTRAST ANALYSIS

One of the possible approaches to reconstruction of 2D and 3D images of tissue structure can be based on the analysis of contrast of laser-induced speckles in the image or diffraction plane. In the case of probe laser beam scattering by system of stationary and moving scatterers as it takes place for *in-vivo* tissue with the developed microcapillary net the dynamic speckle pattern occurs in the observation plane. Being recorded with finite exposure time, the image of such pattern will be characterized by the exposure-dependent contrast and hence can be used for evaluation of the dynamic parameters of erythrocytes travelling through the capillaries. Such technique defined as Laser Activated Speckle Contrast Analysis (LASCA) has been developed by Briers *et al.* [81-85]. Basic arrangement used for monitoring and imaging of blood perfusion level for *in-vivo* tissues is shown in Figure 21.

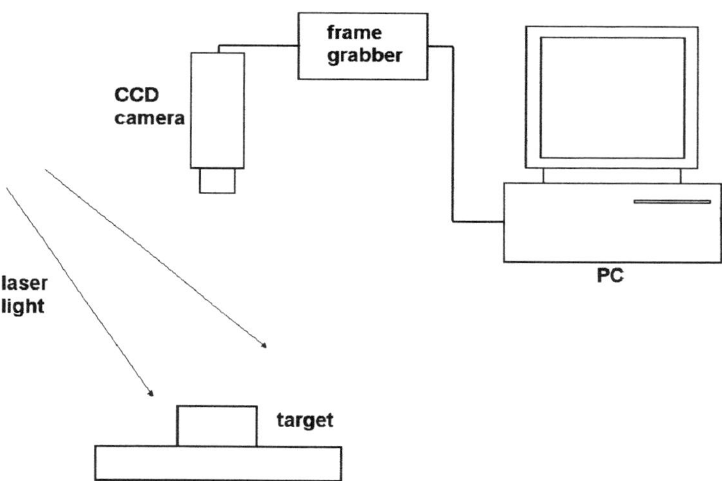

Figure 21. Basic setup for LASCA.

Object (e.g. tissue surface) is illuminated by the broad collimated beam. CCD camera acquires the speckle-modulated image of the illuminated tissue surface with given exposure time T. The modulation depth, which is evaluated as speckle contrast V, depends on T and this dependence can be expressed as [84,85]:

$$V(T) = \frac{\sigma_s}{\langle I \rangle}; \quad \sigma_s^2(T) = \frac{1}{T}\int_0^T \widetilde{g}_2(\tau)\, d\tau \qquad (18)$$

where σ_s^2 is the *spatial* variance of the intensity in the speckle pattern, T is the integration time and $\widetilde{g}_2(\tau)$ is the autocovariance of the *temporal* fluctuations in the intensity of a single speckle. Such parameters of erythrocytes as average velocity and concentration can be evaluated measuring the dependence of $V(T)$ for chosen fragment of image and using the appropriate dynamic scattering model for analytical or numerical representation of $\widetilde{g}_2(\tau)$. Two-dimensional distribution of blood microcirculation parameters, or "blood perfusion map" can be reconstructed carrying out the described above procedure for each fragment of the processed frame and does not require any mechanical scanning. In this case 2D imaging of the dynamic tissue is provided by the acquisition and processing of the sequence of frames with gradually increasing exposure time; such imaging procedure can be defined as the full-field technique.

Another approach based on contrast evaluation for the speckle patterns induced by the object illumination with the broadband light source is considered in Ref. 86. In this case, speckles appear due to random interference of a great number of partial components of optical field induced by multiple scattering of probe light into the tissue volume. Each partial component is characterized by the effective optical path length s. If the pathlength difference between two components is large compared with the coherence length l_c of the used light source, then interference modulation of their superposition will be damped; finally, the contrast value of the resulting speckle pattern will depend on the pathlength statistics, approaching to zero in case $s_{mod} \gg l_c$ and to 1 if $s_{mod} \ll l_c$ (s_{mod} is the modal value of the pathlength distribution). In such a way, distortions of the pathlength statistics caused by the presence of the absorbing or scattering macroinhomogeneity, will be manifested in variations of the contrast value if scattering object is scanned by the light source and detector.

Speckle contrast can be expressed as [86]:

$$V = \left\{ \int_0^\infty \int_0^\infty S(\lambda)S(\lambda'') \left| \left\langle exp\left[-2\pi j s\left(\frac{1}{\lambda} - \frac{1}{\lambda'} \right) \right] \right\rangle \right| d\lambda\, d\lambda' \right\}^{1/2} \Bigg/ \int_0^\infty S(\lambda)\, d\lambda,$$

where $S(\lambda)$ is the spectral density of the light source used and s is the value of the effective optical path of the individual component of the scattered field.

The expected value of the phase term, or characteristic function $\left\langle exp\left[-2\pi js\left(\frac{1}{\lambda}-\frac{1}{\lambda'}\right)\right]\right\rangle$ can be expressed by introducing the probability density function of the effective optical paths $\rho(s)$ as:

$$\left\langle exp\left[-2\pi js\left(\frac{1}{\lambda}-\frac{1}{\lambda'}\right)\right]\right\rangle = \int_0^\infty \rho(s)\, exp\left[-2\pi j\left(\frac{1}{\lambda}-\frac{1}{\lambda'}\right)\right]ds$$

The pathlength statistics described by $\rho(s)$ depends on the illumination and detection conditions as well as on the geometry of the probed scattering system. It is necessary to note that this imaging technique based on the application of the contrast of partially coherent speckles as imaging parameter, will be characterized by the less quality of the reconstructed images of absorbing or scattering inhomogeneities in comparison, e.g., with usual CW transillumination technique [86,87]. This is because of the weak dependence of contrast on the probability density function $\rho(s)$: in case of the "conventional" above described diffusing light technologies the corresponding imaging parameters are expressed as integral transforms of $\rho(s)$. On the contrary, if the contrast value of partially coherent speckles is applied as imaging parameter, it is expressed as the integral transform of self-convolution (or autocorrelation function) of $\rho(s)$ and hence the reconstructed images should be expected as more "blurred" (due to the more smoothed spatial distributions of speckle contrast in comparison with intensity distributions).

ACKNOWLEDGEMENTS

Work on this chapter was supported by the Russian Foundation for Basic Research (grants ## 00-02-81014, 01-02-17493 and 00-15-96667 "Leading Scientific Schools") and by the Civilian Research and Development Foundation (grant # REC-006).

REFERENCES

1. G. Müller, B. Chance, R. Alfano et al. (eds.), *Medical Optical Tomography: Functional Imaging and Monitoring*, SPIE Press, Bellingham, WA, **IS11**, 1993.
2. O. Minet, G. Mueller, and J. Beuthan (eds.), *Selected Papers on Optical Tomography,*

Fundamentals and Applications in Medicine, SPIE Press, Bellingham,WA, **MS 147**, 1998.

3. V.V.Tuchin (ed), *Selected Papers on Tissue Optics: Applications in Medical Diagnostics and Therapy*, SPIE Press, Bellingham, WA, **MS 102**, 1994.

4. H.Podbielska, C.K.Hitzenberger, V.V.Tuchin (eds), Special section on interferometry in biomedicine, *J. Biomed. Optics,* **3**, pp.5-79, pp. 225-266, 1998.

5. V.V.Tuchin, H.Podbielska, C.K.Hitzenberger, (eds), Special section on coherence domain optical methods in biomedical science and clinics, *J. Biomed. Optics,* **4**, pp. 94-190,1999.

6. V.V. Tuchin, *Tissue optics: light scattering methods and instruments for medical diagnosis*, SPIE Tutorial Texts in Optical Engineering, **TT38**, SPIE Press, Bellingham, WA, 2000.

7. K.M. Yoo, Feng Liu, and R.R. Alfano, "When does the diffusion approximation fail to describe photon transport in random media?", *Phys. Rev. Lett.,* **64**, pp. 2647-2650, 1990.

8. A. Ishimaru, *Wave Propagation and Scattering in Random Media*, Academic Press, New York, 1978.

9. D.S. Smith, W.J. Levy, S. Carter, M. Haida, B. Chance, in *Proc. Photon Migration and Imaging in Random Media and Tissues*, B. Chance, R. Alfano, eds., SPIE, Bellingham, WA, p.511, 1993.

10. A. Yodh and B. Chance, "Spectroscopy and imaging with diffusing light", *Physics Today,* **48**, pp. 34-40, 1995.

11. G. Jarry, S. Ghesquierre, J.M. Maarek, S. Debray, Bui-Mong-Hung, and D.Laurent, "Imaging mammalian tissues and organs using laser collimated transillumination", *J. Biomed. Eng.,* **6**, pp. 70-74, 1984.

12. P.C. Jackson, P.H. Stevens, J.H. Smith, D. Kear, H. Key, and P.N.T. Wells, "The development of a system for transillumination computed tomography", *Br. J. Radiol.,* **60**, pp. 375-380, 1987.

13. M. Tamura, Y. Nomura, and O. Hazeki, "Laser tissue spectroscopy - near infrared CT", *Rev. Laser Eng. (Japan),* **15**, pp. 74-82, 1987.

14. I. Oda, Y. Ito, H. Eda, T. Tamura, M. Takada, R. Abumi, K. Nagai, K. Nakagawa, and M.Tamura, "Non-invasive haemoglobin oxygenation monitor and computed tomography by NIR spectrophotometry", *Proc. SPIE,* **1431**, pp. 284-293, 1991.

15. S.R. Arridge, P. Van der Zee, M. Cope, and D.T. Delpy, "New results for the development of infra-red absorption imaging", *Proc. SPIE,* **1245**, pp. 91-103, 1990.

16. S.R. Arridge, P. Van der Zee, M. Cope, and D.T. Delpy, "Reconstruction methods for infrared absorption imaging", *Proc. SPIE,* **1431**, pp. 204-215, 1990.

17. J. Fishkin, E. Gratton, M.J. van de Ven, and W.W. Mantulin, "Diffusion of intensity modulated near infrared light in turbid media", *Proc. SPIE,* **1431**, pp. 122-135, 1991.

18. K.W. Berndt and J.R. Lakowich, "Detection and localization of absorbers in scattering media using frequency domain principles", *Proc. SPIE,* **1431**, pp. 149-158, 1991.

19. D.A. Boas, M.A. O'Leary, B. Chance, and A.G. Yodh, "Scattering of diffuse photon density waves by spherical inhomogeneities within turbid media: analytic solution and applications", *Proc. Natl. Acad. Sci. USA,* **91**, pp. 4887-4891, 1994.

20. M.A. O'Leary, D.A. Boas, B. Chance, and A.G. Yodh, "Refraction of diffuse photon density waves", *Phys. Rev. Lett.,* **69**, pp. 2658-2661, 1992.

21. J.M. Schmitt, A. Knuttel, and J.R. Knutson, "Interference of diffusive light waves", *J. Opt. Soc. Am. A,* **9**, pp.1832-1843, 1992.

22. B.J. Tromberg, L.O. Svaasand, T.T. Tsay, and R.C. Hackell, "Properties of photon density waves in multiply scattering media", *Appl. Opt.,* **32**, pp. 607-616, 1993.

23. W.W. Mantulin, S. Fantini, M. A. Franceschini-Fantini, S. A. Walker, J.S. Maier, and E. Gratton, "Tissue optical parameter map generated with frequency-domain spectroscopy," *Proc. SPIE,* **2396**, pp.323-330, 1995.

24. R.M. Danen, Y. Wang, X.D. Li, et al.,"Regional imager for low-resolution functional imaging of the brain with diffusing near-infrared light," *Photochem. Photobiol.*, **67**, pp. 33-40, 1998.
25. X.D. Li, T. Durduran, A.G. Yodh, et al., "Diffraction tomography for biochemical imaging with diffuse photon-density waves," *Opt. Lett.*, **22**, pp. 573–575, 1997.
26. Y. Aizu and T. Asakura, "Bio–speckle phenomena and their application to the evaluation of blood flow," *Opt. Laser Technol.*, **23**, pp. 205–219, 1991.
27. S. Fantini, M.A. Franceschini, J.B. Fishkin, et al., "Quantitative determination of the absorption and spectra of chromophores in strongly scattering media: a light–emitting-diode based technique," *Appl. Opt.*, **32**, pp. 5204–5212, 1994; M.A. Franceschini, K.T. Moesta, and S. Fantini, "Frequency-domain techniques enhance optical mammography: initial clinical results," *Proc. Natl. Acad. Sci. USA*, **94**, pp. 6468-6473, 1997.
28. J.B. Fishkin, O. Coquoz, E.R. Anderson, et al., "Frequency–domain photon migration measurements of normal and malignant tissue optical properties in a human subject," *Appl. Opt.*, **36**, pp. 10–20, 1997.
29. B. Tromberg, O. Coquoz, J.B. Fishkin, et al., "Non–invasive measurements of breast tissue optical properties using frequency–domain photon migration," *Phil. Trans. R. Soc. Lond. B.*, **352**, pp. 661–668, 1997.
30. A. Knuttel, J.M. Schmitt, and J.R. Knutson, "Spatial localization of absorbing ·bodies by interfering diffusive photon–density waves," *Appl. Opt.*, **32**, pp. 381–389, 1993.
31. B. Chance, M. Cope, E. Gratton, N.Ramanujam, and B.Tromberg, "Phase measurement of light absorption and scatter in human tissue," *Rev. Sci. Instrum.*, **69**, pp. 3457-3481, 1998.
32. B. Chance, K. Kang, L. He, H. Liu, and S. Zhou, "Precision localization of hidden absorbers in body tissues with phased-array optical systems," *Rev. Sci, Instrum.*, **67**, pp. 4324-4332, 1996.
33. M. G. Erickson, J. S. Reynolds, and K. J. Webb, "Comparison of sensitivity for single-source and dual-interfering-source configurations in optical diffusion imaging," *J. Opt. Soc. Am. A*, **14**, pp.3083-3092, 1997.
34. B. Chance, E. Anday, S. Nioka, et al., "A novel method for fast imaging of brain function, non-invasively, with light," *Optics Express*, **2**, pp. 411-423, 1998.
35. J.G. Fujimoto and M.S. Patterson (Eds.), *Advances in Optical Imaging and Photon Migration*, OSA TOPS, **21**, 1998.
36. B.Chance, E.Anday, E.Conant, S.Nioka,S.Zhou, and H.Long, "Rapid and sensitive optical imaging of tissue functional activity, and breast," *OSA TOPS*, **21**, pp. 218-225, 1998.
37. D.J. Papaioannou, G.W. Hooft, S.B. Colak, and J.T. Oostveen, "Detection limit in localizing objects hidden in a turbid medium using an optically scanned phased array," *J.Biomed. Opt.*, **1**, pp. 305–310, 1996.
38. E.B. de Haller, "Time-resolved transillumination and optical tomography," *J.Biomed. Opt.*, **1**, pp. 7–17, 1996.
39. G. Maret and P.E. Wolf, "Multiple light scattering from disordered media. The effect of Brownian motion of scatterers", *Z. Phys. B*, **65**, pp. 409-413, 1987.
40. D.A.Boas and A.G. Yodh, "Spatially varying dynamical properties of turbid media probed with diffusing temporal light correlations", *J. Opt. Soc. Am. A*, **14**, pp. 192-215, 1997.
41. A.G. Yodh, N. Georgiades, and D.J. Pine, "Diffusing-wave interferometry", *Opt. Communications*, **83**, pp. 56-59, 1991.
42. M. Born and E. Wolf, *Principles of Optics*, Pergamon Press, London, 1964.
43. B.J. Ackerson, R.L. Dougherty, N.M. Reguigui, and U. Nobbman, "Correlation transfer: application of radiative transfer solution methods to photon correlation problems", *J. Thermophys. And Heat Trans.*, **6**, pp. 577-588, 1992.
44. D.A. Boas, L.E. Campbell, and A.G. Yodh, "Scattering and imaging with diffusing temporal field correlations", *Phys. Rev. Lett.*, **75**, pp. 1855-1858, 1995.
45. T. Wilson, ed. *Confocal microscopy*, Academic Press, San Diego, CA, 1990.

46. R.H. Webb, "Confocal optical microscopy", *Rep. Prog. Phys.*, **59**, pp. 427-471, 1996.
47. B.R. Masters (ed), *Selected Papers on Confocal Microscopy*, **MS131**, SPIE Press, Bellingham, WA, 1996.
48. M. Bohnke and B.R. Masters, "Confocal Microscopy of the Cornea," *Prog. Retinal Eye Res.*, **18**, pp. 553-628, 1999.
49. M. Rajadhyaksha and J.M. Zavislan, "Confocal laser microscope images tissue *in vivo*", *Laser Focus World*, Febriary, 1997.
50. M. Rajadhyaksha, R. Rox Anderson, and R.H. Webb, "Video-rate confocal scanning laser microscope for imaging human tissues *in vivo*", *Appl. Opt.*, **38**, pp. 2105-2115, 1999.
51. C.J.J. Sheppard and T. Wilson, "Depth of field in the scanning microscope", *Opt. Lett.*, **3**, pp. 115-117, 1978.
52. T. Wilson and A.R. Carlini, "Three-dimensional imaging in confocal imaging systems with finite sized detectors", *J. Microsc.*, **149**, pp. 51-66, 1988.
53. T. Wilson and A.R. Carlini, "Size of the detector in confocal imaging systems", *Opt. Lett.*, **12**, pp. 227-229, 1987.
54. D.R. Sandison, D.W. Piston, R.M. Williams, and W.W. Webb, "Quantitative comparison of background rejection, signal-to-noise ratio, and resolution in confocal and full-field scanning microscopes," *Appl. Opt.*, **34**, pp. 3576-3588, 1995.
55. M. Rajadhyaksha and J.M. Zavislan, "Confocal reflectance microscopy of unstained tissue *in vivo*", *Retinoids*, **14**, pp. 26-30, 1998.
56. A.F. Fercher, "Optical coherence tomography," *J. Biomed. Opt.*, **1**, pp. 157–173, 1996.
57. D. Huang, E.A. Swanson, C.P. Lin, J.S. Schuman, W.G. Stinson, W. Chang, M.R. Hee, T. Flotte, K. Gregory, C.A. Puliafito, J.G. Fujimoto, "Optical coherence tomography," *Science*, **254**, pp. 1178-1181, 1991.
58. V.V.Tuchin and J.Izatt (Eds), Coherence domain optical methods in biomedical science and clinical applications II, *Proc. SPIE*, **3251**, 1998.
59. V.V.Tuchin and J.Izatt (Eds), Coherence domain optical methods in biomedical science and clinical applications III, *Proc. SPIE*, **3598**, 1999.
60. V.V.Tuchin, J.Izatt, and J. Fujimoto (Eds), Coherence domain optical methods in biomedical science and clinical applications IV, *Proc. SPIE*, **3915**, 2000.
61. J.M. Herrmann, C. Pitris, B. E. Bouma, S.A. Boppart, C.A. Jesser, D.L. Stamper, J.G. Fujimoto, and M.E. Brezinski, "High resolution imaging of normal and osteoarthritic cartilage with optical coherence tomography", *The Journal of Rheumatology*, **26**, pp. 627-635, 1999.
62. B.E. Bouma, G.J. Tearney, S.A. Boppart, M.R. Hee, M.E. Brezinski, and J.G. Fujimoto, "High resolution optical coherence tomographic imaging using a modelocked Ti:Al$_2$O$_3$ laser", *Opt. Lett.*, **20**, pp. 1486-1488, 1995.
63. S.A. Boppart, B.E. Bouma, M.E. Brezinski, G.J. Tearney, and J.G. Fujimoto, "Imaging developing neural morphology using optical coherence tomography", *Journal of Neuroscience Methods*, **70**, pp. 65-72, 1996.
64. H.-W. Wang, A.M. Rollins, and J.A. Izatt, "High speed, full field optical coherence tomography", *Proc. SPIE*, **3598**, pp. 204 – 212, 1999.
65. G.J. Tearney, M.E. Brezinski, B.E. Bouma, S.A.Boppart, C. Pitris, J.F.Southern, and J.G. Fujimoto, "In vivo endoscopic optical biopsy with optical coherence tomography", *Science*, **276**, pp. 2037-2039,1997;G.J.Tearney, S.A.Boppart, B.E.Bouma, M.E. Brezinski, N.J.Weissman,J.F.Southern, and J.G.Fujimoto,"Scanningsingle-mode fiber optic catheter-endoscope for optical coherence tomography", *Opt. Lett.*, **21**, pp. 543-545, 1996.
66. S.A. Boppart, B.E. Bouma, C. Pitris, G.J. Tearney, and J.G. Fujimoto, "Forward-imaging instruments for optical coherence tomography", *Opt. Lett.*, **22**, pp. 1618-1620, 1997.
67. G.J. Tearney, M.E. Brezinski, J.F. Southern, B.E. Bouma, S.A. Boppart, and J.G. Fujimoto, "Optical biopsy in human gastrointestinal tissue using optical coherence tomography", *The American Journal of Gastroenterology*, **92**, pp. 1800-1804, 1997.

68. J.M. Herrmann, M.E. Brezinski, B.E. Bouma, S.A. Boppart, C. Pitris, J.F. Southern, and J.G. Fujimoto, "Two- and three-dimensional high-resolution imaging of the human oviduct with optical coherence tomography", *Fertility and Sterility*, **70**, pp. 155-158, 1998.

69. W. Drexler, U. Morgner, F.X. Kartner, C. Pitris, S.A. Boppart, X.D. Li, E.P. Ippen, and J.G. Fujimoto, "*In vivo* ultrahigh resolution optical coherence tomography", *Opt. Lett.*, **24**, pp. 1221-1223, 1999.

70. S.A. Boppart, J. Herrmann, C. Pitris, D.L. Stamper, M. E. Brezinski, and J. G. Fujimoto, "High-resolution optical coherence tomography-guided laser ablation of surgical tissue", *Journal of Surgical Research*, **82**, pp. 275-284, 1999.

71. G. Hausler, J.M. Herrmann, R. Kummer, and M.W. Lindner, "Observation of light propagation in volume scatterers with 10^{11}-fold slow motion", *Opt. Lett.*, **21**, pp. 1087-1089, 1996.

72. A. Eigensee, G. Hausler, J.M. Herrmann, M.W. Lindner, "A new method of short-coherence interferometry in human skin (*in vivo*) and in solid volume scatterers", *Proc. SPIE*, **2925**, pp. 169-178, 1996.

73. M. Brezinski, K. Saunders, C. Jesser, X. Li, and J. Fujimoto, "Index matching to improve optical coherence tomography imaging through blood", *Circulation*, **103**, pp.1999-2003, 2001.

74. V.V. Tuchin, X. Xu, R.K. Wang, "Sedimentation of immersed blood studied by OCT", *Proc. SPIE*, **4241**, pp. 357-369, 2001.

75. R.K. Wang, X. Xu, V.V. Tuchin, J.B. Elder, "Concurrent enhancement of imaging depth and contrast for optical coherence tomography by hyperosmotic agents", *J. Opt. Soc. Am. B*, **18**, pp. 948-953, 2001.

76. D.A. Zimnyakov, V.V. Tuchin, A.A. Mishin "Spatial speckle correlometry in applications to tissue structure monitoring", *Appl. Opt.*, **36**, pp. 5594-5607, 1997.

77. S.M. Rhytov, U.A. Kravtsov, V.I. Tatarsky, *Introduction to Statistical Radiophysics, P.2. Pandom Fields*, Nauka Publishers, Moscow, 1978.

78. J. Feder, *Fractals*, Plenum Press, New York, 1988.

79. D.A. Zimnyakov, V.V. Tuchin, and S.R. Utts, "A study of statistical properties of partially developed speckle fields as applied to the diagnostics of structural changes in human skin", *Opt. Spectrosc.*, **76**, pp. 838-844, 1994.

80. D.A. Zimnyakov, I.L. Maksimova, and V.V. Tuchin, "Controlling optical properties of biological tissues: II. Coherent optical methods for studying the tissue structure", *Opt. Spectrosc.*, **88**, pp. 936-943, 2000.

81. A.F. Fercher and J.D. Briers, "Flow visualization by means of single-exposure speckle photography", *Opt. Commun.*, **37**, pp. 326-329, 1981.

82. J.D. Briers and A.F. Fercher, "A laser speckle technique for the visualization of retinal blood flow", *Proc. SPIE*, **369**, pp. 22-28, 1982.

83. J.D. Briers and S. Webster, "Quasi-real time digital version of single-exposure speckle photography for full-field monitoring of velocity or flow fields", *Opt. Commun.*, **116**, pp. 36-42, 1995.

84. J.D. Briers and S. Webster, "Laser speckle contrast analysis (LASCA): a non-scanning, full-field technique for monitoring capillary blood flow", *J Biomed Opt.*, **1**, pp.174-179, 1996.

85. J.D. Briers, G. Richards and X.W. He, "Capillary blood flow monitoring using laser speckle contrast analysis (LASCA)", *J Biomed Opt.*, **4**, pp. 164-175, 1999.

86. C.A. Thompson, K.J. Webb, and A.M. Weiner, "Imaging in scattering media by use of laser speckle", *J. Opt. Soc. Am. A*, **14**, p.2269-2277, 1997.

87. L.V. Kuznetsova, D.A. Zimnyakov, "Multiple-beam interferometry of turbid media with quasi-monochromatic light", *Proc. SPIE*, **4001**, pp. 217-223, 2000.

Chapter 6

LASERS IN UROLOGY

S.K. Sharma[1] and A.K. Hemal[2]
[1]Post Graduate Institute of Medical Education and Research, Chandigarh, INDIA
[2]All India Institute of Medical Sciences, New Delhi, INDIA

6.1 INTRODUCTION

Although lasers have been widely used in ophthalmology, the field of urology was not left behind in this regard. The first laser used in the field of urology was ruby laser. Since, then various lasers have been used for variety of urological conditions, i.e., prostate, stone disease, strictures, bladder hemangioma and transitional cell carcinoma of lower and upper urinary tract. Photodynamic therapy tissue welding are other uses of laser therapy. Recent technological advancement uses the holmium laser, a multi-functional tool in urology that can be used for intracorporeal lithotripsy, strictures, excision and ablation of urothelial tumours, condylomata and prostate. Use of lasers in treatment of urological disease is discussed in this chapter.

6.2 LASERS IN BENIGN PROSTATIC HYPERPLASIA

Benign prostatic hyperplasia (BPH) is an almost inevitable part of the aging process in men. Symptoms of BPH include slowing and interruption of the urinary stream, incomplete bladder emptying, hesitancy, post-micturition dribbling, frequency and nocturia. These symptoms may not cause an individual any inconvenience, but can lead to considerable interference to quality of life. In more severe cases, and especially if complications such as urinary retention occur, surgical relief of the obstruction is indicated. Traditionally, this relief has been provided by transurethral resection of the prostate (TURP). However, in the past decade, attempts to find alternative treatments to TURP have been stimulated by the desire to avoid the morbidity of TURP. The use of laser energy in this context has been evolving rapidly.

The basic advantage of laser prostatectomy over TURP is safety; none of the serious complications of TURP, i.e., bleeding and transurethral resection syndrome have been reported with laser prostatectomy. Consequently, patients on anticoagulants or with bleeding diatheses, those refusing to undergo transfusion and patients with congestive heart failure are good candidates for a laser procedure.

6.2.1 Laser Prostatectomy

In the early 1980's, the first verifiable attempts were made to harness the energy of the laser beam for transurethral treatment of BPH. McPhee [1] coupled a standard electroresectoscope with a Nd:YAG laser fiber in 1981, using the wire loop electrode to resect tissue and the free beam laser to coagulate and provide hemostasis. This mixed technique proved cumbersome and impractical in actual use for transurethral resection of the prostate. Other investigators attempted to ablate prostate tissue in canine models using simple end-firing fibres emitting a focused, high energy density Nd:YAG laser beam at very high power settings (up to 100 watts) [2]. In 1985, Shanberg *et al.* [3] reported using a similar approach clinically with the Nd:YAG laser to perform TUIP in 10 men with small obstructive prostate, meeting with limited success. By 1991, Smith [4], a pioneering investigator in the field, concluded in a review of lasers for treatment of BPH that there seemed little promise for a free beam laser in the treatment of BPH.

In the late 1980's, the first delivery system purposely designed for the performance of free beam laser prostatectomy was developed [5]. This transurethral ultrasound-guided laser-induced prostatectomy (TULIP ^{TM}, Intra-Sonix, Inc.) device was a uniquely engineered apparatus: a 22 French size rigid urethral probe which combined an intraurethral ultrasound transducer to image the prostate and guide treatment; a Nd:YAG delivery fiber with a distal prism mechanism to deflect the beam laterally into the prostate; and an intraprostatic balloon which, when inflated, created a constant standoff distance between laser and prostatic urethral surface, as well as compressing the periurethral prostate to improve depth of laser penetration into the gland. Clinical outcomes reported with the TULIP system were generally good, perhaps less efficacious than TURP [6]. However, the morbidity associated with this prototypical instrument was greater than seen with subsequent free beam laser approaches [6]. The lack of direct visual control of the TULIP operation with total reliance on intraurethral ultrasound imaging made median lobe treatment difficult. This perhaps explains the occurrence of postoperative stress incontinence in 2 of 89 patients treated with TULIP in the series reported by Schulze *et al.* [6]. Table 1 below exhibits the type of lasers used in BPH.

Table 1. Different types of lasers in use for benign prostatic hyperplasia .

Types	<ul><li>Nd:YAG</li><li>Ho:YAG</li><li>KTP:YAG</li><li>Semiconductor diode</li></ul>
Mechanism	**Coagulation** Occurs at 100^0C 40-70W Protein denatured with consequent necrosis and sloughing • **Vaporization** Occurs at 300^0C Over 70W Tissue water vaporizes with instantaneous debulking of area.

6.2.2 Nd:YAG Laser Prostatectomy

Nd:YAG wavelength offers several specific benefits for transurethral prostatectomy in addition to its widespread availability. It is transmitted by means of flexible delivery fibers to facilitate endoscopic use. Its minimal absorption by water allows use in a fluid medium. It penetrates deeply into tissue and produces superb coagulation and hemostasis.   Johnson *et al.* [7] first reported use of a flexible, side-firing Nd:YAG laser delivery fiber which could be positioned in the prostatic urethra under direct vision through a standard cystoscope. Although the new side-firing fibers facilitate transurethral treatment of laterally placed BPH tissue, the key to the final realization of successful prostatectomy using the free beam Nd:YAG laser was an artifact produced by lateral deflection of the laser beam by these devices; the creation of considerable beam divergence and thus a relatively low energy density beam. Combined with long exposure times, this allows transmission of very large quantities of laser energy into the prostate, in turn converted to heat energy conducted through a large volume of prostate tissue. Thus, maximizing the depth and volume of tissue coagulation, for the first time an adequate extent and efficiency in Nd:YAG laser destruction of BPH tissue by means of coagulation necrosis was achieved [8,9]

Nd:YAG laser prostatectomy is typically performed under regional or general anesthesia. Though, local prostatic block (Periprostatic infiltration with bupivacaine and lidocaine) combined with intravenous sedation has also been reported [10]. A relatively small caliber cystoscope (22 French size or less)will accommodate almost all side firing fibers used for Nd:YAG laser prostatectomy. Because Nd:YAG laser coagulation seals blood vessels, preventing both bleeding and intraoperative fluid absorption, sterile water irrigation is commonly used. Room temperature, rather than warm irrigation, is preferred to help dissipate the significant heat generated at and near the reflecting surfaces of side-firing fibers and prevent premature deterioration of the fiber tip or charring of tissue surfaces, either of which will limit laser energy transmission and efficacy of the operation [11].

In the standard spot coagulation technique used for Nd:YAG prostatectomy, side-firing delivery fiber is held in close apposition without touching obstructing BPH tissue and Nd:YAG laser energy applied continuously for a minimum of 60 to 90 seconds. Power settings between 40 and 60 watts are used, dependent upon the delivery fiber and the degree of divergence of its emitted laser beam [9-12]. Optimal results and maximal tissue coagulation have been obtained with widely divergent laser beams of 30° or more [12]. With each spot laser application, an ellipsoidal volume of prostate tissue is coagulated. Maximal depths of prostatic coagulation of approximately 1.5 cm have been measured under clinical conditions in human histopathologic studies, with an average lateral radius of tissue effect over 1 cm (corresponding to a total lesion width or diameter over 2 cm), producing a total ellipsoidal volume of coagulation necrosis of approximately 4 cc for each spot application. Multiple such spot applications are repeated no more than 2 cm apart and preferably with some overlap, to all obstructing lateral and median lobe tissue along the prostatic urethra. It has been estimated that at least 1000, and preferably 1500 joules Nd:YAG laser energy per gram of BPH should be administered to assure complete coagulation of all obstructing tissue and good voiding outcomes [12-13]. It is this technique which is often referred to as visual laser ablation of the prostate (VLAP) in the literature.

As an alternative to the Nd:YAG spot coagulation technique, a high power longitudinal dragging technique has also been described [14].This technique is better suited to those side-firing fibers which emit laser beams with relatively narrow angles of divergence (approximately 15°) and thus higher energy density, and those fibers with no metallic components [12]. Very high Nd:YAG laser power settings between 60 and 80 watts or more are used. The side firing fiber is held in close apposition or even touching the prostate, although the later technique will cause premature deterioration of the fiber. Beginning at the bladder neck, the laser is activated and the side-firing fiber slowly withdrawn along the length of the prostatic urethra to the verumontanum. Very slow drag rates, only 1cm movement every 20 to 30 second, are recommended to maximize tissue destruction [14]. This is repeated circumferentially along the prostatic urethra until all obstructing lateral and median lobe tissue has been treated. This technique produces extensive coagulation necrosis of periurethral prostate tissue, qualitatively identical to that observed during the spot coagulation or VLAP technique described above, while the total depth of tissue coagulation may be quantitatively somewhat less using this slow drag approach.

Following Nd:YAG laser prostatectomy, there is minimal acute tissue loss due to vaporization, and the extensive coagulation necrosis of BPH tissue causes prostatic swelling which may actually acutely worsen voiding. Although this edema subsides within days, clinically significant voiding improvement is typically not recognized for at least 3 to 4 weeks postoperatively, and maximal voiding outcomes are usually not achieved until 3 to 4 months postoperatively. This corresponds with the time course for the treated BPH tissue, which undergoes coagulation necrosis to dissolve and slough in the urinary stream [7]. Eventually, a significant prostatic tissue defect is realized. Mean prostatic volume losses of 28%, 34% and 37% , respectively, have been documented by transrectal ultrasound following Nd:YAG laser prostatectomy in 3 published reports [14-16]. Although many patients will tolerate early catheter removal even only 1 to 3 days following Nd:YAG laser prostatectomy, most of these men will experience significant voiding symptoms early in the postoperative period. Therefore, most experienced practitioner will leave a small, 16 French size, urethral catheter in place for 5 to 7 days after Nd:YAG laser prostatectomy. This operation is typically performed on an outpatient or same day surgery basis, and patients discharged after surgery with the catheter to leg bag drainage, to be removed in the office setting the following week. However, in our country patient needed hospita-lization for 2-3 days.

The acute operative morbidity of Nd:YAG laser prostatectomy is negligible and much less than encountered with electrocautery resection techniques. TUR-syndrome has never been reported, and significant bleeding or transfusion have been distinctly rare. This may be explained by the physical mechanism of interaction of the Nd:YAG laser with prostate tissue leading to, coagulation and sealing of blood vessels through several mm depth. In 2 large, multi-institution studies reported from the United States and United Kingdom respectively, morbidity of Nd:YAG lasers prostatectomy was compared to standard TURP in randomized prospective trials [17,18]. TURP was associated with serious treatment related complications in more than one third of cases 35.6% and 33.3% in the United States and United Kingdom respectively during one year postoperative follow up, including blood transfusion required in 14 of 134 total men undergoing TURP in the 2 series. By contrast, Nd:YAG laser prostatectomy was associated with serious treatment related complications in only 10.% and 6.6% of men, respectively, in the United States and United Kingdom studies with no transfusion requirement in 132 laser cases. In an Australian single Institution trial, Costello *et al.* [19] randomized 71 men in a prospective comparision of Nd:YAG laser prostatectomy and TURP. Serious treatment-related complications occurred in 35.1% (followed up to 3 years after TURP) with blood transfusions required in 3 of 37 men. For 3 years postoperative follow up, serious treatment-related complications occurred in only 11.8% of laser treated men, with no blood transfusions requirement. These findings are remarkably identical to those in the USand UK multi-center reports. In the most detailed analysis of acute and long term complications for Nd:YAG laser prostatectomy, others have documented a 14.3% total complications in 230 men with minimum post operative follow up of 12 months and a median follow up of 35 months [12,13]. No significant bleeding, transfusion requirement, TUR-syndrome, or prostatic perforation were observed. Postoperative prostatitis occurred in 2.6% of men. The syndrome, in which the laser-coagulated, necrotic prostate tissue mass becomes infected, causes significant dysuric symptoms and requires multiple weeks of oral antibiotics therapies. Perhaps greater care to assure preoperative sterile urine and adequate preoperative antiboitics prophylaxis is required for Nd:YAG laser prostatectomy than with electrocautery resection in order to avoid this prostatitis syndrome.

It is also suggested that chronic or recurrent bacterial prostatitis represents a contra-indication for Nd:YAG laser prostatectomy [13]. Stress related urinary incontinence was not observed in these 230 cases and has been a very rare complication in the worldwide experience with Nd:YAG laser prostatectomy. Urethral strictures and bladder neck contracture occurred in 1.7% and 4.3% of patients respectively, followed over a long period. The incidence of urethral stricture, in particular, is much less than observed in long-term patients undergoing TURP, probably due to shorter operative times and use of smaller caliber endoscopes with less intraoperative manipulation required in Nd:YAG laser.

Impotence has been documented only rarely following Nd:YAG laser prostatectomy in multiple published series. Although many initial papers reported very low rates of retrograde ejaculation following Nd:YAG laser prostatectomy, in more recent series using current aggressive treatements retrograde ejaculation has occurred in as many as 36% to 47% of men [12-19].

One of the most extensively studied of the new alternative surgical therapies for BPH, Nd:YAG laser prostatectomy offers comparable efficacy with greatly reduced complication rates as compared to standard TURP. The major drawback of this operative approach is the prolonged postoperative catheterization requirement compared to TURP and delayed onset of voiding improvement through several weeks after surgery. Time required for laser prostatectomy is longer than TUR(P) for similar size of prostate. We have used Nd:YAG laser prostatectomy in our departments, however due to procedural intricacies, delayed results, associated problems and outcome is inferior to TUR (P). It was not found very attractive and is used infrequently now with its role limited to patients with bleeding diathesis or in a patient on pacemaker. We have also noticed post operative stricture, bladder neck obstruction and the need for TUR (P) in some of the cases.

6.2.3 KTP Laser Prostatectomy

Compared to the Nd:YAG laser, the KTP laser wavelength produces very similar effects in non-pigmented tissues such as the prostate. It is an excellent tissue coagulator with perhaps somewhat greater tissue vaporization than produced with the Nd:YAG laser due to the vascularity and hemoglobin content of prostate tissue. The KTP wavelength is delivered via the same flexible laser fibres as the Nd: YAG wavelength and is readily transmitted through fluid irrigation during endoscopic surgery, like the Nd:YAG laser. The KTP laser has largely been used in an adjunctive role following Nd:YAG laser coagulation of the prostate, most often to incise the bladder neck using a delivery system with narrow beam divergence and high energy density. The KTP laser is commonly packaged with the Nd:YAG laser as a dual wavelength, single laser source, facilitating these combined maneuvers.

In one of the few and certainly the best study wherein solely the KTP wavelength was utilized to perform laser prostatectomy, Shingleton *et al.* [20] entered 70 men with symptomatic BPH into a randomized prospective trial comparing KTP laser prostatectomy with TURP with reasonable benefits.

6.2.4 Interstitial Laser Coagulation of the Prostate

The technique of interstitial laser coagulation (ILC) of the prostate was developed to avoid the sloughing of necrotic material and prolonged irritation. The principle of the technique is to insert a laser fiber with a diffuser tip into the prostatic adenoma either transurethrally under trans-rectal ultrasound guidance. Energy is then delivered to cause coagulative necrosis resulting in cavities up to a 2 cm diameter. This technique was first described by Muschter and Hofstetter [21] who have continued to modify and refine the equipment.

There are various systems for performing ILC. One such system employs a diode laser emitting a wavelength of 830 nm. The fibers end in a diffuser tip made of Teflon, 10mm long and 1.2mm in diameter. The laser generator is controlled by software which lowers the power output as treatment progresses to maintain temperature at the diffuser tip at 100 ° C. Results of trials using ILC have shown improvements in symptom scores and flowrates similar to other forms of laser treatment.

As would be expected, since no tissue is removed during the ILC, relief of obstruction is delayed until resorption of necrotic prostate has occurred. However, the incidence of irritative side effects is much lower than with VLAP. Re-operation rates even with short-term follow up were high (9.6%) [22] and long-term data is clearly awaited.

6.2.5 Ho:YAG Laser Prostatectomy

The Ho:YAG laser wavelength is highly absorbed by tissue water, causing rapid heating with vaporization or incision of irradiated tissues. The Ho:YAG laser can be transmitted through low-water-content flexible delivery fibers which will also transmit the Nd:YAG wavelength. The Ho:YAG wavelength can be effectively transmitted through 1 to 2 mm of liquid medium, and so can be used endoscopically with fluid irrigation if the delivery fiber is held near or against tissues to be treated. The tissue incising and vaporizing ability of the Ho:YAG laser had prompted studies of its potential use to treat bladder outlet obstruction [21,22].

Initial human clinical trials of Ho:YAG laser prostatectomy beginning in Palo Alto in 1994 [21], established its safety in clinical practice and showed the inefficiency of trying vaporize large volumes of BPH with existing delivery systems, which led to the development of a much more practical and efficient technique for laser resection of the prostate (HoLRP) [23].

HoLRP is performed under regional or general anesthesia. Low-water-content Ho:YAG laser transmission fibers are now available in both simple end-firing and lateral firing designs, although the later confer little or no benefit using the HoL for prostatectomy, where efficiency is maximized with the high energy density beam emitted by end-firing fibers. A standard cystoscope and normal saline irrigation are utilized. Using the pulsed Ho:YAG laser at very high energies and pulse rates, cystoscopes which offer some means of fiber fixation, to minimize fiber vibration, facilitate HoLRP.

There are several working bridges, sheaths with directed instrument channels, and so-called "laser resectoscopes," which suit the purpose. Alternatively, the laser fiber can be passed through a 6 French size end hole ureter catheter to provide greater rigidity and passed through a standard cystoscope sheath and working bridge. The Ho:YAG laser is set to deliver at least 2 to 2.5 joules per laser pulse, at pulse rates between 25 and 40 per second (these settings translate to laser power outputs between 50 and 80 watts, and essentially represent maximum settings of currently available

Ho: YAG laser sources) and recently up to 100 watts settings source is also available [21-24].

To perform HoLRP, deep incisions or "grooves" are created through the bladder neck at 5 and 7 O'clock and continued to the level of the verumontanum on either side of the median lobe, thereafter undermining and "resecting" the median lobe tissue.

The lateral lobes are "resected" in a similar fashion, beginning with incisions or "grooves" from the bladder neck to the verumontanum anteriorly (1 and 11 O'clock), and then directed upwards from posteriorly. These grooves are connected at the apex of each lateral lobe at the level of the verumontanum, and the lateral lobe BPH tissue undermined and freed at the level of the prostatic surgical capsule. During resection, the Ho:YAG laser seals tissue planes, providing coagulation for 2 to 3 mm depth beyond the level of vaporization, and thus superior hemostasis compared to electrocautery techniques. Additional spot coagulation can be achieved by increasing the standoff distance between tissue and laser fiber, defocusing the Ho:YAG beam to increase coagulation properties [21-24].

HoLRP appears to combine the minimal morbidity of Nd:YAG laser prostatectomy and the immediate voiding-outcomes associated with standard TURP. Longer follow-up and wider trial of this technique is obviously warranted [25,26], and recent series are coming up with an excellent outcome [27]. HoLRP for small and moderate size, and fibrous prostates are shown in Figures 1 to 3 respectively. Some of the techniques of Ho:YAG laser prostatectomy are mentioned in Table 2

We have limited experience at the moment with HoLRP. However, on personal communications with other colleagues and combining all our experience, the technique appears to be promising, effective and efficient. The complications we have noticed are early and delayed. Early complications included retention of urine (6%), UTI (8%), whereas in delayed group, stricture (5%), and need for TUR(P) in 4%. The enucleation of the prostate using a Holmium in large glands comprising of lateral and median lobes, are first enucleated then morcellated or divided in small pieces with resectoscope and evacuated. The use of mercellation requires an off angle lens to fit the continuous resectoscope or large cystoscope which is not usually available, and often a nephroscope is used.

In a recently published paper by Gilling *et al.* [27], Ho laser enucleation of the prostate (HoLEP) was compared with TURP for large prostate (40-200 gms). 50 patients were enrolled and divided in two groups comprising 25 in each. The rate of tissue removal was 0.7g/min operating room time for each of the two procedures. There was one blood transfusion in TURP group. Five patients in the TURP group required recatheterization compared with 3 in HoLEP group. Post op AUA scores, Qmax values and quality of life scores were similar at 1 and 3 months postoperatively. Thus, concluding that HoLEP plus transurethral tissue morcellation is a safe, efficacious procedure with a shorter catheter time and hospital stay than TURP in larger prostate glands [27]. In another series cost effectiveness and complications of HoLEP were evaluated and it was observed that it saves in hospital costs because of reduced length of stay with acceptable early and late complications [28].

6.3 LASER TREATMENT OF BLADDER AND URETHRAL TUMORS

6.3.1 Bladder Tumor

One of the first and most common applications for laser energy in genitourinary surgery has been in the treatment of tumors of the lower urinary

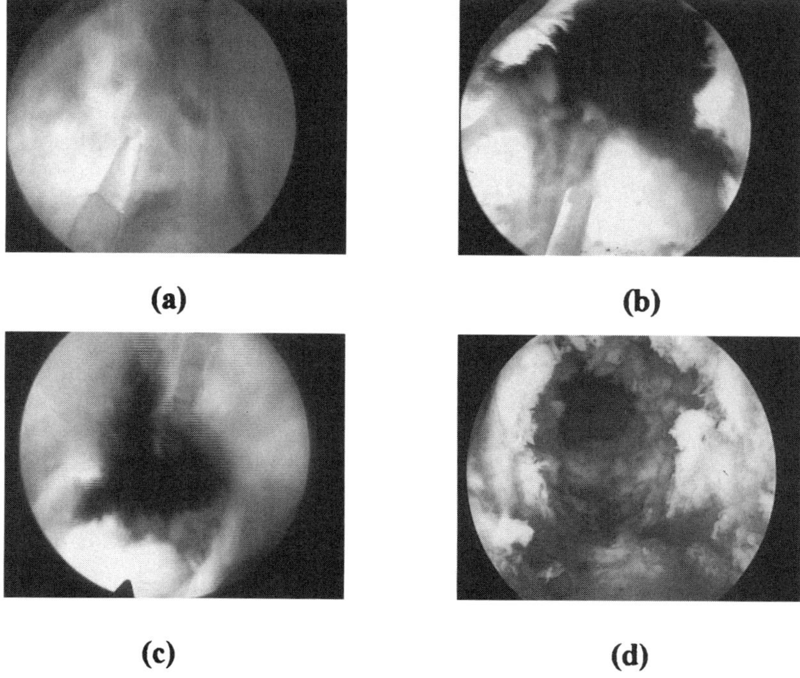

(a) (b)

(c) (d)

Figure 1. Holmium laser resection for small prostate. (a) Endoscopic view demonstrating enlargement of prostate keeping endoscope at the level of Verumontanum, also seen laser fiber in view, (b) Showing resection of prostate with linear incision using laser fiber, (c) Demonstration of cut at 12 O'clock position, (d) Endoscopic view of the prostate after HoLRP (near completion).

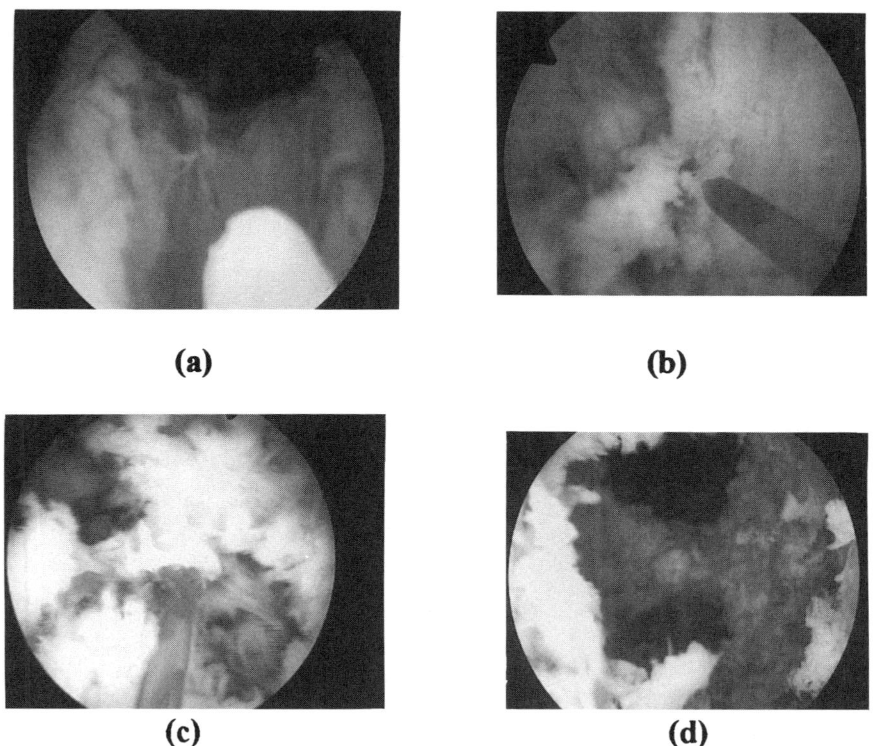

Figure 2. Holmium laser resection for fibrous prostate. (a) Demonstrating laser incision at 6 O'clock position, (b) Demonstration of division of prostate chip with laser fiber, (c) Demonstration of deeper resection showing prostatic tones in view, (d) Demonstrating prostatic fossa and sub-trigo resection of the prostate: a minor complication.

tract. Small tumors of the bladder are most commonly encountered and most amenable to laser ablation [29]. A free beam has been used extensively for this indication. With the Nd:YAG wavelength, the endpoint of treatment is when the tumor and surrounding mucosa assume a pale, gray white discoloration, often with some gross shrinkage but seldom with complete ablation of the exophytic tumor mass occurs. The necrotic, coagulated bladder tumor later sloughs in the urinary stream. Since Nd:YAG light only reliably penetrates with complete tumor necrosis over a depth of a few millimeters, large tumors are not optimally treated with laser, although combination therapies of electrocautery resection for tumor debulking, followed by Nd:YAG laser irradiation to treat the tumor base and achieve hemostasis, have been described. Recently, Johnson [30] has reported using the Ho:YAG wavelength to successfully vaporize bladder tumors, leaving a flush base. We have treated small bladder tumor and bladder recurrence with free beam laser and in cases of large tumors, base was fulgurated after resection of tumor with electrocautery. In primary bladder tumors, the lack of tumor histology with

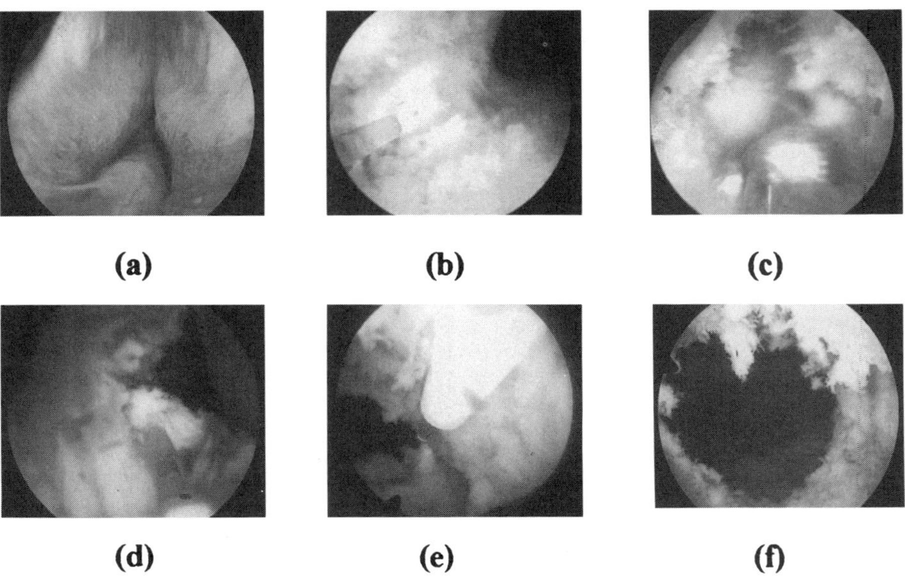

Figure 3. Holmium laser resection of moderate size prostate with trilobar enlargement. (a) Endoscopic view of prostate, (b) Initial incision at 7 O'clock position, (c) Demonstrating resected median lobe with its left over part near apex (verumontanum), (d) Final resection of residual median lobe, (e) Resection of residual prostate tissue, (f) Final view after holmium laser prostectomy.

laser ablation, compared to standard resection techniques, eliminates the ability to assign a grade or pathologic stage and hence accurate prognosis of the lesion. This is a distinct disadvantage of laser treatment. To some degree, this disadvantage may be overcome by cold cup biopsy sampling of the tumor prior to laser treatment. And such sampling may or may not be representative of the grade and depth of invasion of the entire tumor.

The most serious complication of Nd:YAG laser treatment of bladder tumor is injury to adjacent bowel. This rare event is most likely during treatment or over treatment of lesions at the bladder dome, and may occur with or without obvious perforation of the bladder, since significant amounts of thermal energy can be conducted through the intact bladder wall to the bowel during Nd:YAG therapy.

This kind of injury can be avoided by exercising care, especially during treatment of tumors at the bladder dome, and limiting power settings and duration of Nd:YAG laser applications. We have not come across any such injury in our experience.

Table 2. Procedures for Ho:YAG laser prostatectomy.

I.	Ho: YAG Laser ablation of Prostate
	• Slow
	• No tissue for histopathology
II.	Ho: YAG Laser resection of Prostate
	• Adenoma is completely excised till capsule.
	• Pulse rate – 25-40/sec; Energy 2-2.5J/pulse
	• Safe, effective
	• Tissue available for histopathology
	• Fewer irritative symptoms
III.	Ho: YAG Laser enucleation of Prostate
	• Can be used for large adenoma.
	• Median and lateral lobes are dissected retrogradely
	• Morcellation and evacuation of adenoma
	• Tissue for histopathology
	• Safe, efficacious
	• No bleeding and TUR syndrome
	• Can be used in bleeding diathesis, patients with congestive heart failure
	• Shorter catheter time and hospital stay.
	• Contraindicated in chronic prostatitis

It has been suggested that laser therapy might prove advantageous in the management of transitional cell carcinoma of the bladder by reducing recurrence rates following resection. Theoretically, the no-touch approach using laser light without physical disruption of the tumor and potential spread of malignant cells through the irrigating medium, as well as the possibility that the thermal energy produced by the laser might seal local lymphatic and blood vessels draining the tumor, are attractive. In practice, this potential reduction in tumor recurrence rates has not been clearly demonstrable. Beisland and Seland [31] prospectively randomized patients to electrocautery resection and Nd:YAG laser ablation of their bladder tumors. They observed a diminished rate of local tumor recurrence following laser treatment.

Patients can be treated with little or no anesthesia, which may be particularly advantageous in the older and sicker individual. The hemostasis achievable with laser allows treatment of anticoagulated patients. Thus, very small papillary lesions, which are almost inevitably superficial and low grade, are most suitable to laser therapy. Small tumor recurrences, where the histologic diagnosis has been obtained at prior resection, may also prove good candidates for laser ablation. Multiple small tumors, lesions overlying the ureteral orifice or obturator nerve, difficult to reach lesions directly behind the bladder neck, and tumors occurring in chronically ill patients who are either not suitable candidates for anesthesia or are systemically anticoagulated, may be particularly suitable for laser ablation. Transmural bladder lesions from endometriosis may also be candidates for Nd:YAG laser coagulation.

6.3.1.1 Photodynamic Therapy

Photodynamic therapy (PDT) is a fasci-nating application of laser light for the treatment of transitional cell carcinoma of the bladder [32]. In this modality, a photosensitizing agent is systemically administered to the patient prior to therapy. Hemato-porphyrin derivatives have been commonly used as senstizers, and tend to be selectively concentrated in neoplastic growths. When exposed to laser light of the appropriate wavelength, singlet oxygen and superoxide radicals are produced in sensitized tissue and these cytotoxic agents result in cell death. Thus, this approach relies upon biochemical reactions induced by laser light, rather than the thermal effects which characterize most laser tissue interactions in typical surgical applications. The most common laser source used for photodynamic therapy in the bladder has been a tunable dye laser coupled with an argon laser source, producing visible red light at a wavelength of 630 nanometers. The delivery system consists of a transurethral probe which emits light in a spherical distribution, capable of irradiating the entire bladder mucosal surface.

The primary clinical indication for photodynamic therapy has been the treatment of diffuse disease of the bladder mucosa, whether carcinoma in situ or large numbers of papillary lesions. This modality may also have some value as a prophylactic treatment following resection of bladder tumours. The ability to achieve total bladder irradiation, as opposed to treating just focal areas of the mucosa, makes photodynamic therapy particularly attractive in these situations [33]. However, this operative approach is technically cumbersome and the necessary equipments are relatively expensive and of limited availability compared to the now readily available and very effective intravesical agents for immunotherapy and chemotherapy. Complications of photodynamic therapy include cutaneous photosensitivity, sterile cystitis, and bladder contracture. We have used in some cases, however cost of sensitizer and cumbersome technique makes it not a popular alternative in our department.

6.3.2 Urethral Tumors

Benign condylomata, caused by the human papillomavirus, probably represent the most common tumors of the male urethra, occurring in approximately 5 per cent of men with external genital lesions from the virus. Treatment of these benign urethral tumors can be problematic, but is greatly facilitated by laser. Both Nd:YAG and Ho:YAG laser wavelengths may be used to ablate these lesions, with precision and hemostasis, and with minimal risk of postoperative urethral stricture compared to electrocautery excision. These are covered later in the chapter.

6.3.2.1 Urethral Hemangioma

Hemangioma of the urethra is seldom described in the literature. These are usually seen in age range from 3 to 68 years with predominance in 3rd decade of Life. Although Nd:YAG laser fulguration has been described for treatment of bladder hemangioma, however its use in urethral hemangioma has not been reported until our case [34]. Though two cases of laser treatment of urethral hemangioma with Argon laser or KTP laser have been described. The advantage is precise fulguration with good chances of control and lesser chances of urethral stricture and procedure can be repeated as per need [34].

6.3.3 Upper Urinary Tract Tumors

The ability to transmit laser light through thin, flexible delivery fibers makes laser a particularly advantageous instrument for ablation of tumors of the upper urinary tract. During retrograde access to the upper urinary tract via a flexible ureteroscope, a flexible laser fiber may be the only useful tool for tumor ablation. Both free beam Nd:YAG and Ho:YAG laser wavelengths can be utilized in this application. Small, papillary transitional cell tumors of the ureter or renal pelvis, or the occasional upper tract hemangioma which causes gross hematuria, are the most common lesions of the upper urinary tract which might be suitable for laser ablation.

The same disadvantages of laser therapy described for treatment of bladder tumors are magnified in the treatment of upper urinary tract lesions. In particular, the muscular walls of the ureters and renal pelvis are much thinner than the bladder wall. Thus, conservative management of transitional cell carcinoma of the upper urinary tract, including laser ablation, must be undertaken only with caution and in carefully selected patients [35]. The patient with a solitary kidney or very limited global renal function is the most suitable candidate.

6.4 STRICTURE OF URINARY TRACT

Urethral stricture and bladder neck contracture are relatively common obstructing lesions of the lower urinary tract. These consist of concentric, constricting fibrous scar, and may result from a variety of inflammatory and traumatic insults. Today, urethral catheterization and other iatrogenic manipulations are responsible for many urethral strictures. Transurethral resection of the prostate may produce stricture or contracture of the bladder neck and contracture of the bladder neck anastomosis is not uncommon following radical prostatectomy. The primary treatment for such lesions is generally transurethral incision, and this may be effectively performed with lasers.

6.4.1 Internal Uretherotomy for Stricture of Urethra

Operating through a small gauge cystoscope, strictures of the anterior urethra can be incised under direct vision. Dorsal (12 o'clock position) incision of the urethra is recommended to avoid inadvertent creation of a urethrocutaneous fistula. For internal urethrotomy to be effective, regardless of the incising instrument used, it is generally felt that incisions must be carried through the entire depth and length of the fibrous plaque which forms the stricture. Almost all common surgical laser wavelengths and instruments have been used at one time or another to incise urethral strictures.

Both the Nd:YAG and KTP lasers can be used, but the absorption of these wavelength results in very significant heat transfer to surrounding tissues, and there is concern that the resulting thermal injury may infact promote recurrence of the stricture. True incising or vaporizing laser tools are thus, at least theoretically, better suited for this operation. The Nd:YAG laser has been used successfully [36-38]. While slower than transurethral incision with a cold knife, laser internal urethrotomy offers improved control and precision with superior hemostasis. Laser internal urethrotomy has been performed in fully anticoagulated patients with good hemostasis. During laser incision, because of this hemostasis and the careful, layer-by-layer dissection through the fibrous urethral plaque which laser allows, the operator can directly visualize both the extent of the plaque and the soft tissue layers beyond the plaque when the incision is completed.

Vaporizing lasers such as the Ho:YAG may actually ablate part of this fibrous plaque as well, rather than simply incising it. Although, in theory, these combined advantages may reduce stricture recurrence following laser therapy as compared with standard cold knife techniques, this has not yet been demonstrable in clinical trials [37]. We have substantial experience in the management of stricture urethra with Nd:YAG laser. In an initial evaluation, we found the results for stricture of penile, bulbar and posterior of urethra satisfactory. Subsequent, long term follow up over a period of 3 years, led us to believe that sequale following initial laser OIU causes less fibrosis and recurrence in comparision to cold or hot knife [38,39]. Another important use of this modality is core-through internal urethrotomy, where one has to make passage in choked urethra such as traumatic stricture. In these cases, often one encounter bleeding while using cold knife in such cases, whereas use of Nd:YAG or Ho:YAG laser obviates the bleeding and help in proceeding to complete surgery under relatively clear vision. A HO:YAG Laser can be used for the purpose of incision.

6.4.2 Bladder Neck Incision

Contractures of the bladder neck can be similarly incised with laser instruments, regardless of etiology (see Figure 4). They may be performed at any position around the circumference of the bladder neck, but paired lateral incisions (3 and 9 O'clock) or a single anterior or posterior incision (12 O' or 6 O'clock) are probably most commonly utilized. The fiborous contracture should be incised deeply and completely, exposing perivesical fat, to ensure efficacy. The Nd:YAG contact laser, utilizing a large sapphire chisel tip, is well-suited to this operation. A free beam Ho:YAG laser is also very effective in this application, and high pulse energies can be used to incise even the dense fibrous contracture of the bladder neck.

6.4.3 Incision of Ureteral Strictures

Stricture of the ureter may be congenital, as is the case in primary ureteropelvic junction (UPJ) obstruction, or acquired following trauma (such as passage of a stone) or iatrogenic manipulations (ureteroscopy). The resulting narrowing and obstruction of the ureter typically produces higher pressures and gradual dilation in the upper urinary tract, often progressing to renal deterioration if uncorrected. In the past, most treatments involved open surgical correction of the ureteral lesion, but recently, development of relatively delicate rigid and flexible ureteroscopes allows endoscopic access to any segment of the ureter. This access, combined with flexible, small caliber cutting instruments, now allows many of these strictures to be incised endoscopically (endoureterotomy).

The Ho:YAG laser, transmitted through a small, flexible fiber, can be employed through even the smallest working flexible ureteroscope and utilized to incise stricture anywhere along the ureter. The delicacy and flexibility of the available fiberoptic transmission devices, combined with the precision and control with which laser incisions can be performed, make laser light a particularly useful tool for endoureterotomy (see Figure 5). Ideally, full thickness incision of the ureter, until retroperitoneal fat or extravasation of injected contrast material can be visualized, is recommended to achieve optimal results and limit recurrence of the stricutre. Obviously, the operating surgeon must posses a keen knowledge of the local retroperitoneal vascular anatomy in the region of the ureteral stricture so that such an incision does not precipitate a major vascular injury [40]. Following endoureterotomy, a large caliber (at least 8 French size) ureteral stent is left in place for a few weeks to limit urinary extravasation and facilitate healing [40,41].

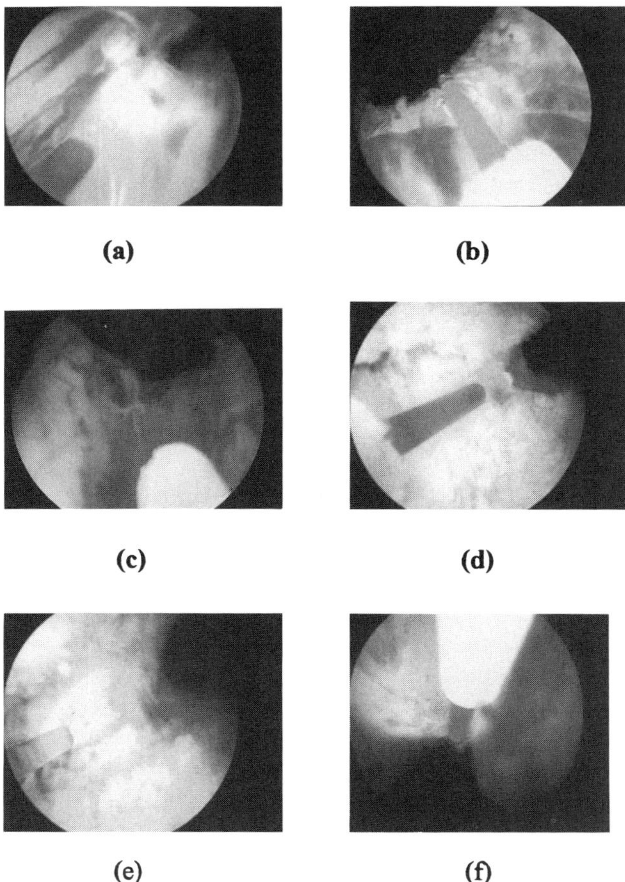

(a)   (b)

(c)   (d)

(e)   (f)

Figure 4. Holmium laser bladder neck incision(a)Demonstration of incision at 7 O'clock, (b)Demonstration of incision at 5 O'clock, (c)Demonstration of incision at 6 O'clock, (d)Demonstrating deeper cut with laser fiber showing prostate tissue in bladder neck area.
(e)Further deeper cut demonstrating various layers and fibrous capsule, (f) Demonstration of cut at 12 O'clock position.

6.4.3.1 Uretero-Enteric Stricture

Following urinary diversion, strictures may commonly occur at the anastomosis of ureter to bowel. Again, such uretero-enteric strictures have generally required open revision in the past, but now can be accessed endoscopically with modern flexible instruments; and a cutting laser wavelength such as the Ho:YAG transmitted through a flexible fiber is particularly well-suited for incision of these lesions. Because the ureter lies in a non-anatomic location following diversion to bowel, even greater care must be taken to assess the local vascular anatomy prior to these incisions, often necessitating intensive radiographic study [41].

6.4.4 Incision for Ureteropelvic Junction Obstruction, Calyceal Diverticulum, Infundibular Stenosis and Renal Cyst

While an endoscopic cold knife has been used most often to incise the ureteropelvic junction (endopyelotomy), a cutting laser instrument is also suited to this task, and may offer advantages of precision and improved hemostasis. The Ho:YAG laser has been employed successfully for endopyelotomy [36]. Because a larger caliber, rigid nephroscope can be placed with percutaneous access, a Nd:YAG contact laser with a small chisel headpiece might also be suitable for this indication. The incision for endopyelotomy is typically placed posterolaterally along the ureter to avoid major blood vessels, and should be full-thickness with visualization of perirenal fat and/or contrast extravasation through the incision. Ureteral stents up to 14/7 French size have been specifically designed for use after endopyelotomy or a regular double J stent can be used. Similarly retro-grade endopyelotomy can also be performed.

Rarely, the infundibulum to a renal calyx may become strictured. If this infundibular stenosis assumes clinical significance, it may be incised using either antegrade (percutaneous) or retrograde (ureteroscopic) approaches. The Ho:YAG laser, with its flexible fiber transmission, may be used in either approach. A Nd: YAG contact laser with a small saphire chisel tip may be used through a rigid nephroscope to perform an infundibulotomy. Another relatively rare renal lesion is the calyceal diverticulum. The diverticulum harbor stones or infection. Treatment via percutaneous access typically included opening of the narrow neck of the diverticulum, and an incising laser instrument may facilitate this maneuver [42]. Laser lithotripsy (Section 6.5) may facilitate treatment of stones contained within the diverticulum. The Ho:YAG laser wavelength is capable of both incising the diverticular neck and performing lithotripsy in such a case. Finally, definitive treatment of a calyceal diverticulum requires ablation of its epithelial lining. A free beam Nd:YAG laser can be used for this application. Thus, HoLaser can be utilized for making incision at UPJ with either antegrade or retrograde approach [43].

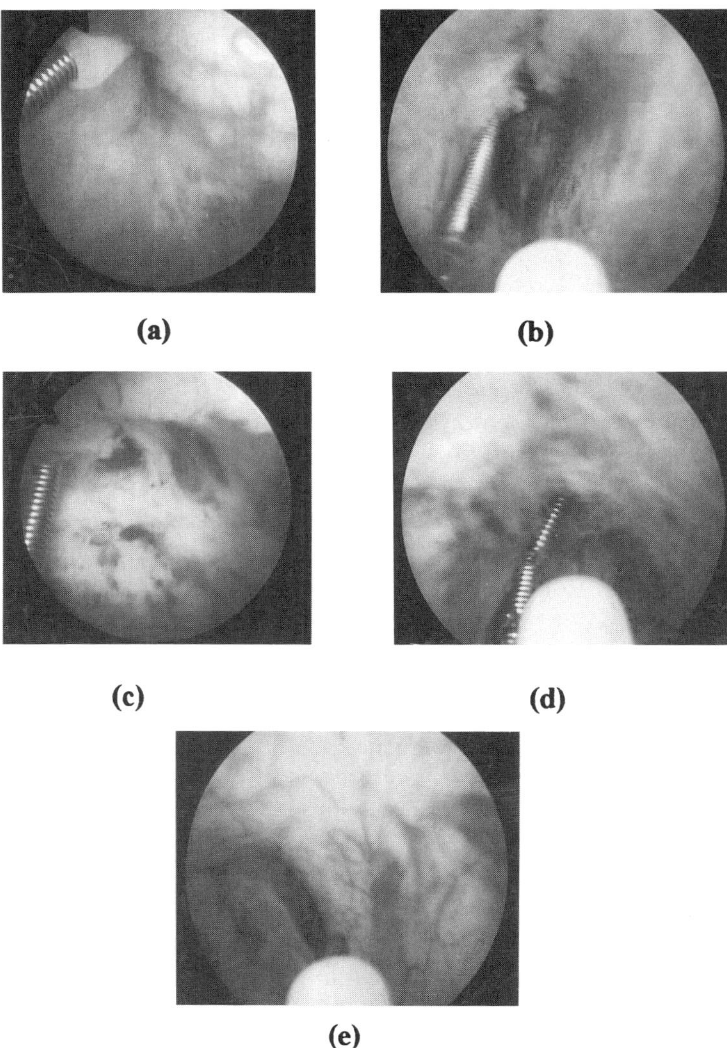

Figure 5. Holmium Laser Endopyelotomy. (a) Ureteral access catheter with stainless steel guide wire inside it emerging from ureteropelvic junction (UPJ), (b) Initial cut at UPJ, (c) Deeper cut demonstrating peripelvic tissue, (d) Further deeper cut, also seen damaged stainless steel guide wire which was placed across (universal), (e) Final view demonstrating clear vision with minimal bleeding.

The treatment of the rarely symptomatic benign renal cyst may involve a similar percutaneous approach with drainage and ablation of the epithelial lining of the cyst to prevent recurrence, and a coagulating laser wavelength such as the Nd:YAG can be used to "paint" the interior of the cyst for this purpose.

6.5   LASER LITHOTRIPSY

The character of laser energy to be transmitted through flexible fiber has created interest. Mulvancey and Beck [44] innovated the technique for stone disintegrations. They used long pulsed ruby laser for disintegration of stone, though it was never used in clinical practice due to thermal damage produce by it. Later, carbon dioxide laser and the continuous wave neodymium: yttrium-aluminium garnet (Nd:YAG) laser were used , but the problem that remained was the delivery of laser.

Pulsed laser light can be used as an effective device for fragmentation of urinary calculi [45,46]. It has been postulated that laser energy creates local plasma at the surface of a calculus, with rapid expansion and collapse for the plasma "bubble" producing shock waves capable of physical disruption of the stone. However, it is not clear that this is indeed the actual or only mechanism of laser lithotripsy, and furthermore the mechanisms may actually vary between different laser wavelengths, laser pulse durations, and other physical characteristics of the laser light. The most common laser source used for lithotripsy has been a pulsed dye laser with a wavelength of 504 nanometers. More recently, the Ho:YAG laser wavelength has also proven to be an excellent lithotriptor. Other laser sources, including the Alexandrite and Q-switched Nd:YAG lasers, have demonstrated lesser clinical utility for this application [46-49]. Laser lithotripsy is based on pulsatile light delivered through small, flexible quartz fibre to the stone through the working channel of flexible or semirigid ureteroscopes.

The pulsed-dye laser commonly was used for endoscopic lithotripsy in the early 1990s. This laser is thermal fire and breaks stone along the fracture plains of stone with a photoacoustic effect [46]. The pulsed-dye laser fragments all stone compositions with the exception of cystiene. The laser can also be used in benign and malignant tumor of genitalia [47,52,54-56]. Different types of lasers, with their characteristics, used in urolithasis are given in Table 3.

Table 3. Different types of lasers in urolithasis

Type	Wave length nm	Energy mJ/ pulse	Mecha-nism	Fibre size um	Fragmen -tation rate	Draw-backs	Remarks
Q-switched Nd:YAG laser	1064	20-80	Plasma medi-ated event	400-600	55-83%	Calcium oxalate monohy-drate and brushite stone, fragile delivery systems, large fibre	Fibre kept at distance
Tunable pulsed dye laser	504	140	Oscill-ation of Cavita-tion bubble	200-400	77-99%	Calcium oxalate monohy-drate and Cysteine stones, high cost	Direct contact, -more strong, wide safety
Q-switched Alexandrite	755	30-120	Plasma and Cavita-tion bubble	200-300	60-97%^	-Tissue injury, -Technical problems	Strong
Ho:YAG Laser	2100	200-4000	Photo-therma	200-1000	90-100%	-Cyanide produc-tion with uric acid stone, -slow -cost, tissue injury	-Fibre tip in direct contact, -very strong should be kept 1mm away from tissue.

6.6 SOME USEFUL LASER DEVICES FOR LITHOTRYPSY

6.6.1 Pulsed Q-switched Nd:YAG Laser

This emits at a wavelength of 1064 nm, with pulse duration of 8 ns and a pulse energy of 20 to 80 mJ. The mechanism for action is that laser pulse absorbed by the pigments in the stone and heat is generated. As a result, material is vaporized, free electrons are liberated, and a plasma is formed. Plasma absorbs heat and it expands between the tip of the laser fiber and the stone surface. The rapid expansion leads to stone fragmentation. The size of fibers range from 400 to 600 um. Stone fragmentation rates range from 55% to 83% [45]. The Hofmann and Hautung [48] demonstrated safely but main drawbacks are inability to fragment calcium oxalate monohydrate (COM) and brushite stones, fragile delivery system and large fiber.

6.6.2 Tunable Pulsed-dye Laser

The tunable pulsed dye laser has pulse duration in microseconds as opposed to nanoseconds for Nd:YAG laser. As energy reaches the stone-fluid interface, the pulse energy is absorbed primarily by the stone, leading to formation of cavitation bubble and its expansion and collapse results in the generation of mechanical shock waves. This shock wave is more powerful than plasma based [50]. Stone fragmentation rates of 77% to 99% have been reported [51]. The drawbacks are failure to break COM and cystine stones and high cost.

6.6.3 Q-Switched Alexandrite Laser

It operates at a wavelength of 755nm, pulse duration of 150 to 1000ns, and energy output of 30 to 120mJ per pulse. Since its pulse duration lies between the Nd:YAG and pulse laser, therefore, both plasma and cavitation bubble form.

The plasma is responsible for fiber consumption, whereas cavitation bubble leads to stone fragmentation [52] It is delivered with a 200-300um quartz fiber. Stone fragmentation success rate of 60-97% have been reported [53]. It produces tissue injury and single purpose Alexandrite laser may not be cost effective.

6.6.4 Ho:YAG Laser

The Ho:YAG laser is based on 2150-mm wavelength of light energy, which when applied through a lower water density quartz fiber and in a water based medium, creates a vaporization bubble at the tip. This vaporization bubble produces no shock wave effect but does destabilize stones, quickly creating fine dust and small fragments [46,54]. The energy can be delivered by any size of fibre as small as 200-um fiber. The larger the Ho laser fiber diameter, however, the greater the size of the vaporization bubble and the more efficient and expeditious the treatment. The most common technique used for Ho laser lithotripsy is to first core out the central portion of the stone, converting it to fine dust, while fragmenting the remaining shell into small, possible pieces that are less than 2mm [46.50].

The laser settings used for ureteroscopic lithotripsy begin with 0.6 J of energy and 5 Hz frequency of pulsation. The energy and frequency of pulsation then are increased gradually to obtain the desired effect. Higher frequency of pulsation increases the kinetic effect on the stone and may decrease the efficiency of treatment, which is particularly true when small fragments are considered. For large stone use higher energy to core central portion then convert to lower settings to fragment center shell.

Compared to instruments for mechanical stone fragmentation or ultrasonic lithotripsy, the ability to transmit pulsed dye or Ho:YAG laser light through a thin, flexible fiber confers a significant advantage to laser for intracorporeal lithotripsy, especially for calculi located in the ureter and upper urinary tract. These laser fibers can be easily employed through either small caliber rigid ureteroscopes or flexible ureteroscopes. The wavelength of pulsed dye laser is particularly innocuous to tissue, and therefore poses almost no risk of laser injury to the ureter or renal pelvis compared to other techniques.

The Ho: YAG wavelength is quite capable of tissue vaporization, but for ureteral lithotripsy is used at very low pulse energies and frequencies, and actually produces significantly less mucosal trauma than typically observed with electrohydraulic lithotripsy. Both pulsed dye and Ho:YAG laser lithotripsy produce a much less pronounced mechanical pulse during stone fragmentation than do non-laser lithotripsy instruments, and thus cause much less of a tendency for the stone to "bounce" or migrate up in the ureter. In this regard, the Ho:YAG wavelength probably results in less stone propulsion than the pulsed dye laser.

The Ho:YAG laser appears capable of fragmenting all known calculi, regardless of composition or color. Furthermore, the Ho:YAG laser can be used to pulverize most calculi into very small fragments or powder, and thus can eliminate the concern and possible need to mechanically retrieve or remove residual stone fragments (see Figure 6). Additionally, at higher power settings, beyond what might be considered unsafe for routine use in the ureter, the Ho:YAG can prove an efficient lithotriptor even for treatment of relatively large calculi in the bladder or renal pelvis. Variety of Laser Fibres (200-1000um) are available for endoscopic use. Utilize helium/ neon targeting beam for precise laser placement and maintain fiber at least 1mm from ureteral wall to avoid injury. The energy setting for soft Calculi (Calcium oxalate dihydrate, Strutive) and hard calculi (Calcium oxalate monohydrate, cystine) are laser energy (mj) 200-600; 600-1200 and laser frequency (Hz) 6-8; 8-10 respectively [50]. As mentioned earlier various techniques for achieving stone fragmentation may be employed: working along fracture planes/create holes in the stone and join the dots or create central cavity at high power, then vaporize the remaining shell at low power.

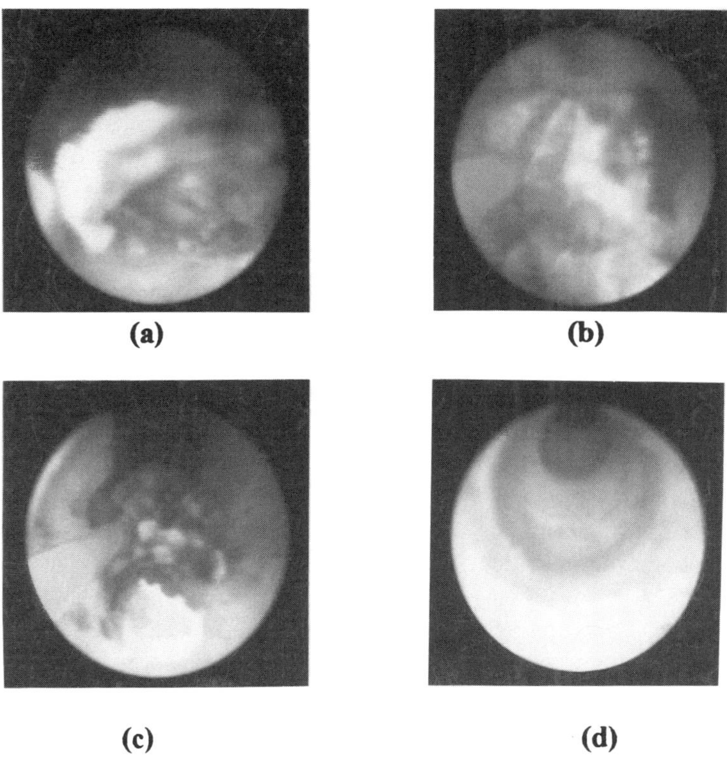

(a)   (b)

(c)   (d)

Figure 6. Holmium Laser Ureteroscopic Lithotripsy. (a) Ureteroscopic view of uretric stone, (b) Disintegration of uretric stone with laser fiber, (c) Fragmented stones with laser energy, (d) Final view of ureteral following Ureteroscopic Lithotripsy with any damage.

6.7   OTHER USES

6.7.1   Malignant Tumors of Penis

Rothenberger and Hofsetter [47] treated 23 patients of the stages T_1 and T_2 [NoMo] as well as 4 cases of T_3 lesions or metastases. In terms of average post observation interval of 7 years only 1 patient died. Four cases of local recurrence were retreated successfully with good cosmesis. Laser treatment may be considered as an alternative to partial penectomy for localized CaPenis up to stage T_2 [54].

6.7.2   Benign Lesion of Penis and Condyloma Acuminata

Benign lesions of the penis or premalignant lesions can be well treated with the laser with good cosmesis. The laser is often used for condyloma accuminata and, if it is CO_2 laser, then vapour must be sucked off, because it can contain active virus [55]. Thus, Nd:YAG laser is to be preferred for urethral condyloma and in case of external warts urethra must be examined because coaffection is frequent [56].

6.7.3   Incision and Ablation of Parenchyma

Partial nephrectomy was done with the Nd:YAG laser with only small blood loss. This laser has been tested with different tips and in combi-nation both with the CO_2 laser and an ultrasonic cutting system [57]. The CO_2 laser was also employed for ablating tissue in subcapsular orchiectomy [58].

6.7.4   Tissue Welding

The field of tissue welding, however, provides a more novel use for lasers in that it is reconstructive rather than destructive. By definition, laser tissue welding is the use of focused laser energy in order to obtain tissue approximation.   This concept of alternative, "suture-less" tissue closure evolved following some success with electrocautery in surgery.   Sigel et al used electrocurrent to close 'venotomy sites [59]. More than 20 years ago this success of electrocautery was followed with the innovations of Yahr and Strully [60] who described the use of laser reapproximation of tissue edges in an unsuccessful vascular anastomosis using laser energy.

The ultimate goal of tissue welding, as with most techniques of tissue closure, is to obtain approximation with minimal scar formation and good tensile strength. The mechanism for the laser weld involves laser delivery of thermal energy that induces changes in the collagen substructure, followed by covalent and electrostatic bonding upon renaturation of the tissue proteins. The technique for surgical welding is fairly straightforward. During the initial phases of solder development there was great concern about the clinical application of a human-based protein solder that might have potential for viral transmission, including hepatitis and HIV. Recent developments, however, have made possible a purified protein solder that carried no risk of viral transmission. In a recent study comparison of different concentrations of protein solders to determine the optimal albumin concentration, it was determined that a 50% human albumin-based solder was optimal for developing maximum acute weld strength [61]. Laser tissue welding has been applied conceptually to every organ and tissue in the genitourinary tract. Clinically, however, laser welding has limited, although expanding, usefulness as mentioned in Tables 4 and 5. Urologic surgery necessitates water-tight, nonlithogenic closures in view of the continuous flow of urine within its borders. Tight anastomotic closures are of even greater importance in urology than in vascular surgery because urine lacks the clotting ability of blood and cannot aid in sealing off any microscopic leak points. Laser welding provides a technology that affords an opportunity for an immediate water-tight, nonlithogenic anastomosis with tensile strength that exceeds that of traditional closure techniques.

Table 4. Applications of laser tissue welding in open urologic surgery.

1. Vasovasostomy
2. Urethral reconstruction (hypospadias repair)
3. Pyeloplasty
4. Augmentation cystoplasty
5. Continent urinary diversion.

Table 5. Potential applications for future.

- Primary anastomosis
  Ureteroureterostomy
  Pyeloplasty
  Ureteroneocystostomy
- Anastomotic closure or reinforcement of
  Bowel
  Bladder
  Urethrocystostomy
  Ureteroenterostomy

In an attempt to apply solder material and to deliver laser energy laparoscopically, a laparoscopic laser-solder delivery system has been developed [62]. The potential for laparoscopic laser welding is expanding and such procedures as pyeloplasties and ureteroneocystotomies among many others are certainly within the realm of future possibilities.

6.7.5 Bladder Hemangioma

This condition can exist independently or as part of the congenital Klippel-Trenaunay-Weber syndrome. Endoscopic resection of such lesions can cause uncontrollable hematuria and thus this therapeutic modality is inadvisable. The management of bladder haemangioma therefore seems to be a good indication for the use of the laser. The Nd:YAG laser applied in noncontact mode can effectively coagulate these lesions, with no complications [63]. We have treated cases of bladder hemangioma with Nd:YAG Laser [63,64].

6.7.6 Suture Removal

A rare complication of urological surgery is the unintended placement of nonabsorbable sutures through the urinary tract. The intraluminal segment of these sutures serves as a nidus for stone formation or can cause obstruction. Within the urinary bladder, these sutures can be easily removed endoscopically, using scissors and graspers. However, for sutures within the ureter, the use of these instruments through the narrow lumen of a ureteroscope is impossible and a small quartz fiber can be used instead [65]. The Nd:YAG and Ho:YAG laser have been used to divide sutures and they are equally effective on all materials. The only exception was Goretex^{TM}, against which the Ho:YAG is ineffective.

REFERENCES

1. McPhee MS; "Prostate". In Lasers in Urologic Surgery, Smith. JA, Jr. ed. St. Louis, Mosby-Year Book. 1989, pp. 41-49.
2. Kandel LB, Harrison LH, McCullough DL, et al. Transurethral Laser prostatectomy: creation of a technique for using the Neodymium:Yttrium Aluminum Garnet (YAG) laser in the canine model. J Urol 1986; 135: 110A.
3. Shanberg Am, Tansey LA, Baghdassarian R. The use of the Neodymium YAG laser in prostatectomy. J Urol , 1985;133:331A.
4. Smith JA, Jr. Laser treatment of the urethra and prostate. Semin Urol : 1991;3:180.
5. Roth RA, Aretz HT. Transurethral ultrasound-guided laser-induced prostatectomy (TULIP procedure): a canine prostate feasibility study. J Urol, 1991; 146: 1128.
6. Schulze H, Pannek J, Martin W, et al. 1128-1135: Transurethral ultrasound –guided laser-induced prostatectomy: clinical outcome and data analysis. Urology 1995 ; 45:241.
7. Johnson DE, Levinson AK, Greskovich FJ etal. Trans urethral laser prostatectomy using right-angle delivery system. SPIE Proceedings 1991;36:1421.
8. Costello AJ, Bolton DM, Ellis D, Crowe H: Histopathological changes in human prostatic adenoma following Neodymium: YAG laser ablation therapy. J Urol 1994;152:1526.
9. Kabalin JN, Terris MK, Mancianti ML, Fajardo LF: Dosimetry studies utilizing the Urolase right angle firing Neodymium: YAG laser fiber in the human prostate. Lasers Surg Med 1996; 18: 72.
10. Leach GE, Siris L, Ganabathi K, et al.: Outpatient visual laser-assisted prostatectomy under local anesthesia. Urology 1994; 43: 149.
11. Van Swol CFP, te Slaa E, Verdaasdonk RM, et al. Variation in output power of laser prostatectomy fibers: a need for power measurements. Urology 1996; 47:672.
12. Kabalin JN: Laboratory and clinical experience with Neodymium: YAG laser prostatectomy. SPIE Proceedings 1996; 2671:274.

13. Kabalin JN, Bite G, Doll S: Neodymium: YAG laser coagulation prostatectomy: 3 years of experience with 227 patients. J Urol 1996; 155: 181.
14. Narayan P, Fournier G, Indudhara R et al. evaporation of the laser using a contact Free beam technique :results in 61 patients with benign prostatic hyperplasia. Urology 1994;43:813.
15. Kabalin JN, Gill HS, Bite G, Wolfe V: Comparative study of laser versus electrocautery prostatic resection: 18-month follow up with complex urodynamic assessment. 1995; J Urol 153:94,
16. Van Erps P, Schapmans S, Cortvriend J, et al. Urodynamic effects of Prolase 2 laser prostatectomy in benign prostatic hyperplasia. Acta Urol Belg 1995; 63:39.
17. Cowles RS, III, Kabalin JN, Childs S, et al. A prospective randomized comparison of transurethral resection to visual laser ablation of the prostate for the treatment of benign prostatic hyperplasia. Urology 1995; 46: 155.
18. Anson K, Nawrocki J, Buckley J, et al. A multicenter, randomized prospective study of endoscopic laser ablation versus transurethral resection of the prostate. Urology 1995; 46: 305.
19. Costello AJ, Crowe HR, Asopa R. Long term results of randomized laser prostatectomy vs TURP: modification of laser prostatectomy technique with biodegradable stent insertion. J Urol, 1996; 155: 316A.
20. Shingleton WB, Terrel F, Fowler JE, Jr. A randomized study of transurethral resection of the prostate versus laser ablation of the prostate in patients with benign prostatic hyperplasia. J Urol 1996; 155: 317A.
21. Muschter R, Hofstetter A. Interstitial laser therapy outcomes in benign prostatic hyperplasia . J Endourol 1995; 9 (2) : 129-135.
22. Suzuki Y, Arai Y, Ishitoya K. Transurethral interstitital laser coagulation for benign prostatic hyperplasia:treatment outcome and quality of life. Br J. Urol 1996;78 (1): 93-98.
23. Johnson DE, Cromeens DM, Price RE. Transurethral incision of the prostate using the Holmium: YAG Laser. Lasers Surg Med 1992; 12: 353.
24. Kabalin JN. Clinical development of Holmium: YAG laser prostatectomy. SPIE Proceedings 1996; 2671: 292.
25. Kabalin JN. Holmoium: YAG laser prostatectomy: results of U.S. pilot study J Endourol, 1996; 10: 453.
26. Gilling PJ, Cass CB, Cresswell MD, Fraundorfer MR. Holmium laser resection of the prostate: preliminary results of a new method for the treatment of benign prostatic hyperplasia. Urology 1996; 10: 453.
27. Gilling PJ, Kennett KM, Fraunderfer MR. Holmium laser enucleation of the prostate (HoLEP) vs Transurethral Resection of the prostate (TURP) for large prostate glands (40-200g): Early results. J Endourol 2000;14(1) Suppl. P5-3, A35.
28. Krahn HP, Glezerson G. Cost effectiveness and complications of Holmium laser enucleation of the prostate (HoLEP). J Endourol 2000;14(1) Suppl. P5-2, A35.
29. Hofstetter A, Kriegmair M, Baumgartner R. "Evaluation of laser treatment of bladder cancer". In: smith Jr JA, Stein BS, Benson Jr RC, editors. Lasers in urologic Surgery. St. Louis: Mobsy-Year Book, Inc., 1994;114-125.
30. Johnson DE. Use of the Holmium: YAG (Ho:YAG) laser for treatment of superficial bladder carcinoma. Lasers surg Med 1994;14:213-218.
31. Beisland HO, Seland P. A prospective randomised study of Nd: YAG laser irradiation versus TUR in the treatment of urinary bladder cancer. Scand J Urol Nephrol 1986;20:209-212.
32. Nseyo UO. Photodynamic therapy. Urol Clin N Am 1992;19:591-599.
33. Kriegmair M, Baumgartner R, Knuchel R, Stepp H, Hofstetter A. Detection of early bladder cancer by 5-Aminolevulinic acid induced porphyrin Fluroscence. J Urol 1996;155:105-110.

34. Khaitan A, Hemal AK. Urethral lemangioma: Laser treatment. Int. Urol Nephrol 2000;
35. Jabbour ME, Smith AD. Primary percutaneous approach to upper urinary tract transitional cell carcinoma. UCNA 2000;27(4), 739-750.
36. Webb DR, Kockelburgh R, Johnson WF. The Versapulse Holmium surgical laser in clinical urology: A pilot study. Minimally Invasive Therapy 1993; 2:23-26.
37. Smith JR JA. Treatment of benign urethral strictures using a sapphire tipped Neodymium:YAG lasers. J Urol 1989;142:1221-1222.
38. Dogra PN, Aron M, Rajeev TP. Core through urethrotomy with the Nd: YAG Laser for post traumatic obliterative stricutre of the bullbomemberanous urethra.   J. Urol 1999;161:81-84.
39. Hemal AK, Kumar R, Gupta NP. Nd:YAG Laser Urethrotomy for Stricture of Anterior Urethra. (Submitted for publication)
40. Schmeller NT, Hofstetter AG. Laser treatment of ureteral tumors. J Urol 1989;141:840-843.
41. Meretyk S, Albaba D, Clayman R, Denstedt J, Kavoussi L. Endoureterotomy for treatment of Ureteral Strictures. J Urol 1992;147:1502-1505.
42. Chong TW, Bui MHT, Fuchs GJ. Calyceal Diverticula : Ureteroscopic management. UCNA 2000;27(4): 647-654.
43. Razvi HA, Chun SS, Denstedt JD, Sales JL. Soft tissue application of Holmium:YAG laser in Urology. J Endourol 1995;9:387-391.
44. Mulvancey WP, Beck CW. The laser beam in Urology. J Urol 1968;99:112.
45. Tanahashi Y, Orikasa S, Ciba R,etal. Distribution of Urinary calculi by laser beam: Drilling experiment in extracted urinary stones. Tohoku J Exp Med 1979;128:189.
46. Dretler SP. An evaluation of ureteral laser lithotripsy: 225 consecutive patients. J Urol 1990; 143:267-272.
47. Rothenberger KH, Hofstetter A: Lasertherapie des Peniskarzinoms. Urologe 1994; (A) 33: 291-294.
48. Hofmann R, HautungR. Use of pulsed Nd: YAG laser in the ureter. Urol clin North Am 1988;15:369
49. Watson GM, Murray S, Dretler SP et al. The pulse-dye laser for Fragmenting urinary Calculi. J Urol 1987;138:195-198.
50. Rink R, Delacretaz, Salathe RP. Fragmentation process of current laser lithotriptors. Laser Surg Med 1995; 16:134.
51. Fugelso P, Neal PM. Endoscopic laser lithotripsy: safe, effective therapy for ureteral calculi. J Urol 1991;145:949.
52. Hofmann R, Hautung R, Schmidt-Kloiber H et al. First clinical experience with a Q-Switched neodymium;YAG laser for urinary calculi. J Urol 1989;141:275
53. Pearle MS, Sech SM, Cobb CG et al. Safety and efficacy of the Alexandrite laser for the treatment of renal and ureteral calculi. Urology 1998;51:33.
54. Rothenberger KH, Hofstetter A. YAG-Laser-Behandlung maligner Tumoren des Penis. Fortschr Med 1982;100: 1806-1808.
55. Garden JM, O'Banion MK, Shelnitz LS: Papillomvirus in the vapor of carbonxyoxide laser treated verrucae. JAMA 1988;259:1199-1202.
56. Schneede P, Muschter R. Laseranwendung bei condyloma acuminata.. Urologe [A] 1994; 33: 299-302.
57. Landau S, Wood TS, Melzer RB et al. Renal evaluation after C.USA. + Nd:YAG Laser partial nephrectomy. Lasers surg. Med 1986;6 :146-149.
58. Bolton DM, Costello AJ: CO_2 Laser subcapsular orchiectomy in the treatment of metastatic prostate cancer. Lasers surg med 14 (1994) 88-89.
59. Siegel B, Acevedo F: Vein anactomosis by electrocoaptive union. Surg forum, 1962; 13:291.

60. Yahr W, Strully K:blood vessel anastomosis by laser and other medical application. JAAMI 1966;1: 28.
61. Poppas D, Wright E, Guthrie P, et al : Women albumiu shoulders for clinical operation during laser tissue welding. Lasers surg med 1995; 7:22.
62. Wolf S, Soble J, Nakada S, et al : Comparison of fibrin glue, laser weld, and mechanical suturing devise for the laparoscopic closure of ureterotomy in a porcine model. J Urol 1997;157:1487-1492.
63. Smith JJ. Laser treatment of bladder haemagnioma. J Urol 1990;143:282-4.
64. Hemal AK, Gupta NP. Fulguration of Bladder Hemangioma with Nd: YAG laser. (Submitted for publication)
65. Bagley DH. Schultz E, Conlin KJ. Laser division of intraluminal sutures. J Endourol 1998;12:355-7.

Chapter 7

LASER LITHOTRIPSY

Tim A. Wollin and Ronald B. Moore
Division of Urology, Department of Surgery, University of Alberta, CANADA

7.1 INTRODUCTION

Over the past two decades, the surgical management of renal and ureteral stones has undergone tremendous change. In contrast to the traditional techniques of open surgery and blind stone basket manipulation, the mainstays of treatment today include extracorporeal shockwave lithotripsy (SWL) and endoscopic intracorporeal lithotripsy. Laser energy has been used clinically to treat urinary tract stones for almost two decades. It is now one of the most common and most popular methods used by urologists for the treatment of renal, ureteral, and bladder calculi. This chapter will review the natural history of stones, the background of managing urinary tract stones and outline the role of lasers in their treatment, comparing them to lithotripsy modalities.

7.1.1 Epidemiological Aspects of Urinary Lithiasis

Archeological excavations in the early twentieth century demonstrated that humans have been afflicted with urinary lithiasis since at least 7000 BC [1]. Despite significant advances in the diagnosis and especially in the therapy of renal stone disease, the incidence of this disorder has increased by more than 60 per cent over the past 25 years and continues to rise, especially in industrialized nations [2]. Prior to industrialization, bladder calculi were the most frequent urinary stone, commonly composed of uric acid and magnesium ammonium phosphate (struvite) [3]. However, today in North America and other industrialized countries, the upper urinary tract is the most common site of stone formation and these stones are composed predominantly of calcium oxalate [3].

Large population-based epidemiologic studies have shown the incidence of calcium urinary lithiasis to be 0.7 to 1.6 per cent in the U.S. [4-6]. The incidence occurs more commonly in males than females with a ratio between 2:1 and 3:1 [7]. Age-adjusted incidence rates are highest in the third to fifth decades and the disease is uncommon in those under 15 years [7-9]. Children seem to be protected by their relatively low excretion of calcium and perhaps because of a higher excretion of polyanionic inhibitors [9].

The etiology of urinary stone disease is multifactorial and the relationships involved in the development of urinary lithiasis in any individual are complex. Genetics, [7,10] geographic location and ambient air temperatures, [7,9,11] socioeconomic status, [9] diet, [8] and one's occupation [7,9,12] have all been suggested as possible etiologic factors for nephrolithiasis.

7.2 SURGICAL MANAGEMENT OF URINARY STONES

As noted above, there has been unparalleled progress in the management of stone disease in the past two decades. When intervention is required, noninvasive or minimally invasive therapy can now be performed successfully in greater than 95% of patients. Open surgical procedures to extract or fragment stones in the kidney and ureter are now required in only one to two percent of patients [13,14]. Extracorporeal shockwave lithotripsy, percutaneous nephrolithotripsy (PCNL) and ureteroscopic techniques are now the mainstays of surgical therapy.

7.2.1 Indications for Surgical Intervention

The decision of when and how to treat a urinary tract stone is largely dependent on the size of the stone, the location of the stone in urinary tract and whether or not it is causing symptoms and/or obstruction for the patient. The accepted indications for surgical intervention include: an obstructing stone in a patient with a solitary kidney, bilateral ureteral obstruction, infection behind an obstructed system, continuous unrelenting pain, or a ureteral stone that is either greater than six to eight millimeters or fails to pass spontaneously with conservative management [15]. The treatment of asymptomatic renal stones is somewhat controversial. However, data suggests that these calculi have approximately a 50% chance of becoming symptomatic within five years, [16] therefore, many urologists will treat asymptomatic stones in an attempt to prevent these symptomatic episodes. Furthermore, some investigators believe these "asymptomatic" caliceal stones are a source of intermittent symptoms and thus should be treated [15,17-19]. Finally, there are certain social situations, such as patients who work as airline pilots, where a stone-free state is mandatory regardless of stone size or symptoms [20]. These patients also require surgical treatment for their stones.

When none of these indications are present, conservative management, by waiting for spontaneous passage of the stone is indicated as first-line treatment. Seventy to ninety per cent of all stones less than or equal to four millimeters in size will pass spontaneously in approximately two to three weeks time [8,21-23]. Only ten to fifteen per cent of stones greater than six millimeters will pass spontaneously and essentially none will pass that are greater than eight millimeters in diameter [22].

7.2.2 Extracorporeal Shockwave Lithotripsy

The development of SWL was born out of a collaborative research in the 1970's between Dornier Aerospace and the University of Munich. This group began investigating the physics of shock waves and their possible use for lithotripsy. Chaussy *et al.* [24] described the first report of shock wave lithotripsy in humans. By October 1984, the Dornier HM-3 (Human Model-three) became commercially available after more than 1000 patients had been treated in Munich and Stuttgart [25]. By 1986, more than 130 Dornier units were operational worldwide and by 1990, at least nine manufacturers were developing second-generation machines [15]. Today, hundreds of thousands of patients worldwide have been treated.

Extracorporeal shockwave lithotripsy uses shock waves generated outside of the body to fragment renal and ureteral calculi. Shock waves created within a shock tube or chamber are propagated through the body tissues where they are focused onto the stone. Since the fluid content of the body is high, little energy loss occurs until the wave reaches the stone [26]. Stone fragmentation is believed to occur as a result of the compressive, reflective, and tensile forces acting on the anterior, interior, and posterior surfaces of the stone [27,28].

The indications for SWL include the standard indications for surgical stone removal. The only absolute contraindications to treatment are pregnancy, febrile urinary tract infection, and coagulopathies that cannot be corrected [29]. In some situations, patient weight is also considered a contraindication because the machine warranty is not effective beyond a certain weight limit and the body habitus precludes aligning the focal point of the shock wave with the stone.

The clinical outcome with SWL is dependent on the stone size, stone location, and stone composition. In general, SWL monotherapy for renal stones less than 1.5 cm results in stone-free rates of 85 per cent with a retreatment rate of approximately 15 per cent [30-33]. As the stone size increases above 2 cm, stone-free rates diminish to less than 50 per cent at three months [31]. In these cases, percutaneous nephrolithotripsy is the preferred treatment.

Concerning stone location, stone-free rates are 60 to 70 per cent for stones in the lower calyces, 75 to 80 per cent for the middle and upper calyces, and 85 to 92 per cent for renal pelvic and upper ureteral stones [34]. In the ureter below the pelvic brim, stone-free rates are reported to be 40 to 96 per cent [35-41]. However, the majority of these studies also report retreatment and ancillary treatment rates of 7 to 40 per cent. Therefore, because ureteroscopic extraction of these stones has a success rate of greater than 95 per cent, some authors suggest that ureteroscopy should be the first choice of therapy for lower ureteral calculi [41-43].

Stone composition also has a role in the clinical effectiveness of SWL. It is well known that stones made up of calcium oxalate monohydrate (COM), calcium phosphate dihydrate (CPD), and cystine, require more shock waves at a higher intensity to achieve fragmentation [30,44]. Basic analysis has shown that these stones have a higher density than other common stones making them "harder" and more difficult to fragment [44]. In situations where a stone fails to fragment with SWL, either PCNL or ureteroscopy with intracorporeal lithotripsy will be required to achieve a stone-free status.

7.2.3 Percutaneous Nephrolithotripsy (PCNL)

Fernström and Johansson [45] described the first percutaneous extraction of a renal stone through a percutaneously established nephrostomy tract in 1976. By the early 1980's, percutaneous nephrolithotomy eventually replaced open surgical lithotomy as the treatment of choice for renal and upper ureteral calculi. At the same time, however, the technology for extracorporeal shock wave lithotripsy was also being developed. By 1984, the "golden age" of percutaneous nephrolithotomy ended as shock wave lithotripsy was introduced to the world [46].

However, widespread use of SWL has not rendered the technique of percutaneous nephrolithotomy obsolete. Instead, the indications for percutaneous stone surgery have been refined. Percutaneous nephrolithotripsy is considered appropriate management for patients with a large stone volume (stone diameter > 2 cm), cases involving specific stone compositions (cystine, calcium oxalate monohydrate), patients with body habitus precluding SWL (morbid obesity), those with collecting system abnormalities that would not allow stone fragments to pass (ureteral-pelvic junction obstruction, caliceal diverticulum), or SWL failures [47,48]. Finally, there is also new evidence that lower caliceal calculi may be better treated initially with PCNL to achieve better stone-free rates [49,50].

The technique of percutaneous nephrolithotripsy involves three interdependent procedures: percutaneous renal access using either fluoroscopy or ultrasound guidance, tract dilatation, and stone fragmentation and extraction. The details of these techniques have been described in detail elsewhere [46,51,52]. Stones that are one centimeter in diameter or less can usually be extracted intact with grasping forceps. Larger calculi require intracorporeal fragmentation using various lithotripsy devices that will be discussed below. Stone-free rates for large staghorn stones range from 60 to 93% with retreatment rates of 21 to 80%. The majority of these retreatments are second-look flexible nephroscopy procedures performed during the same admission to hospital [52].

7.2.4 Ureteroscopy and Intracorporeal Lithotripsy

Although SWL is now used to treat the majority of patients with ureteral stones, like PCNL, there continues to be a subset of patients with ureteral stones that is often managed more effectively with ureteroscopy. This includes patients with calculi located over the sacral ala, those with cystine stones or radiolucent stones, stones greater than one centimeter in size, patients with ureteral anatomy or body habitus precluding SWL, and finally those stones that have failed to fragment with SWL [14,47].

Young [53] is credited with performing the first ureteroscopy in 1929 when he passed a rigid cystoscope into the dilated ureter of a pediatric patient with posterior urethral valves. However, it wasn't until the late 1970's when Goodman [54] and Lyon *et al.* [55] independently reported using techniques to dilate the distal ureter that routine endoscopic evaluation of the ureter became practical. First-generation ureteroscopes were rigid and ranged in size from 9 to 16.0 French (F) (1 French = 0.33 mm) [56]. As a result, early experiences with ureteroscopic stone extraction were challenging and often associated with complication rates of greater than seven to ten percent [57-59].

Over the past decade, improvements in fiber optic technology have brought about a significant decrease in the size of scopes. Ureteroscopes ranging in size from 4 to 8F are now available (1.2 to 2.6 mm diameter). As a result, these miniature scopes can be passed through the ureteral orifice with greater ease and in most cases, without ureteral dilatation [60]. Finally, flexible and actively deflecting instruments are also available that allow one to maneuver the instrument into regions of the ureter and kidney that would be impossible with rigid endoscopes. Consequently, modern ureteroscopic experience is associated with success rates of greater than 95% and major complication rates of less than 2% [59,61].

7.2.5 Intracorporeal Lithotripsy Devices

Stones that are approximately five to six millimeters in size may be extracted intact under direct vision using a variety of baskets or grasping instruments. This will usually require dilatation of the ureteral orifice and intramural portion of the distal ureter prior to extraction. Calculi greater than six millimeters generally will need to be fragmented prior to their removal. A variety of stone-fragmenting instruments or intracorporeal lithotripsy devices are currently available. These can be broadly classified into those that are rigid in nature and therefore operate through a direct mechanical effect on the calculus (ultrasonic and pneumatic lithotripsy; Figure 1) and those that are flexible and usually operate through a shock wave effect (electrohydraulic lithotripsy and some lasers, Figure 2).

7.2.5.1 Ultrasonic Lithotripsy

The ultrasonic lithotriptor consists of a high-frequency generator that applies a current to a piezoceramic crystal causing it to expand and contract at a frequency of greater than 20,000 cycles/sec (Figure 1).

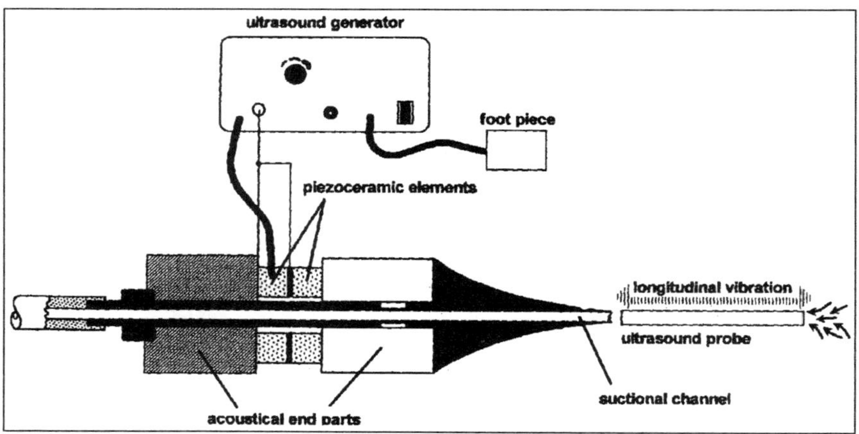

Figure 1. Schematic drawing of ultrasonic lithotripter. Reprinted from Smith AD. Smith's Text book of Endourology. St. Louis: Quality Medical Publications, Inc. [62]

The ultrasonic energy is transmitted down a metal probe and is converted to vibration at the probe tip. When placed in direct contact with a stone, this vibration produces a grinding and drilling effect that ultimately fragments the stone. Probes range in size from 2.5F to 11.5F (0.8 mm to 4.0 mm diameter) with the larger probes having a hollow center that permits simultaneous aspiration of stone particles during lithotripsy [62].

Ultrasonic lithotripsy has proven itself to be a very safe method for stone fragmentation. Animal studies have shown that even when the ultrasonic probe is applied directly to the urothelium, only edema and superficial changes occur [63]. The initial clinical experience with ultrasonic lithotripsy was in the treatment of bladder stones. However, with the development of smaller probe sizes, the use of ultrasonic lithotripsy has expanded to include stones in the upper urinary tract. This device is one of the most common used today during PCNL because of its ability to fragment and clear large stone burdens in an extremely efficient manner. On the whole, the advantages of ultrasonic lithotripsy include its proven safety, the ability to simultaneously evacuate stone material during fragmentation when using hollow probes, and its relatively low cost of operation. Current start-up costs for the generator and associated equipment are approximately $12,000 (US$) [47]. Moreover, there are no disposable components. One shortcoming of the ultrasonic device is related to the rigid design of the probes. As such, this device can only be used in association with rigid and semi-rigid endoscopes.

7.2.5.2 Pneumatic Lithotripsy

The pneumatic lithotriptor fragments stones using mechanics that are similar to a jackhammer. The unit consists of a generator, handpiece, and a direct-contact, solid probe that is powered by a standard electrical source and a clean, dry source of compressed air (Figure 2).

The generator is coupled to the handpiece with flexible rubber tubing, and when it is activated with the foot pedal, compressed air enters the handpiece and propels a small metal projectile against the base of the metal probe at a pressure of 3 atmospheres and a frequency of 12 Hz [64]. With the probe tip in direct contact with the stone, the ballistic energy is transmitted down the probe and fragmentation occurs once the tensile forces of the stone are overcome. No heat is generated with activation of the device. Like ultrasound, the rigid nature of the probes limits its use to rigid endoscopes. However, newer more flexible probes capable of being passed through a flexible ureteroscope are in the developmental stage.

The versatility, efficacy, and safety of pneumatic lithotripsy have been well documented [65-67]. This device is able to fragment all stones regardless of stone composition. However, treatment failure can occur from forward propulsion and migration of the stone in a capacious, dilated ureter. An advantage of pneumatic lithotripsy is that the technology is simple and it provides a reliable, effective, safe, and inexpensive means for performing intracorporeal lithotripsy. The cost of the generator is approximately $21,500 (US$) and each reusable probe costs approximately $150 [47]. Similar to ultrasonic lithotripsy devices, no disposable items are used.

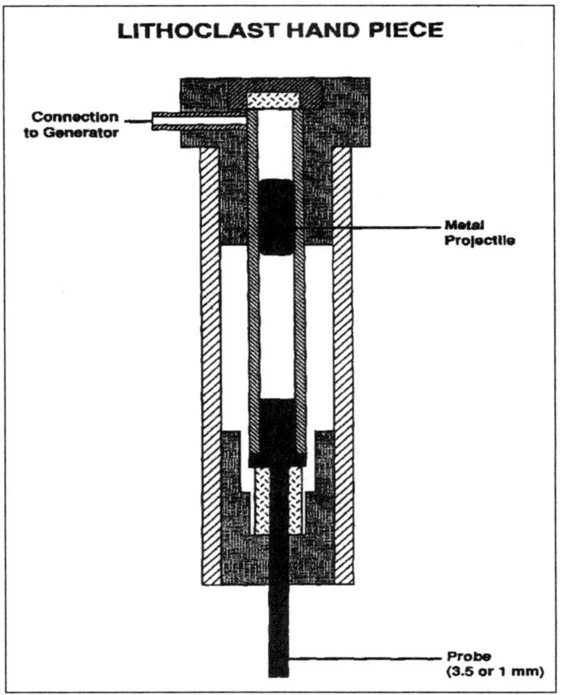

Figure 2. Schematic drawing of pneumatic lithotripsy device. Reprinted from Smith AD. Smith's Text book of Endrourology, St. Louis, Mo: Quality Medical Publishing, Inc. [62]

7.2.5.3   Electrohydraulic Lithotripsy (EHL)

The electrohydraulic lithotriptor consists of an electrical generator, a cable that connects to a flexible EHL probe, and a foot pedal that activates the probe. When the device is activated, an electric current is propagated down the probe and a spark is generated between the insulated metal cores of the probe. The heat from the spark vaporizes a small amount of the surrounding fluid and forms a cavitation bubble. The rapid expansion and subsequent collapse of this bubble results in a strong hydraulic shock wave that is able to achieve stone fragmentation [68].

Reuter and Kern [69] were the first to report treatment of ureteral stones with EHL. Initial experience was fraught with complications because probe size was large (9F) and the procedure was performed blindly by passing the probes up the ureter to the stone and then discharging the instrument. Ureteral perforation was common and stone fragmentation was inconsistent. Today however, intraureteral EHL is performed under direct endoscopic control with smaller caliber probes. Using 1.9 to 3F probes, successful fragmentation rates of 79% to 98% have been reported [70,71]. Ureteral perforations secondary to the electrohydraulic lithotripter energy are reported in 0% to 2% of cases.

The main advantages of EHL are related to its cost, and the small size and flexibility of the probes. The initial cost of the generator and cables range from $11,000 to $18,000 (US$), while probes cost approximately $150 for 9F electrodes to $300 for the smaller 1.9F probes [47]. The small-diameter probe sizes make this device especially suited for use in small caliber ureteroscopes and flexible instruments. Disadvantages of EHL include its relatively narrow margin of safety because of the high pressures generated and the fact that some calculi will not fragment with this device.

7.3 LASER LITHOTRIPSY

The above intracorporeal lithotripsy devices have proved to be effective and safe for clinical use. However, the search for an energy or device that can be used for both ureteral and renal calculi, may be passed through small-caliber endoscopes, and has the ability to reliably and consistently fragment all stone compositions without causing surrounding tissue damage has stimulated the study of lasers for intracorporeal lithotripsy [72].

7.3.1 The History of Laser Lithotripsy

The first attempt at using laser energy to fragment urinary calculi was in 1968. In an *in vitro* study, Mulvaney and Beck [73] demonstrated that ruby and CO_2 lasers were capable of fragmenting urinary stone. However, the ruby laser's thermal effects and the inability to deliver CO_2 laser energy through an endoscope prevented the development of these devices for practical clinical use. Little work in the area of laser lithotripsy was reported over the next decade until 1978 when Fair described fragmentation of urinary calculi using shock waves generated by an optico-acoustic transducer [74]. A thin film of aluminum confined between glass and brass was irradiated with a high-intensity pulsed laser and this produced shock waves of sufficient energy to easily fragment calculi. It was also noted that by shortening the laser pulse, higher peak pressures were generated.

In 1981, Tanahashi *et al.* [75] and Pensel *et al.* [76] independently reported using a continuous wave Nd:YAG laser to fragment bladder calculi in dogs. However, like the ruby laser over a decade earlier, the thermal effects associated with stone fragmentation prevented its development into the clinical realm. For this reason, attention was turned to the study of pulsed laser energy for fragmenting stones.

In 1983, Watson *et al.* [77] reported on the stone fragmenting properties of the Q-switched Nd:YAG (neodymium:yttrium-aluminum-garnet) laser. When a series of 15 ns, 1 J pulses repeated at 10 Hz were focused on a calculus, all types of stones could be fragmented regardless of color or composition. However, a major limitation to this laser was that the high powered Q-switched pulses could not be transmitted through flexible glass fibers without consistently damaging the fibers. In the same study, a non-Q-switched Nd:YAG laser with a pulse duration approximately 10,000 times longer was examined. Using 800 mJ pulses of 100 μsec duration at 40 Hz, Watson *et al.* demonstrated that dense oxalate stones fragmented in 30 seconds. However, fragmentation was associated with charring of the stone surface suggesting that some heating of the stone did occur. When the laser was focused directly on a cadaveric renal pelvis, it caused a visible burn after 30 seconds and perforation after 50 seconds. Therefore, this laser appeared to be intermediary in its effect between the Q-switched pulsed laser and the continuous wave laser.

The authors concluded that lasers could be used for calculus fragmentation without injuring the urinary tract provided that they were not aimed directly at the tissue for longer than a few seconds and if they had short enough pulses that would not allow excessive heat build up.

Therefore, by 1983, some basic principles and problems of using the laser for stone fragmentation were known [72]. Continuous wave lasers were inappropriate for laser lithotripsy because they created too much heat and caused thermal tissue damage; pulsed lasers appeared to act on stones by creating a shock or a stress wave that overcame the tensile strength of the stone; the shorter the laser pulse duration, the higher the pressure of the stress waves; and effective use of lasers for calculi depended on the ability to transmit the energy through optical fibers.

In order to find a laser with more ideal characteristics, Watson and colleagues began studying the pulsed dye lasers. They believed that these lasers had potential because their wavelengths could be adjusted. An ideal wavelength would be one where there was maximal absorption by the pigments in the stone with a lesser degree of absorption by tissue pigments. Theoretically, this would minimize the risk of injury to tissue while maintaining the stone-fragmenting qualities of the laser. Consequently, study of the pulsed dye laser began by measuring the effectiveness of *in vitro* stone fragmentation while varying the wavelength, pulse duration, and fiber size [78]. Optimal stone fragmentation occurred when coumarin green dye was used as the active medium to produce a wavelength of 504 nm, with a pulse duration of 1 μsec, using a 200 micron diameter silica coated quartz fiber.

Once the efficacy of this laser was established, the same researchers investigated the safety of the pulsed dye laser in an *in vivo* animal study [79]. When the fiber tip was abutted against the ureteral wall of a pig and discharged at energies of 25 to 30 mJ per pulse, tissue injury was minimal with only mild inflammatory changes occurring at the site of fragmentation and extending to the superficial muscle fibers. Nishioka *et al.* [80] performed a similar *in vivo* study. This group used the same pulsed dye laser but fragmented biliary calculi within the common bile duct of pigs. They also found minimal tissue injury that consisted microscopically of mild to moderate inflammatory infiltrate composed of lymphocytes, eosinophils, and polymorphonuclear leukocytes.

Clinical experience using the pulsed dye laser for intracorporeal lithotripsy began in the mid-1980's [81-83].In these initial studies, investigators used the coumarin dye laser with a 200-250 μm fiber and energies ranging from 25-40 mJ per pulse. The fiber was placed in contact with the stone through a 9 to 11.5F ureteroscope. Dretler *et al.* [83] reported successfully fragmenting 16 of 17 ureteral calculi for an overall success rate of 94 per cent.

Eight calculi were fragmented with the laser alone, while seven required stone basket extraction of the fragments and one required subsequent ESWL when fragments were flushed into the renal pelvis. During the procedure, the laser was inadvertently discharged onto the ureteral wall in six patients with no sequelae. Watson and Wickham [82] described an 89 per cent successful fragmentation rate of 37 ureteral calculi. No complications were reported.

The development of the coumarin pulsed dye laser ushered in the current era of laser lithotripsy and made it a practical and viable modality for treating urinary tract stones. Since the initial experience with the pulsed dye laser, other lasers have now been used for intracorporeal lithotripsy. These include the Q-switched Nd:YAG laser, the Alexandrite laser, and most recently, the Ho:YAG (holmium:YAG) laser. The mechanism of stone fragmentation, safety, clinical results, and advantages and disadvantages of each of these laser systems is discussed in greater detail below.

7.3.2 Pulsed-dye Laser

Until the mid to late 1990's, the coumarin pulsed dye laser was the most common laser used for laser lithotripsy. It's use clinically and reports of its use in the literature have fallen off considerably since the introduction of the Ho:YAG laser. Nevertheless, it still represents a safe and reliable method for treating upper urinary tract stones for those centers that have the pulsed dye laser at their disposal.

7.3.2.1 Mechanism and Technique of Pulsed-dye Laser Stone Fragmentation

The pulsed-dye laser fragments calculi through a photoacoustic phenomenon called a "plasma". This interaction occurs in lasers that operate in the microsecond or nanosecond domain. Nishioka *et al.* [84] have demonstrated that when the pulsed-dye laser is directed onto a calculus, microscopic heating occurs on the stone surface causing the liberation of free calcium ions. These ions form a cloud or plasma-bubble that expands and contracts with each subsequent laser pulse. With each collapse of the bubble, a photoacoustic shockwave is generated that has sufficient kinetic energy to cause stone fragmentation of most urinary calculi.

To perform pulsed-dye laser lithotripsy, the laser fiber is placed against the stone and the laser discharged. A high-pitched ticking sound is generated during the procedure that occurs as a result of the photoacoustic shockwaves produced from the absorption of the laser energy. On account of the kinetic energy associated with the plasma-mediated shockwave, it is not uncommon to experience proximal stone migration in a dilated ureter during treatment. If this becomes problematic, a stone basket can be used to immobilize the stone while laser lithotripsy is performed.

7.3.2.2 Clinical Results of Pulsed-dye Laser Lithotripsy

There have been numerous clinical series reporting the outcomes with pulsed dye laser lithotripsy. The results of studies that have patient populations greater than 50 patients are summarized in Table 1. Stone-free rates of 70 to 100% are reported. The mean stone-free rate in these patients is 83.6% (2095/2505 patients).

Stone composition and proximal stone migration were the most common causes for treatment failure. Stones composed of calcium oxalate monohydrate, cystine, and calcium phosphate dihydrate (brushite) were the most difficult to fragment. Technical difficulty with the pulsed dye laser was an infrequent cause of failure and was only reported in one early series when a prototype machine was being used [86].

In 1990, a larger 320 µm fiber was introduced for clinical use. Since more energy can be transmitted through a larger fiber, it was believed that the 320 µm fiber might achieve better fragmentation than the standard 200 µm and 250 µm fibers. Several investigators compared the success of stone fragmentation using the different fiber diameters [91,94,97,101,102]. These studies showed no significant differences in the overall success of fragmentation.

However, the authors of these studies repeatedly stated that the increased energy transmitted through the larger fiber improved the efficiency of the

Table 1. Results of Pulsed Dye Laser Lithotripsy

	No. Patients Treated	Stone-Free Rate(%)	Complications (%)
Coptcoat et al., 1988 [85]	120	91/107 (85)	11/120 (9) - stricture (1.6); ureteral perforation (7.5)
Dretler, 1988 [86]	157	106/157 (68)	11/157 (7.0) -sepsis (0.6); DVT (0.6)
Watson and Wickham, 1989 [87]	250	240/250 (96)	2/250 (0.8) -sepsis (0.8)
Dretler, 1990 [88]	222	171/222 (77)	27/222 (12) - ureteral perforation (10.3)
Gautier et al., 1990 [89]	325	238/325 (73)	46/278 (16) - ureteral perforation (6); UTI (5)
Govier et al., 1990 [90]	50	46/50 (92)	1/50 (2) - stricture (2)
Dretler and Bhatta, 1991 [91]	72	59/72 (82)	1/72 (1) - ureteral perforation (1)
Fugelso and Neal, 1991 [92]	204	139/204 (68)	20/204 (10) -sepsis (5); ureteral perforation (2.5)
Grasso et al., 1991 [93]	80	80/80 (100)	0/66 (0)
Vandeursen et al., 1991 [94]	104	85/104 (82)	N/A
Psihramis, 1992 [95]	122	107/122 (88)	3/122 (2) - stricture (0.8); ureteral perforation (1.6)
Ng et al, 1992 [96]	100	97/100 (97)	5/95 (5) - ureteral perforation (3); UTI (2)
MacDermott and Clark, 1993 [97]	175	134/175 (77)	7/175 (4) -sepsis (1.1); ureteral perforation (2.3)
Schmidt and Eisenberger, 1993 [98]	54	38/54 (70)	5/54 (9) -all mild ureteral trauma
Grasso and Bagley, 1994 [99]	176	172/176 (97)	N/A
Boline and Belis, 1994 [100]	248	235/248 (95)	2/248 (0.8)
Turk and Jenkins, 1999 [41]	59	57/59 (97)	5/96 (5)* - ureteral perforation (4.2); stricture (1)

Abbreviations: N/A (not available)
*Complication rate based on total population.

pulsed dye laser for stone fragmentation without compromising the margin of safety [91,94]. In an effort to show this objectively, the number of pulses to achieve fragmentation was compared for the two sizes of fiber. Dretler and Bhatta [91] found that for COM calculi 51-100 mm^2 in size, 2371 pulses were required for fragmentation with a 200 μm fiber at 60 mJ compared to 522 pulses when a 320 μm fiber at 140 mJ was used. Similarly, Vandeursen *et al.* [94] demonstrated that the mean number of pulses to fragment COM stones greater than 4 mm with the 200 μm/60 mJ fiber was 3500 compared to 1053 for the 320 μm/140 mJ fiber.

The wavelength characteristics of the pulsed-dye laser give it a very wide margin of safety. As noted previously, animal studies have shown that minimal tissue injury occurs during pulsed-dye laser lithotripsy [79]. These findings have been confirmed clinically where it is widely held that pulsed-dye laser lithotripsy is the safest form of intracorporeal lithotripsy. The cumulative complication rate for pulsed-dye laser lithotripsy in the studies summarized in Table 1 was 6.7% (148/2209 patients). The most common problem encountered was ureteral perforation that occurred in one to 10.3% of patients.

In almost all cases, the perforations occurred as a result of the ureteroscopic equipment (scopes and guidewires) and not from the laser itself. All patients were treated conservatively with ureteral stenting or percutaneous nephrostomy drainage.

The other most frequently encountered complications in order of decreasing frequency were sepsis/infection (0.6 to 5%), ureteral stricture formation (0.8 to 2%), and miscellaneous others (deep vein thrombosis, mild ureteral abrasions, temperature elevation). Concerning the problem of stricture formation, all of these occurred at the ureterovesical junction of the ureter, well below the site of laser fragmentation.

None were felt to occur as a direct result of the laser energy on the ureter but as a result of ureteral balloon dilatation and ureteroscopy with larger diameter endoscopes. Since the introduction of smaller caliber ureteroscopes (7.0 to 8.0F) where ureteral dilatation is often not required, only one stricture has been reported in a patient following balloon dilatation of the ureterovesical junction [95].

The primary advantage of the pulsed-dye laser is that it has the lowest potential for causing urothelial injury compared to all other forms of lithotripsy. As such, it has shown particular benefit in the management of difficult stone problems such as impacted ureteral stones, submucosal stones, and Steinstrasse (a line of impacted ureteral stones or stone fragments most often seen following SWL). In addition, the laser fibers are reusable. This is in contradistinction to EHL probes, which have a very limited life expectancy.

The major drawback of this device is its high cost. A new pulsed-dye laser unit will cost approximately $100,000 (US$) to purchase and will also require a service contract to cover regular maintenance. Another hindrance is that because cystine stones do not absorb the pulsed-dye laser energy, they are uniformly resistant to fragmentation. Other dense calculi, such as calcium oxalate monohydrate and brushite stones, will fragment with the laser but results are inconsistent, even with the larger diameter laser fibers that deliver higher energies.

7.3.3 Q-Switched Neodymium:YAG Laser

The Q-switched Nd:YAG laser is a pulsed laser capable of generating very high peak powers because of its nanosecond-range pulse duration. Despite the initial encouraging results of Watson and colleagues in 1983, this laser was limited clinically by the fact that the high-powered Q-switched pulses could not be transmitted through laser fibers without consistently damaging the fiber tips.

Further work with this laser did not occur until 1988 when Hofmann and associates were able to transmit the powerful pulses through specially designed fibers that focused the laser energy at the fiber tip [103]. These investigators also showed that no significant macroscopic or microscopic tissue damage occurred when the laser was discharged directly onto pig urothelium. Like the pulsed dye laser, stone fragmentation occurs through a plasma-mediated response.

The technique of lithotripsy is achieved in the same fashion as the pulsed dye laser. The tip of the fiber is placed on or very near the stone and the laser is then discharged. The reported clinical experience with the Q-switched Nd:YAG laser is not extensive, but fragmentation rates of 55% to 85% have been reported in small series of patients [104-108]. Hofmann and Hartung [106] have described the outcome in 189 patients treated with this laser. Using a 8 ns pulse duration with single pulse energies of 20-80 mJ, they were able to achieve a stone-free rate of 95% (179/189). The laser failed to achieve stone fragmentation in 10/189 patients (5%).

Complications occurred in 14/189 (7.4%) patients. These consisted of ureteral perforation in two patients and mild to moderate hematuria in the remaining twelve patients. A total of ten additional patients were felt to have had unintentional direct irradiation of the ureter with the laser without any adverse effect. Failures were associated with calcium oxalate monohydrate stone composition and difficulties related to the large diameter of the laser fiber (600 μm). There have been no clinical reports describing the use of this laser in the literature since 1993.

7.3.4 Alexandrite Laser

The alexandrite laser is a pulsed solid-state laser that emits light at 750 nm. Like the pulsed-dye and Q-switched Nd:YAG lasers, stone fragmentation occurs through a plasma-mediated shock wave. Initial experimental studies with the alexandrite laser were reported in the early 1990's. In an *in vitro* and *in vivo* study, Mattioli *et al.* [109] demonstrated effective stone fragmentation with no evidence of tissue injury when the laser was fired directly onto the ureter and bladder of rabbits.

However, in another *ex vivo* study using pigs, the 250 μm quartz fiber was demonstrated to easily fragment with pieces of the fiber becoming embedded in the ureteral wall when a short pulse duration (350 ns) was used [110]. With a longer one-microsecond pulse, fiber fragmentation did not occur, but histological damage was seen to the level of the muscularis mucosa. Therefore, depending on the pulse energy and pulse width used, tissue effects from the alexandrite laser range from little to no injury, [109] to hematoma formation and perforation of the bladder or ureteral walls [111]. Like the Q-switched Nd:YAG laser, clinical experience with the alexandrite laser is somewhat limited. Reported clinical results have been variable with fragmentation rates ranging from 46% to 88% [111-114].

7.3.5 Holmium:YAG Laser

The holmium laser represents the most recent addition to the armamentarium of laser lithotripsy devices. This is a pulsed, solid-state laser that operates at a wavelength of 2100 nm in the near infrared portion of the electromagnetic spectrum. The laser's active medium is the rare earth element, holmium. It is usually combined with a yttrium-aluminum-garnet (YAG) crystal (holmium:YAG), but yttrium-scandium-gallium-garnet (holmium:YSGG) has also been employed [115]. The pulse duration of the holmium laser ranges from 250 to 350 μsec, the pulse energy from 0.2 to 5.0 J/pulse, the frequency from 5 to 50 Hz, and the average power from 2.0 to 100 Watts (Figure 3). Laser fiber size ranges from 200 μm up to 1000 μm (Figure 4).

As a result of the holmium laser's wavelength characteristics, it is not only an excellent laser lithotripter, but it is also able to cut and coagulate tissue making it a multi-purpose surgical laser. This is in contradistinction to the pulsed dye laser, which is single-purpose, stone-fragmenting laser. In addition to its stone-fragmenting properties, the holmium laser has been used in urology for resection of the prostate, [116,117] incision of ureteral strictures, [118,119] and treatment of transitional cell carcinoma of the bladder and upper urinary tracts [118,120,121]. The laser has also been used in orthopedics, [122] ophthalmology, [123] otolaryngology, [124,125] cardiology, [126,127] oral/maxillofacial sugery, [128] gastroenterology, ([129,130] and pulmonary medicine [131].

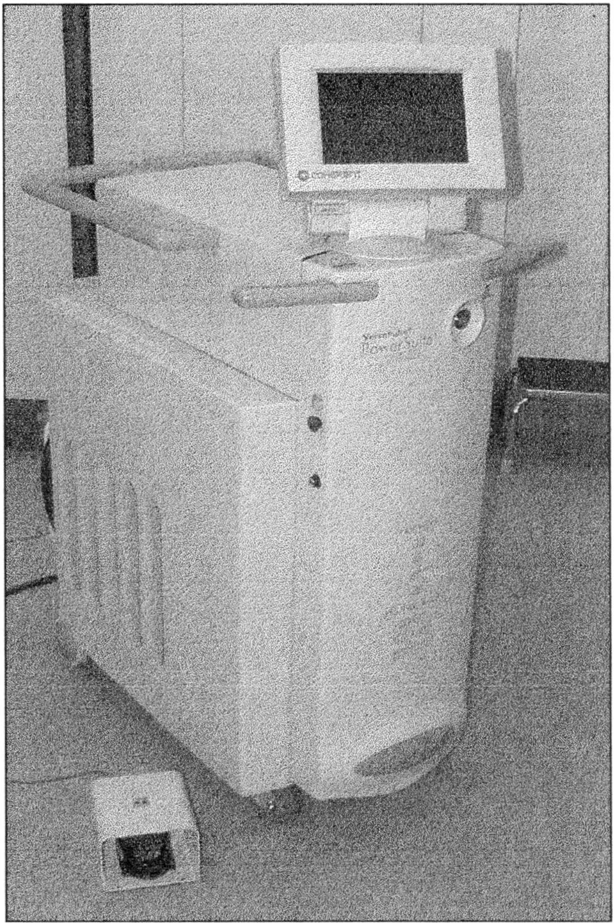

Figure 3. Holmium:YAG laser system.

7.3.5.1 Holmium Laser Tissue Interactions

The optical absorption coefficient for water at 2100 nm is approximately 40 cm^{-1}, which means that the holmium wavelength is significantly absorbed by water. When used in water, 95% of the holmium energy will be absorbed within approximately 0.5 mm [118,132,133]. Since tissue is composed mainly of water, the majority of the holmium energy is absorbed superficially and this results in superficial cutting or ablating laser-tissue interactions. Tissue studies with the holmium laser have shown that the zones of thermal injury associated with tissue ablation range from 0.5 to 1.0 mm [132,134]. With this amount of surrounding thermal injury, hemostasis for blood vessels larger than 1.0 mm in diameter occurs, making it possible to safely perform soft tissue applications. Animal studies have demonstrated excellent hemostasis with the holmium laser when used to perform partial nephrectomy [132]. The current clinical experience with holmium laser resection of the prostate gland also demonstrates the holmium laser's excellent hemostatic properties [116,117]. This traditionally vascular procedure can be done virtually in a bloodless field when performed with the holmium laser.

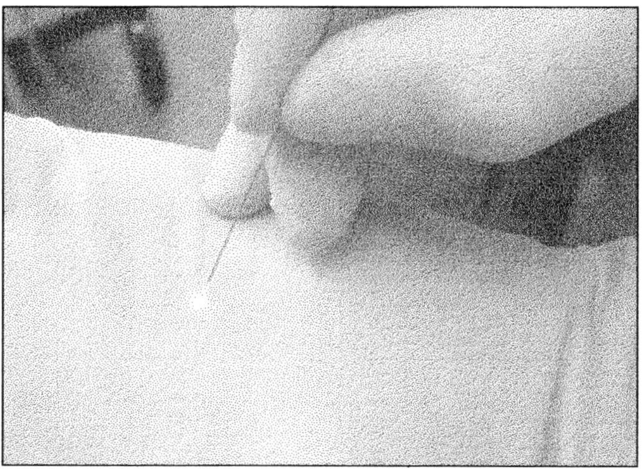

Figure 4. A 365 µm holmium laser fiber.

7.3.5.2 Mechanism of Holmium Laser Stone Fragmentation

As a result of its longer pulse duration (>200µsec), the holmium laser *does not* fragment urinary calculi through a plasma-mediated interaction but through a thermal-mediated interaction. Initial evidence for this concept came from work by Zhong *et al.* [135]. These investigators used high-speed photography and acoustic pressure measurements to compare stone fragmentation with the pulsed-dye laser and the holmium laser. Compared to the spherical cavitation bubble and strong shockwave emission produced by the pulsed-dye laser, the longer pulse duration of the holmium laser produced an elongated bubble with a much weaker shockwave emission. This finding has been confirmed by other investigators who have shown that as the pulse duration of the laser increases, the cavitation bubble produced in the liquid medium becomes more elongated and cylindrical in shape; and this leads to a decreased magnitude in the subsequent pressure wave compared to the spherical bubble produced by short-pulsed lasers [133]. Therefore, because the shockwave associated with the holmium laser is relatively weak, stone fragmentation must be more dependent on a thermal effect that causes "stone vaporization".

This hypothesis has now been proved by an elegant five-part experimental study performed by Vassar *et al.* in 1999 [136]. In the first segment of the study, it was shown that holmium laser lithotripsy caused greater stone mass loss for stones that were dry in air compared to stones that were fragmented wet in air or in water. This suggested that holmium laser lithotripsy requires direct absorption of laser energy by stone compared to a plasma-mediated mechanism where water is required to create the cavitation bubble. Next, like Zhong *et al.* [135], high-speed photography was used to demonstrate that holmium laser stone fragmentation occurs before collapse of the vapor bubble. Thirdly, stone mass loss was compared for stones at different temperatures. Stone mass loss was greater for stones fragmented at room temperature compared to stones that had been kept at $-80°$ C. Next, stone composition analysis and analysis of the irrigant in which lithotripsy was performed demonstrated that thermochemical reactions had occurred as a result of the holmium laser lithotripsy. Calcium oxalate monohydrate yielded calcium carbonate, cystine yielded cysteine and free sulfur, calcium hydrogen phosphate dihydrate (brushite) yielded calcium pyrophosphosphate, magnesium ammonium phosphate yielded ammonium carbonate and magnesium carbonate, and uric acid stones yielded cyanide. These thermal by-products can only be generated from stone surface temperatures that are hot enough for thermochemical reactions ($100°$ C to $264°$ C) [136]. Finally, the pressure waves associated with holmium laser lithotripsy were measured using needle hydrophones and peak pressures were consistently less than 20 bars. This pressure level is considered too low to have any significant effect on stone fragmentation.

The finding of cyanide being produced as a result of holmium laser lithotripsy of uric acid calculi is an interesting discovery and obviously has potential clinical implications related to the safety of holmium laser lithotripsy of uric acid stones. To date, there have been no reported cases of cyanide toxicity in adults and children who have had their uric acid stones treated with the holmium laser [137,138]. The actual risk of cyanide toxicity is not known but is apt to be very low since the majority of the cyanide produced is likely not absorbed systemically but evacuated from the body in the irrigation fluid. Further *in vitro* testing has revealed that cyanide production varies with holmium pulse energy [139]. Therefore, when it is known beforehand that a patient has uric acid stones, it is recommended that holmium laser lithotripsy be performed at a pulse energy of less than or equal to 1.0 Joules/pulse to minimize cyanide production [139]. Interestingly, in this same study, cyanide production was also demonstrated following lithotripsy with the pulsed dye laser and the alexandrite laser. Significantly less cyanide was produced, so the margin of safety would be even greater.

7.3.5.3 Technique of Holmium Laser Lithotripsy

The technique of holmium laser lithotripsy is relatively straightforward and involves placing the fiber on the stone surface and then activating the laser. Compared to some of the soft-tissue applications of the laser, the overall power used for stone fragmentation is considerably less (Table 2). In general, pulse energies of 0.8 to 1.2 J and pulse rates of 6 to 10 Hz are more than adequate to achieve effective fragmentation. Stone fragmentation occurs in a "drilling" fashion in that the laser fiber bores down into the stone while emitting a fine spray of stone dust. One can either create multiple holes within the stone surface or work away at creating a larger superficial cavity. Either way, as the main calculus breaks apart, laser lithotripsy is continued until fragments are less than 2 to 3 mm. At this size, the fragments can be left to pass spontaneously or they can be retrieved with baskets or grasping forceps.

Table 2. Holmium laser parameters for various applications.

	Pulse Energy (Joules/pulse)	Frequency (Hz)	Power (Watts)
Incision of strictures	1.0 to 2.0	10 to 15	10 to 30
Ablation of TCC	0.6 to 1.2	6 to 15	3.6 to 18
Prostate resection	2.4 to 2.6	25 to 50	60 to 100
Laser lithotripsy	0.5 to 1.2	5 to 15	2.5 to 20

Since the holmium wavelength is able to cut and coagulate tissue, it is very important that certain guidelines be followed to avoid intra-operative complications. First, the entire procedure must be done under video monitoring or direct vision with the fiber in contact with the stone at all times. In situations where stone dust begins to obstruct the operator's vision, lithotripsy should be halted until the irrigation has a chance to clear the field. One must also be cautious about drilling through the stone to the backside where tissue damage can then occur blindly. Finally, because the holmium wavelength is capable of cutting through metal, it is important not to direct the laser energy directly at the safety guidewire or stone baskets. Moreover, the laser fiber should always be extended at least 3 to 5 mm beyond the tip of the endoscope to avoid damage to the lens system of the scope. Failure to adhere to these principles can lead to unwanted effects in the surrounding tissue or to endourologic equipment.

7.3.5.4 Clinical Results of Holmium Laser Lithotripsy

The first published reports of holmium laser lithotripsy appeared in 1995 [140,141]. Since that time there have been over 75 reports in the scientific literature describing the technique and results of stone fragmentation with the holmium laser. The clinical results from these studies have been uniformly excellent. As a result, the holmium laser is now a well-established modality for performing intracorporeal lithotripsy and is the most common laser in use for this application.

Table 3 summarizes the clinical results of holmium laser lithotripsy for series having greater than 50 patients. Successful fragmentation with stone-free rates of 90 to 97% is achieved in the majority of cases. The mean stone-free rate is 95.0% (1489/1568 patients). Unlike the pulsed dye laser, the final determinant of success is not the laser's ability to fragment the stone, but non-laser factors such as stone location, stone size, and situations of difficult access because of associated anatomic abnormalities or ureteral stenosis. The holmium laser will fragment all calculi regardless of composition, including cystine, calcium oxalate monohydrate, and brushite.

The average complication rate with holmium laser lithotripsy is 4.1% (66/1619 patients). Almost all complications reported were due to the ureteroscopic procedure itself and not as a direct result of the laser energy. Due to the tissue effects of the holmium laser, there could be concern about the potential for long-term ureteral tissue injury. However, the reported stricture rate is low (0.3 to 3%) and is comparable to the stricture rate reported for non-laser ureteroscopic stone treatment [59,60,71,142]. Sofer *et al.* [138] have the largest reported series of holmium laser lithotripsy. Concerning stricture formation, a total of eight patients developed strictures post-operatively in their series. For six of these cases, there was either a past history of iatrogenic injury that occurred during previous attempts at stone fragmentation or a long duration of stone impaction with ureteral narrowing and fibrosis noted at the time of ureteroscopy. It was not believed that the laser contributed to stricture formation in any of these cases. Nonetheless, the potential for this type of injury exits and careful attention to technique must be maintained in order to avoid ureteral complications.

Holmium laser lithotripsy for renal calculi used either as an adjunct during percutaneous nephrolithotripsy or as a primary intracorporeal lithotripsy device during retrograde ureteroscopy has also been reported [138,143-148]. During percutaneous surgery, the holmium laser is most helpful in clearing small volumes of stone when flexible instruments are required to access stones in a calyx remote from the nephrostomy tract. For larger stone burdens, using the laser as a sole modality is often too time-consuming and not as efficient as other devices like ultrasonic or pneumatic lithotripsy. However, with the development of flexible ureteroscopes, retrograde ureteroscopy is being expanded into the proximal ureter and kidney and several centers are reporting using ureteroscopy as a primary procedure for patients with renal calculi [138,143,144,146-148]. When the smaller 200 μm fiber is used, almost any stone in any region of the renal collecting system can be accessed in a retrograde fashion and then fragmented with the laser. Grasso *et al.* [143] currently have the largest experience treating intra-renal calculi in a retrograde manner with the holmium laser. Out of 99 patients, 80% had their stones fragmented and cleared with one single procedure. This rate increased to 90% after a second ureteroscopy.

Like the other laser lithotripsy devices, the main drawback to the holmium laser would seem to be the overall cost. The purchasing cost of a new holmium system ranges from \$80,500 to \$132,000 (US\$), depending on the power output of the laser desired. However, because of the laser's overall clinical effectiveness, its re-usable laser fibers, and the laser's expanding

Table 3. Results of ureteral holmium laser lithotripsy

	No. Stones Treated	Stone-Free Rate(%)	Complications (%)
Devarajan et al, 1998 [149]	300	270/300 (90)	12/300 (4) stricture (3.3); sepsis (0.6); peritonitis (0.3)
Schroff et al, 1996 [150]	114	99/114 (87)	6/114 (5) stricture (2.5); perforation (2.5)
Scarpa et al, 1999 [151]	150	139/150 (93)	0/150 (0)
Grasso et al, 1998 [143]	106	103/106 (97)	2/106 (2) pyelonephritis (1); hemature (1)
Gould, 1998 [152]	127	123/127 (97)	9/127 (7) febrile UTI (7)
Yip, et al, 1998 [153]	69	63/69 (91)	7/69 (10) stricture (1.4); fever (2.8); stent migration (4.2)
Sofer et al, 2001 [138]	542	531/542 (98)	24/598 (4)[*] stricture (0.3); UTI (0.6); ureteral perforation (1.2);
Matsuoka et al, 1999 [145]	88	80/88 (91)	-
Tawfiek et al, 1999 [147]	82[†]	81/82 (99)	6/51 (4)[†] fever (3.2)

[*]   includes an additional 56 patients with treated with renal calculi.

[†]   holmium laser used in 93% of patient population. Complications based on addition 73 patients with renal calculi.

applications in urology and other surgical specialities, holmium laser lithotripsy may be more cost-effective in the long term than some of the other devices. In our institution, using variable costs only, we have found that the average stone case treated with EHL costs approximately \$425.00 (US\$) compared to approximately \$70.00 (US\$) for the holmium laser. Therefore, even though the start-up costs of the laser are higher, the day-to-day expenses associated with non-laser treated cases are significant. With time, these higher variable costs will offset the higher capital cost of the laser. More importantly, the overall effectiveness of the holmium laser in dealing with routine and difficult stone patients makes this instrument invaluable without even considering the economic impact.

7.4   SUMMARY

From the early *in vitro* studies of Mulvaney and Beck [73], to the multiple clinical reports currently describing the success of stone fragmentation with the holmium laser, laser lithotripsy has developed from a mere possibility to a successful reality in just over 30 years (72). The holmium:YAG laser and the coumarin pulsed dye laser are the most common laser systems used today for laser lithotripsy. Stone-free rates are excellent, ranging from 70 to 100% and treatment is associated with a major complication rate of only 0.3 to 3%.

The holmium laser is a multi-purpose laser that has soft tissue applications in addition to its stone-fragmenting abilities. Its 2100 nm wavelength allows it to fragment all stone compositions. Conversely, the pulsed dye laser is limited to lithotripsy as its only application. Although dense calculi are sometimes resistant to fragmentation, its lack of tissue effects means that the pulsed dye laser has the largest margin of safety of all the laser systems for laser lithtripsy.

The only significant disadvantage for using lasers to treat urinary stones is the high start-up costs associated with purchasing a laser system. However, when one considers the high variable costs associated with some non-laser lithotripsy devices from the disposable equipment required, and the decreased success rates with these devices, laser lithotripsy may be more cost-effective in the long-term for some centers.

REFERENCES

1.   Goldman IL, Resnick MI, Buck AC. In: Wickham JEA, Buck AC, editors. Renal tract stone. Metabolic basis and clinical practice. London: Churchill Livingstone, 1990.
2.   DeVita MV, Zabetakis PM. Laboratory investigation of renal stone disease. Clinical Laboratory Medicine 1993; 13:225-234.

3. Pak CYC, Resnick MI. Introduction. In: Resnick MI, Pak CYC, editors. Urolithiasis. A medical and surgical reference. Philadelphia: W.B. Saunders Company, 1990.

4. Johnson CM, Wilson DM, O'Fallon WM, Malek RS, Kurland LT. Renal stone epidemiology: A 25-year study in Rochester, Minnesota. Kid Int 1979; 16:624-631.

5. Hiatt RA, Dabs LG, Friedman GD. Frequency of urolithiasis in a pre-paid medical care program. Am J Epid 1982; 115:255.

6. Sierakowski R, Finlayson B, Landes RR. The frequency of urolithiasis in hospital discharge diagnoses in the United States. Invest Urol 1987; 15:438-441.

7. Frangos DN, Rous SN. Incidence and economic factors in urolithiasis. In: Rous SN, editor. Stone disease. Diagnosis and management. Orlando: Grune and Strutton, Inc., 1987.

8. Menon M, Parulkar BG, Drach GW. Urinary lithiasis: Etiology, diagnosis, and medical management. In: Walsh PC, Retik AB, Vaughan ED, Jr., Wein AJ, editors. Campbell's urology. Philadelphia: W.B. Saunders company, 1998: 2661-2733.

9. Robertson WG. Epidemiology of urinary stone disease. Urol Res 1990; 18(Supplement):S3-S8.

10. Boyce WH, Garvey FK, Strawcutter HE. Incidence of urinary calculi among patients in general hospitals, 1948 to 1952. JAMA 1956; 161:1437.

11. Prince CL, Scardino PL. A statistical analysis of ureteral calculi. J Urol 1960; 83:561.

12. Scott R. The epidemiology of urolithiasis. In: Wickham JEA, Buck AC, editors. Renal tract stone. Metabolic basis and clinical practice. London: Churchill Livingstone, 1990.

13. Assimos DG, Boyce WH, Harrison LH, McCullough DL, Kroovand RL, Sweat et al. The role of open stone surgery since extracorporeal shock wave lithotripsy. J Urol 1989; 142(2 Pt 1):263-267.

14. Begun FP. Modes of intracorporeal lithotripsy: Ultrasound versus electrohydraulic lithotripsy versus laser lithotripsy. Semin Urol 1994; 12:39-50.

15. Spirnak JP, Resnick MI. Extracorporeal shockwave lithotripsy. In: Resnick MI, Pak CYC, editors. Urolithiasis. A medical and surgical reference. Philadelphia: W.B. Saunders company, 1990.

16. Glowacki LS, Beecroft ML, Cook RJ, Pahl D, Churchill DN. The natural history of asymptomatic urolithiasis. J Urol 1992; 147:319-321.

17. Mee SL, Thuroff JW. Small caliceal stones: Is extracorporeal shoce wave lithotripsy justified? J Urol 1988; 139:908-910.

18. Andersson L, Sylven M. Small caliceal calculi as a cause of pain. J Urol 1983; 130:752.

19. Brannen GE, Bush WH, Lewis GP. Caliceal calculi. J Urol 1986; 135:1142.

20. Zheng W, Denstedt JD, Segura JW. Urinary calculi in aviation pilots: What to do? Canadian Journal of Urology 6[3], 794. 1999. Ref Type: Abstract

21. Marberger M, Hofbauer J, Turk C, Hobarth K, Albrecht W. Management of ureteric stones. Eur Urol 1994; 25(4):265-272.

22. Morse RM, Resnick MI. Ureteral calculi: natural history and treatment in an era of advanced technology. J Urol 1991; 145(2):263-265.

23. Ueno A, Kawamura T, Ogawa A, Takayasu H . Relation of spontaneous passage of calculi to size. Urol 1977; 10:544-546.

24. Chaussy C, Brendel W, Schmiedt E. Extracorporeally induced destruction of kidney stones by shock waves. Lancet 1980; 2:1265-1268.

25. McCullough DL. Extracorporeal shock wave lithotripsy. In: Walsh PC, Retik AB, Stamey TA, Vaughan ED, Jr., editors. Campbell's Urology. Philadelphia: W.B. Saunders Company, 1992.

26. Segura JW. Surgical management of urinary calculi. Semin Nephrol 1990; 10(1):53-63.

27. Martin TV, Sosa RE. Shock-wave lithotripsy. In: Walsh PC, Retik AB, Vaughan ED, Jr., Wein AJ, editors. Campbell's urology. Philadelphia: W.B. Saunders Company, 1998: 2735-2752.

28. Chuong CJ, Zhong P, Preminger GM. A comparison of stone damage caused by different modes of shock wave generation. J Urol 1992; 148:200.

29. Streem SB. Contemporary clinical practice of shock wave lithotripsy: a reevaluation of contraindications. J Urol 1997; 157(4):1197-1203.

30. Zhong P, Preminger GM. Differing modes of shock-wave generation . Semin Urol 1994; 12:2-14.

31. Drach GW, Dretler SP, Fair W, Finlayson B, Gillenwater JY, Griffith DP et al. Report of the United States cooperative study of extracorporeal shock wave lithotripsy. J Urol 1986; 135:-1127.

32. Lingeman JE, Newman D, Mertz JH, Mosbaugh PG, Steele RE, Kahnoski RJ et al. Extracorporeal shock wave lithotripsy: the Methodist Hospital of Indiana experience. J Urol 1986; 135(6):1134-1137.

33. Graff J, Diederichs W, Schulze H. Long-term follow up in 1,003 extracorporeal shock wave lithotripsy patients. J Urol 1988; 140(3):479-483.

34. Wilson WT, Preminger GM. Extracorporeal shock wave lithotripsy. An update. Urol Clin North Am 1990; 17:231-242.

35. Rauchenwald M, Colombo T, Petritsch PH, Vilits P, Hubmer G. In situ extracorporeal shock wave lithotripsy of ureteral calculi with the MPL-9000X lithotriptor. J Urol 1992; 148(3 Pt 2):1097-1101.

36. Thomas R, Macaluso JN, Vandenberg T, Salvatore FT. An innovative approach to management of lower third ureteral calculi. J Urol 1993; 149(6):1427-1430.

37. Mobley TB, Myers DA, Jenkins JM, Grine WB, Jordan WR. Effects of stents on lithotripsy of ureteral calculi: treatment results with 18,825 calculi using the Lithostar lithotriptor [see comments]. J Urol 1994; 152(1):53-56.

38. Eden CG, Mark IR, Gupta RR, Eastman J, Shrotri NC, Tiptaft RC. Intracorporeal or extracorporeal lithotripsy for distal ureteral calculi? Effect of stone size and multiplicity on success rates. J Endourol 1998; 12(4):307-312.

39. Biri H, Kupeli B, Isen K, Sinik Z, Karaoglan U, Bozkirli I. Treatment of lower ureteral stones: Extracorporeal shockwave lithotripsy or intracorporeal lithotripsy? J Endourol 1999; 13(2):77-81.

40. Pardalidis NP, Kosmaoglou EV, Kapotis CG. Endoscopy vs. extracorporeal shockwave lithotripsy in the treatment of distal ureteral stones: Ten years' experience. J Endourol 1999; 13(3):161-164.

41. Turk TMT, Jenkins AD. A comparison of ureteroscopy to in situ extracorporeal shock wave lithotripsy for the treatment of distal ureteral calculi. J Urol 1999; 161(1):45-47.

42. Segura JW. Ureteroscopy for lower ureteral stones. Urol 1993; 42(4):356-357.

43. Peschel R, Janetschek G, Bartsch G. Extracorporeal shock wave lithotripsy versus ureteroscopy for distal ureteral calculi: a prospective randomized study. J Urol 1999; 162(6):1909-1912.

44. Dretler SP. Stone fragility. A new therapeutic distinction. J Urol 1988; 139:1124-1127.

45. Fernstrom I, Johansson B. Percutaneous pyelolithotomy. A new extraction technique. Scand J Urol Nephrol 1976; 10(3):257-259.

46. Spirnak JP, Resnick MI. Percutaneous management. In: Resnick MI, Pak CYC, editors. Urolithiasis. A medical and surgical reference. Philadelphia: W.B. Saunders Company, 1990.

47. Wollin TA, Denstedt JD. Intracorporeal lithotripters: function and features. Contem Urol 1997; 9(10):63-84.

48. Segura JW. Role of percutaneous procedures in the management of renal calculi. Urol Clin North Am 1990; 17(1):207-216.

49. Lingeman JE, Siegel YI, Steele B, Nyhuis AW, Woods JR. Management of lower pole nephrolithiasis: a critical analysis. J Urol 1994; 151:663-667.

50. Elbahnasy AM, Clayman RV, Shalhav AL, Hoenig DM, Chandoke P, Lingeman JE et al. Lower-pole caliceal stone clearance after shockwave lithtripsy, percutaneous nephrolithotomy, and flexible ureteteroscopy: impact of radiographic spatial anatomy. J Endourol 1998; 12(2):113-119.
51. Lingeman JE, Smith LH, Woods JR, Newman D. Bioeffects and long-term results of ESWL. In: Moster MB, editor. Urinary calculi: ESWL, endourology, and medical therapy. Philadelphia: Lea and Febiger, 1989.
52. Clayman RV, McDougall EM, Nakada SY. Endourology of the upper urinary tract: percutaneous renal and ureteral procedures . In: Walsh PC, Retik AB, Vaughan ED, Jr., Wein AJ, editors. Campbell's Urology. Philadelphia : W.B. Saunders Company, 1998: 2789-2874.
53. Young HH, McKay RW. Congenital valvular obstruction of the prostatic urethra. Surg Gynecol Obstet 1929; 48:409.
54. Goodman TM. Ureteroscopy with pediatric cystoscope in adults. Urol 1977; 9:394.
55. Lyon ES, Kyker JS, Schoenberg HW. Transurethral ureteroscopy in women: a ready addition to urologic armamentarium. J Urol 1978; 119:35.
56. Huffman JL. Ureteroscopy. In: Walsh PC, Retik AB, Vaughan ED, Jr., Wein AJ, editors. Campbell's Urology. Philadelphia: W.B. Saunders Company, 1998: 2755-2787.
57. Goodfriend R. Ultrasonic and electrohydraulic lithotripsy of ureteral calculi. Urol 1984; 23(1):5-8.
58. Lytton B, Green DF, Green DF. Complications of ureteral endoscopy. J Urol 1987; 137(4):649-653.
59. Harmon WJ, Sershon PD, Blute ML, Patterson DE, Segura JW. Ureteroscopy: current practice and long-term complications. J Urol 1997; 157:28-32.
60. Stoller ML, Wolf JS, Jr., Hofmann R, Marc B. Ureteroscopy without routine balloon dilation: An outcome assessment. J Urol 1992; 147:1238-1242.
61. Watson GM, Landers B, Nauth-Misir R, Wickham JEA. Developments in the ureteroscopes, techniques and accessories associated with laser lithotripsy. World J Urol 1993; 11:19-25.
62. Denstedt JD. Intracorporeal lithotriptors. In: Smith AD, Badlani GH, Bagley DH, Clayman RV, Jordan GH, Kavoussi LR et al., editors. Smith's Textbook of Endourology. St. Louis: Quality medical publishing, Inc., 1996: 60-77.
63. Howards SS, Merill E, Harris S, Cohn J. Ultrasonic lithotripsy. Laboratory evaluations. Invest Urol 1974; 11:273-277.
64. Denstedt JD, Eberwein PM, Singh RR. The Swiss Lithoclast: a new device for intracorporeal lithotripsy. J Urol 1992; 148:1088-1090.
65. Denstedt JD. Use of Swiss Lithoclast for percutaneous nephrolithotripsy. J Endourol 1993; 7(6):477-480.
66. Schulze H, Haupt G, Piergiovanni M, Wisard M, von Niederhausern W, Senge T. The Swiss Lithoclast: a new device for endoscopic stone disintegration.J Urol 1993;149:15-18.
67. Tawfiek ER, Grasso M, Bagley DH. Initial use of Browne Pneumatic Impactor. J Endourol 1997; 11(2):121-124.
68. Clayman RV. Techniques in percutaneous removal of renal calculi. Mechanical extraction and electrohydraulic lithotripsy. Urol 1984; 23:11-19.
69. Reuter HJ, Kern E. Electronic lithotripsy of ureteral calculi. J Urol 1973; 110:181-183.
70. Denstedt JD, Clayman RV. Electrohydraulic lithotripsy of renal and ureteral calculi. J Urol 1990; 143(1):13-17.
71. Elashry OM, DiMeglio RB, Nakada SY, McDougall EM, Clayman RV. Intracorporeal electrohydraulic lithotripsy of ureteral and renal calculi using small caliber (1.9F) electrohydraulic lithotripsy probes. J Urol 1996; 156(5):1581-1585.
72. Dretler SP. Laser lithotripsy: A review of 20 years of research and clinical applications. Lasers Surg Med 1988; 8:341-356.

73. Mulvaney WP, Beck CW. The laser beam in urology. J Urol 1968; 99:112-115.
74. Fair HD. In vitro destruction of urinary calculi by laser-induced stress waves. Medical Intrumentation 1978; 12:100-105.
75. Tanahashi Y, Numata I, Kambe K, Harada K, Chiba Y, Toyota S et al. Transurethral disintegration of urinary calculi by the use of the laser beam. In: Kaplan I, editor. Laser surgery IV. Proceedings of the fourth international symposium on laser surgery. Jerusalem: Academic Press, 1981: 30-33.
76. Pensel J, Frank F, Rothenberger K, Hofstetter A, Unsold E. Destruction of urinary calculi by neodymium-YAG laser irradiation. In: Kaplan I, editor. Laser surgery IV. Proceedings of the fourth international symposium on laser surgery. Jerusalem: Academic Press, 1981: 4-6.
77. Watson G, Wickham JEA, Mills TN, Brown SG, Swain P, Salmon PR. Laser fragmentation of renal calculi. Br J Urol 1983; 55:613-616.
78. Watson G, Murray S, Dretler SP, Parrish JA. The pulsed dye laser for fragmenting urinary calculi. J Urol 1987; 138:195-198.
79. Watson G, Murray S, Dretler SP, Parrish JA. An assessment of the pulsed dye laser for fragmenting calculi in the pig ureter. J Urol 1987; 138(1):199-202.
80. Nishioka NS, Kelsey PB, Kibbi AG, Delmonico F, Parrish JA, Anderson RR. Laser lithotripsy: Animal studies of safety and efficacy. Lasers Surg Med 1988; 8:357-362.
81. Dretler SP, Watson G, Murray S, Parrish JA. Laser fragmentation of ureteral calculi: Clinical experience. Lasers Surg Med 1986; 6:191.
82. Watson GM, Wickham JE. Initial experience with a pulsed dye laser for ureteric calculi. Lancet 1986; 1(8494):1357-1358.
83. Dretler SP, Watson G, Parrish JA, Murray S. Pulsed dye laser fragmentation of ureteral calculi: initial clinical experience. J Urol 1987; 137:386-389.
84. Nishioka NS, Teng P, Deutsch TF, Anderson RR. Mechanism of laser-induced fragmentation of urinary and biliary calculi. Lasers Life Sci 1987; 1:231-245.
85. Coptcoat MJ, Ison KT, Watson G, Wickham JE. Lasertripsy for ureteric stones in 120 cases: lessons learned. Br J Urol 1988; 61 (6):487-489.
86. Dretler SP. Techniques of laser lithotripsy. J Endourol 1988; 2:123-129.
87. Watson GM, Wickham JEA. The development of a laser and a miniaturised system for ureteric stone management. World J Urol 1989; 7:147-150.
88. Dretler SP. An evaluation of ureteral laser lithotripsy: 225 consecutive patients. J Urol 1990; 143(2):267-272.
89. Gautier JR, Leandri P, Rossignol G, Caissel J, Quintens H. Pulsed dye laser in the treatment of 325 calculi of the urinary tract. Eur Urol 1990; 18(1):6-9.
90. Govier FE, Gibbons RP, Correa RJ, Brannen GE, Weissman RM, Pritchett et al. Pulsed dye laser fragmentation of ureteral calculi: a review of the first 50 cases performed at Virginia Mason Medical Center. J Urol 1990; 143(4):685-686.
91. Dretler SP, Bhatta KM. Clinical experience with high power (140 mj.), large fiber (320 micron) pulsed dye laser lithotripsy. J Urol 1991; 146(5):1228-1231.
92. Fugelso P, Neal PM. Endoscopic laser lithotripsy: safe, effective therapy for ureteral calculi. J Urol 1991; 145(5):949-951.
93. Grasso M, Shalaby M, el Akkad M, Bagley DH. Techniques in endoscopic lithotripsy using pulsed dye laser. Urol 1991; 37(2):138-144.
94. Vandeursen H, Pittomvils G, Boving R, Baert L. High energy pulsed dye laser lithotripsy: management of ureteral calcium oxalate monohydrate calculi. J Urol 1991; 145(6):1146-1150.
95. Psihramis KE. Laser lithotripsy of the difficult ureteral calculus: results in 122 patients. J Urol 1992; 147(4):1010-1012.
96. Ng FC, Ravi T, Lim PH, Chng HC. Pulsed dye laser lithotripsy--the Toa Payoh Hospital experience. Br J Urol 1992; 69(4):358-362.

97. MacDermott JP, Grove J, Clark PB. Laser lithotripsy with the Candela MDL-2000 LaserTripter. Br J Urol 1993; 71(5):512-515.
98. Schmidt A, Eisenberger F. Lasertripsy of ureteral calculi using pulsed-dye laser with automatic shut-off after tissue contact. J Endourol 1993; 7(3):201-204.
99. Grasso M, Bagley DH. Endoscopic pulsed-dye laser lithotripsy: 159 consecutive cases. J Endourol 1994; 8(1):25-27.
100. Boline GB, Belis JA. Outpatient fragmentation of ureteral calculi with mini-ureteroscopes and laser lithotripsy. J Endourol 1994; 8(5):341-343.
101. Baba S, Asanuma H, Tazaki H. Pulsed dye laser lithotripsy for ureteral stone fragmentation. Keio J Med 1993; 42(4):209-211.
102. Boline GB, Belis JA. Lasertripsy of upper urinary tract calculi after unsuccessful extracorporeal lithotripsy or ureteroscopy: Comparison with primary lithotripsy. J Endourol 1993; 7:473-476.
103. Hofmann R, Hartung R, Geissdorfer K, Ascherl R, Erhardt W, Schmidt-Kloiber H et al. Laser induced shock wave lithotripsy- biologic effects of nanosecond pulses. J Urol 1988; 139:1077-1079.
104. Thomas S, Pensel J, Engelhardt R, Meyer W, Hofstetter AG. The pulsed dye laser versus the Q-switched Nd:YAG laser in laser- induced shock-wave lithotripsy. Lasers Surg Med 1988; 8(4):363-370.
105. Hofmann R, Hartung R, Schmidt-Kloiber H, Reichel E. First clinical experience with a Q-switched neodymium:YAG laser for urinary calculi. J Urol 1989; 141(2):275-279.
106. Hofmann R, Hartung R. Laser lithotripsy of ureteral calculi. Urol Res 1990; 18 Suppl 1:S49-55.
107. Maghraby H, Knipper A, Muschter R, Hofstetter AG. Laser lithotripsy: Further experience with Nd:YAG laser. J Endourol 1990; 4(2):161-167.
108. Benizri E, Wodey J, Amiel J, Toubol J. Comparison of 2 pulsed lasers for lithotripsy of ureteral calculi: report on 154 patients. J Urol 1993; 150(6):1803-1805.
109. Mattioli S, Cremona M, Benaim G, Ferrario A. Lithotripsy with a Q-switched alexandrite laser system. Eur Urol 1991; 19:233-235.
110. Strunge C, Brinkmann R, Flemming G, Engelhardt R. Interspersion of fragmented fiber's splinters into tissue during pulsed alexandrite laser lithotripsy. Lasers Surg Med 1991; 11(2):183-187.
111. Weber HM, Miller K, Ruschoff J. Alexandrite laser lithotripter in experimental and first clinical application. J Endourol 1991; 5:51-55.
112. Pertusa C, Albisu A, Acha M, Blasco M, Llarena R, Arregui P. Lithotripsy with the alexandrite laser: our initial 100 clinical cases. Eur Urol 1991; 20(4):269-271.
113. Denstedt JD, Chun SS, Miller MD. Intracorporeal lithotripsy with the alexandrite laser. Lasers Surg Med 1997; 20(4):433-436.
114. Pearle MS, Sech SM, Cobb CG, Riley JR, Clark PJ, Preminger GM et al. Safety and efficacy of the Alexandrite laser for the treatment of renal and ureteral calculi. Urol 1998; 51(1):33-38.
115. Nishioka NS, Domankevitz Y. Reflectance during pulsed holmium laser irradiation of tissue. Lasers Surg Med 1989; 9:375-381.
116. Gilling PJ, Cass CB, Malcolm A, Cresswell M, Fraundorfer MR, Kabalin JN. Holmium laser resection of the prostate versus neodymium:yttrium-aluminum-garnet visual laser ablation of the prostate: a randomized prospective comparison of two techniques for laser prostatectomy. Urol 1998; 51(4):573-577.
117. Moody JA, Lingeman JE. Holmium laser enucleation of the prostate with tissue morcellation: initial United States experience. J Endourol 2000; 14(2):219-223.
118. Erhard MJ, Bagley DH. Urologic applications of the holmium laser: preliminary experience. J Endourol 1995; 9(5):383-386.

119. Singal RK, Denstedt JD, Razvi HA, Chun SS. Holmium:YAG laser endoureterotomy for treatment of ureteral stricture. Urol. In press.
120. Razvi HA, Chun SS, Denstedt JD, Sales JL. Soft-tissue applications of the holmium:YAG laser in urology. J Endourol 1995; 5:387-390.
121. Johnson DE. Use of the holmium:YAG (Ho:YAG) laser for treatment of superficial bladder carcinoma. Lasers Surg Med 1994; 14:213-218.
122. Janis LR, Kravitz RD, Wagner SS. The pulsed holmium:yttrium-aluminum-garnet laser. Applications to ankle arthroscopy. Clin Podiatr Med Surg 1994; 11:483-498.
123. Koch DD, Abarca A, Villarreal R. Hyperopia correction by noncantact holmium:YAG laser thermal keratoplasty. Clinical study with two-year follow-up. Ophthalmology 1996; 103:731-740.
124. Gleich LL, Rebeiz EE, Pankratov MM, Shapshay SM. The holmium:YAG laser-assisted otolaryngologic procedures. Arch Otolaryngol Head Neck Surg 1995; 121(10):1162-1166.
125. Panwar SS, Martin FW. Trans-nasal endoscopic holmium: YAG laser correction of choanal atresia. J Laryngol Otol 1996; 110(5):429-431.
126. White CJ, Ramee SR, Collins TJ, Mesa JE, Murgo JP. Holmium: YAG laser-assisted coronary angioplasty with multifiber delivery catheters. Cathet Cardiovasc Diagn 1993; 30(3):205-210.
127. de Marchena EJ, Mallon SM, Knopf WD, Parr K, Moses JWM-CD, Myerburg RJ . Effectiveness of holmium laser-assisted coronary angioplasty. The Holmium Laser Coronary Registry. American Journal of Cardiology 1994; 73(2):117-121.
128. Koslin MG, Martin JC. The use of the holmium laser for temporomandibular joint arthroscopic surgery. J Oral Maxillofac Surg 1993; 51(2):122-123.
129. Das AK, Chiura A, Conlin MJ, Eschelman D, Bagley DH. Treatment of biliary calculi using holmium: yttrium aluminum garnet laser. Gastrointestinal Endoscopy 1998; 48(2):207-209.
130. Monga M, Gabal-Shehab LL, Kamarei M, D'Agostino H. Holmium laser lithotripsy of a complicated biliary calculus. J Endourol 1999; 13(7):505-506.
131. McCaughan JS, Jr., Heinzmann HG, McMahon D. Impacted broncholiths removed with the holmium: YAG laser. Lasers Surg Med 1996; 19(2):230-232.
132. Johnson DE, Cromeens DM, Price RE. Use of the holmium:YAG laser in urology. Lasers Surg Med 1992; 12(4):353-363.
133. Jansen ED, Asshauer T, Frenz M, Motamedi M, Delacretaz G, Welch AJ. Effect of pulse duration on bubble formation and laser-induced pressure waves during holmium laser ablation. Lasers Surg Med 1996; 18(3):278-293.
134. Nishioka NS, Domankevitz Y, Flotte TJ, Anderson RR. Ablation of rabbit liver, stomach, and colon with a pulsed holmium laser. Gastroenterology 1989; 96(3):831-837.
135. Zhong P, Tong HL, Cocks FH, Pearle MS, Preminger GM. Transient cavitation and acoustic emission produced by different laser lithotripters. J Endourol 1998; 12:371-378.
136. Vassar GJ, Teichman JMH, Glickman RD, Weintraub SE, Chan KF, Pfefer TJ et al. Holmium:YAG lithotripsy: photothermal mechanism. J Endourol 1999; 13:181-190.
137. Teichman JM, Champion PC, Wollin TA, Denstedt JD. Holmium:YAG lithotripsy of uric acid calculi . J Urol 1998; 160(6 Pt 1):2130-2132.
138. Sofer M, Watterson JD, Wollin TA, Nott L, Razvi HA, Denstedt JD. Holmium:YAG laser lithotripsy for upper urinary tract calculi in 598 patients. Accepted for publication, J Urol. 2001.
139. Corbin NS, Teichman JM, Nguyen T, Glickman RD, Rihbany L, Pearle MS et al. Laser lithotripsy and cyanide. J Endourol 2000; 14(2):169-173.
140. Denstedt JD, Razvi HA, Sales JL, Eberwein PM. Preliminary experience with holmium: YAG laser lithotripsy. J Endourol 1995; 9(3):255-258.
141. Matsuoka K, Iida S, Nakanami M, Koga H , Shimada A, Mihara T et al. Holmium: yttrium-aluminum-garnet laser for endoscopic lithotripsy. Urol 1995; 45(6):947-952.

142. Fuchs GJ. Ultrasonic lithotripsy in the ureter. Urol Clin North Am 1988; 15(3):347-359.
143. Grasso M, Chalik Y. Principles and applications of laser lithotripsy: experience with the holmium laser lithotrite. Journal of Clinical Laser Medicine & Surgery 1998; 16(1):3-7.
144. Grasso M, Conlin M, Bagley D. Retrograde ureteropyeloscopic treatment of 2 cm. or greater upper urinary tract and minor Staghorn calculi. J Urol 1998; 160(2):346-351.
145. Matsuoka K, Iida S, Inoue M, Yoshii S, Arai K, Tomiyasu K et al. Endoscopic lithotripsy with the holmium:YAG laser. Lasers Surg Med 1999; 25(5):389-395.
146. Gould DL. Retrograde flexible ureterorenoscopic holmium-YAG laser lithotripsy: the new gold standard. Tech Urol 1998; 4(1):22-24.
147. Tawfiek ER, Bagley DH. Management of upper urinary tract calculi with ureteroscopic techniques. Urol 1999; 53(1):25-31.
148. Mugiya S, Ohhira T, Un-No T, Takayama T, Suzuki K, Fujita K. Endoscopic management of upper urinary tract disease using a 200-microm holmium laser fiber: initial experience in Japan. Urol 1999; 53(1):60-64.
149. Devarajan R, Ashraf M, Beck RO, Lemberger RJ, Taylor MC. Holmium: YAG lasertripsy for ureteric calculi: an experience of 300 procedures. Br J Urol 1998; 82(3):342-347.
150. Shroff S, Watson GM, Parikh A, Thomas R, Soonawalla PF, Pope A. The holmium: YAG laser for ureteric stones. Br J Urol 1996; 78(6):836-839.
151. Scarpa RM, De Lisa A, Porru D, Usai E. Holmium:YAG laser ureterolithotripsy. Eur Urol 1999; 35(3):233-238.
152. Gould DL. Holmium:YAG laser and its use in the treatment of urolithiasis: our first 160 cases. J Endourol 1998; 12(1):23-26.
153. Yip KH, Lee CW, Tam PC. Holmium laser lithotripsy for ureteral calculi: an outpatient procedure. J Endourol 1998; 12(3):241-246.

Chapter 8

LASER DERMATOLOGY

Geoffrey Dougherty[1] and Terence Ryan[2]
[1]Faculty of Allied Health Sciences, Kuwait University, KUWAIT
[2]Oxford Brookes University, Oxford, U.K.

8.1 INTRODUCTION

The impact of lasers in the field of dermatology has been quite large, whether as a tool to measure blood supply or as a means of destroying specific structures within the skin. The technology of the laser is a major advance. Nevertheless, there is probably - even with current technology - some fine tuning yet to be done, based not on the properties of the laser but on a greater understanding of the skin. There is a tendency to consider the skin as a homogeneous organ, without recognition of its great variety and the influence of site, age and pathology.

In order to understand as to why in recent years laser technology has been embraced by the dermatology profession, it is necessary to review the functions of the skin. Most textbooks in the past emphasized that the skin was for protection and that the epidermis was a barrier layer between one's inside and the environment. Its innervation allowed one to sense danger and its blood supply was more for thermoregulation than for anything else. In recent years, there has been more emphasis on the skin as an organ of display. In the sense of "love at first sight" or "color prejudice" it is an organ of communication. When the World Health Organization embraced well-being within the term "health", it allowed the "look good, feel good" factor to come to the fore and justified the work of the cosmetic surgeon and the marketing of the cosmetic industry to restore disfigurement, to manage the consequences of aging and to destroy unwanted pathology.

There was, in the past, one snag - which was that to remove one component of the skin without damaging adjacent tissues was an impossibility, and especially the epidermis was in the way in all maneuvers aimed at the destruction of a dermal component. To be able to focus, with lasers, on the dermis without destroying the epidermis was a major advance, but mistakes were made because the technician regarded anything that looked pink as being a blood vessel and anything that looked brown as being a melanocyte, and there was an assumption that the anatomy of these components of the skin varied only a little.

With respect to pigment, most pigment is produced by the melanocytes, which lie in the basal cell layer of the epidermis and pump melanin into the epidermal cells. Sometimes, however, there is incontinence and the pumping system results in melanin passing into the dermis, where it is taken up by macrophages and can remain at various depths within the dermis for years. Obviously, therefore, to remove melanin from the epidermis or from the dermis requires at least some investigation as to its siting. Usually, Wood's light is helpful in this respect, this being the range of ultra-violet rays which border on the blue. When it is shone on the skin, it is quite easy to detect whether the melanin is in the most superficial layers of the skin - such as the epidermis - or whether it resides at a deeper level.

With respect to the vascularity of the skin, pinkness is due to hemoglobin and usually this resides within a blood vessel, which if it is compressed empties and this results in blanching. Blood that has leaked outside the blood vessel, known as purpura, does not blanch on pressure. Similarly, if there is a relationship between the epidermis and its blood vessel, such that loops of vasculature are surrounded by epidermis, they will not always empty on compression. The anatomy of normal vasculature includes capillary loops draining into a horizontal venous plexus. Blood vessels in the skin may have a diameter as large as 100-300 μm, and in disease states they may be considerably larger than this. Blue light reflected from the deeper layers of the skin passes through the epidermis with greater facility than red light. This is why some deep elements like veins or blue nevi appear to be blue - whereas in fact they have red blood and reddish-brown pigment. While some of the pinkness of the skin can be reflected from quite deep layers, most of the color of the skin comes from the horizontal sub-papillary plexus of venules. If, however, the capillary loops are elongated and tortuous - as they may be in port wine birthmarks, or in psoriasis and some congestive disorders of the lower legs due to venous diseases - then these vessels lying in the uppermost dermis may contribute most of the color. That which can be seen on the surface of the skin depends on the thickness of the epidermis and, to some extent, the amount of tissue fluid lying between the vessel and the epidermis. In certain inflammatory conditions, cell infiltrates can also prevent the color penetrating through to the surface: thus, edema fluid can produce pallor, and melanin can produce a brown screen.

Fine tuning of laser therapy probably requires knowledge of the exact relationship of the elements of the skin. The use of a magnifying lens of between 12 to 25 X can be helpful in this respect, but it is also necessary to indent the skin with some form of probe to see whether edema fluid is playing a part in paling the pink. The modern dermal scans using high frequency ultrasound are a great advance with respect to identifying the exact depth of the skin, and an important observation is that such equipment can measure the thickness of the epidermis and also the relative water component in the upper dermis.

It is a new finding that much of the variability of the upper dermis is dependent on its water content. There is diurnal variation. Water collects when any part of the body is dependent, due to the effects of gravity: elevation can make some of the water disappear. Water in the upper dermis is held within the ground substance, but the balance between delivery by the blood vessel system and removal by the lymphatics plays some part. Those who use lasers should understand how small are the distances being discussed. Almost everything lies in a level less than 1 mm in depth and usually less than 0.3 mm. Certainly when one is dealing with pathology the depths increase, but one is still talking in terms of a few millimeters, and most cosmetic work is less than 1 mm in depth.

Patient satisfaction is not proportional to the amount of destruction that has occurred in the skin. Patients want to look young without scarring. In order to do this, a full assessment of the lesion by contemporary technology is required. It is always best to under-do destructive processes, and some camouflage may also be a supplement to management. It is a fact that most men do not like to put camouflage on, but all women use lipstick and equivalents of foundation creams and rouge. The difficulties become much greater in the pigmented Asian or Middle Eastern skin. The size, shape, depth and distribution of the chromophore and its surrounding tissues are variables that influence the pattern and degree of response to laser therapy. Skin is not homogenous: pigment size, depth and distribution varies with region, age and pathology. The visibility of the damaged chromophore also is dependent on the density and reflection of the tissues intervening between it and the observer. A knowledge of wound healing and factors predisposing to keloids is desirable. The upper arm, chest and legs are the most common sites for keloids. Deeper and infected wounds are more likely to heal with hypertrophy, and a family history of keloids should always be considered.

8.2 BASIC PRINCIPLES AND CONCEPTS

8.2.1 Laser Beam

Laser light can be delivered as continuous (CW), "pseudo-continuous" or pulsed beams. The continuous wave lasers, such as the carbon dioxide, argon, krypton, and argon dye lasers, emit a beam that is at constant energy. "Pseudo-continuous" wave lasers, such as the copper lasers, emit a beam in which the pulses are so rapid that the light appears to be continuous. Pulsed lasers can be subdivided into long pulsed (~ microseconds) and short-pulsed (~ nanoseconds) lasers, depending on their pulse durations. The flashlamp-pumped pulsed dye laser (PDL) is a long-pulsed laser emitting a beam with a pulse duration of 450 μs. The Q-switched lasers have photooptical shutters that allow extremely short bursts of high-energy laser light in the nanosecond range. This high power output (~ 10^9 W) is delivered to the tissue in nanoseconds. The energy is transformed into heat so rapidly, causing temperature rises of ~ 300° C in tens of nanoseconds, that tissue treated, be it melanosomes or tattoo pigment, explodes [1].

8.2.2 Some Characteristic Features of Laser Light

Laser light has physical properties that are therapeutically useful. In particular, it is

(i)   spatially and temporally coherent

The light waves comprising laser light are aligned with each other (i.e. coherent), travelling in exactly the same parallel direction over large distances with very little divergence, a property known as collimation. This makes the light extremely focusable, allowing a high intensity to be applied over a small area.

(ii)   monochromatic

i.e., it comprises a very narrow range of wavelengths. This enables appropriate laser sources to be chosen to selectively target particular chromophores (a chromophore is a group of atoms that imparts a color to a substance and absorbs a specific wavelength of light). For example, oxyhemoglobin has absorption peaks at 400 nm (violet), 541 mm (green) and 577 nm (yellow). Theoretically, light at or near these wavelengths will be selectively absorbed into blood vessels and will spare adjacent structures. (In practice, however, wavelength selection is rarely sufficient to produce selective damage because blood vessels are relatively large (100 - 300 μm) and because heat is conducted to contiguous structures [2].

The most importance characteristics of laser light are irradiance, energy fluence, and exposure time. Irradiance, or power density, is the power per unit area incident on the skin during a single pulse and is given by:

$$\text{Irradiance (W/cm}^2) = \frac{\text{Laser power output (W)}}{\text{Laser beam cross-sectional area (cm}^2)}$$

For example, a carbon dioxide laser with a power output of 50 W and spot size with a diameter of 0.5 cm produces an irradiance of about 250 W/cm^2. If the beam is focused to a smaller spot size (diameter 0.2 cm), the irradiance increases to about 1500 W/cm^2.

Energy fluence, or energy density, is the energy per unit area incident on the skin for a specified length of time. For a single laser pulse of constant power, the energy fluence is the product of the irradiance and the time of exposure.

$$\text{Fluence (J/cm}^2) = \frac{\text{Laser power output (W) x Exposure time (sec)}}{\text{Laser beam cross-sectional area (cm}^2)}$$

Fluence can be adjusted on many of the newer pulsed and Q-switched lasers. Increasing the fluence increases the energy to which the skin is exposed if beam diameter and exposure time are constant.

Divergence of the laser beam occurs when the cross-sectional area of the spot size increases as the handpiece is moved away from its focal point. The beam can be focused by holding the handpiece close to the skin, narrowing the diameter of the spot size and decreasing the divergence. Carbon dioxide lasers have different applications depending on the divergence of the beam. The focused beam of the carbon dioxide laser can be used as a cutting tool. The defocused beam is used for ablation or superficial destruction, as in the treatment of verruca [3,4].

The wavelength of the light produced by a laser depends on the active medium. Carbon dioxide lasers produce an invisible infrared beam of wavelength 10.6 μm: and the argon laser produces a 488 nm wavelength, blue-green beam. Depth of penetration of laser light through skin increases directly with the wavelength of the light. Therefore, the longer wavelength of the Q-switched ruby laser (694 nm) is more likely to lighten deeper dermal pigmented processes than the shorter wavelength visible light lasers [5] (Table 1).

8.2.3 Basic Elements of Laser-Tissue Interaction

The interaction of laser light with the skin is complex and dependent on many factors. The clinical and histologic response of skin to laser light varies

Table 1. Laser systems in dermatology

Laser system	Wavelength (nm)	Output mode	Absorption characteristics
Argon (blue-green)	488-514	CW	Hemoglobin, melanin
Dye (pigment)	500 - 520	Pulsed	Melanin
Copper (green)	511	Pulsed	Hemoglobin, melanin
Krypton (green)	521,530	CW	Hemoglobin, melanin
Frequency doubled: Nd:YAG (green)	532	Q-switched	Melanin, tattoos (red), hemoglobin
Krypton (yellow)	568	CW	Hemoglobin
Copper (yellow)	578	Pulsed	Hemoglobin
Argon ion-pumped dye (yellow, red)	585, 630	CW	Hemoglobin, melanin
Dye (vascular)	577, 585	CW, Pulsed	Hemoglobin
Ruby	694	Q-switched	Melanin, tattoos
Alexandrite	755	Q-switched	Tattoos, melanin
Nd: YAG (infrared)	1064	CW, Q-switch	Protein, tattoos
Er: YAG (infrared)	2940	Pulsed	H_2O
CO_2 (infrared)	10, 600	Pulsed	H_2O

considerably depending on the type of laser used, viz. whether pulsed, continuous-wave, or "pseudo-continuous" and the energy fluence.

Skin characteristics, however, are less well defined. Chromophores absorb the majority of laser light incident on the skin. The primary chromophores of the skin are oxyhemoglobin (with three main absorption peaks at 418, 542 and 577 nm) and melanin (which has a very broad range of absorption). Although not a true chromophore, intracellular and extracellular water is another component of skin that can determine the specificity of laser-tissue interaction, especially for the infrared lasers. The water content influences the quality of the thermal effect produced by some lasers, which can range from protein denaturation at temperatures of 40°C, to coagulation at temperatures of 60°C, vaporization at 100°C, and carbonization at 300°C.

Selective heat damage (photothermolysis) makes it possible to selectively target and destroy specific cellular and subcellular structures, a process of denaturing protein coagulation and vaporizing or charring the tissues whilst sparing normal structures. It occurs only if the wavelength of the laser light is appropriate and the time to heat the target is less than the time it takes for heat to diffuse from the target [6] (the thermal relaxation time). In other words, large objects take longer to cool. Thermal relaxation time decreases with decreasing target size: it is 1 - 10 ms for a blood vessel (diameter, 50 - 100 μm) in a port wine stain, but only 1μs for a subcellular particle 0.5 μm in size, such as a tattoo pigment granule or a melanosome [7].

The early lasers used in dermatology (e.g. argon, argon dye-tunable and copper vapor lasers) produced light as a continuous beam: their shuttering mechanisms were unable to produce pulses shorter than 20 ms - much longer than the thermal relaxation time of blood vessels in a pale port wine stain. However, subsequent technological developments - from the flashlamp-pumped dye laser, through fast-shuttered scanning vascular lasers, to Q-switched lasers - have resulted in much shorter pulses enabling treatment for vascular and pigmentary tissue targets.

Laser light can have a tissue effect only if it penetrates deeply enough to be absorbed by the target chromophore. Skin penetration increases with the wavelength of the light; vascular lasers penetrate no more than 1.2 mm at a wavelength of 565 nm, whilst the Q-switched Nd: YAG laser (at 1064 nm, in the near-infrared) penetrates about 2 mm. Longer wavelengths are needed for targets deeper in the dermis. However, as wavelength moves into the far-infrared range, tissue water becomes the major absorber and penetration decreases sharply. Clearly, chromophores will not be treatable if they lie deeper than the penetration of their most absorbed wavelength [8].

The use of lasers is safe when common sense and preventive measures are practiced [9]. It is usual to treat a small, representative area as a test site and review in eight weeks before proceeding to treatment of the whole lesion. A laser is not in direct contact, and therefore is less likely to spread viruses and other infections through contagion. The steam produced by vaporization does have the potential for spreading viruses that are present in the patient's tissue. Appropriate protection and vaccination against hepatitis viruses is an advisable precaution. Appropriate safety goggles that filter specific wavelengths of laser light should be worn at all times while the laser is in operation. When a carbon dioxide laser is used, flammability around the treatment site is of great concern. Cloth drapes should be wet with sterile water or saline solution. Metal instruments are usually burnished or ebonized to decrease reflection of laser light. Protective cylinders and shields are available that attach to the end of the handpiece to contain fumes, vaporized particles, and splattered blood and tissue. These vaporized particles may contain fragments of human papillomavirus DNA from verrucas treated with the carbon dioxide laser [10]. HIV p24 gag antigen has also been detected in plume smoke: however, infectivity is unknown [11]. Suction pumps and vacuum exhaust systems with submicron filters are employed to remove the plume and any potential infectious agents.

8.3 DERMATOLOGICAL APPLICATIONS OF LASERS

8.3.1 Therapeutic

The unique properties of lasers create an enormous potential for specific therapy of skin diseases. An immediate improvement in appearance is desirable, but this cannot always be expected. In the early days of this technology, there was always considerable purpura and major immediate discoloration of the skin. Of course, the major Hippocratic principle of "do not harm" must over-ride efficacy. Complete removal of the lesion is not always compatible with absence of scarring. The time taken to destroy unwanted tissue is a limiting factor. Advances are therefore aimed at speeding up the process, and to make treatment of large lesions a more rapid process a series of lasers is now available. The goal is to allow the physician to match optimally the laser and the treatment protocol to particular conditions such as abnormalities of skin surface topography and texture, vascular lesions, and pigmented lesions. The laser can cut like the sharpest of scalpels while, at the same time, it can coagulate and therefore prevent bleeding and leakage of lymph, sealing all cut vessels as it passes through the tissues.

8.3.1.1　Surface Problems

The carbon dioxide (CO_2) laser operates at a wavelength of 10.6 μm (in the far infrared) which is absorbed by water. As water is the main component of skin, this laser is non-selective, ablating all tissue in its path to an even depth. It is useful for treating disorders of skin surface texture and tomography (wrinkles, scars, sun damage, benign skin appendages and thickening of the tissues such as rhinophyma, a condition in which the skin of the nose produces a grossly bulbous enlargement).

In the focused mode, the CO_2 laser is used as a hemostatic cutting tool (useful for patients with bleeding disorder or those taking anticoagulants). It does not use a fiber optic cable and acts close to the skin. In its defocused mode, lying further from the skin with a wider beam diameter, it is used as a skin surface ablative tool. In this mode , it produces a bloodless field destruction as it seals small blood vessels. It was a significant advance for conditions such as actinic cheilitis (precancerous change in the lips produced by ultra-violet light), some benign cutaneous tumors and recalcitrant warts [12-16].

The early CO_2 lasers had significant side effects. Heating of target tissues and consequent heat transmission to non-target tissues, such as dermal collagen, led to unacceptable levels of scarring and hypopigmentation in tattoo removal and skin resurfacing [17]. Many variables were difficult or impossible to quantify and varied between operators.

Noteworthy advances have been made in CO_2 lasers for treating the surface of the skin ("skin resurfacing"). Technology has reduced operator dependence, improving reproducibility of results. Two distinct approaches have been used to achieve char-free tissue ablation.

(i)   High-Energy, Short Pulsed CO_2 Lasers

This involves very high energy, short-pulsed CO_2 lasers, delivering peak pulse powers of 500 W, with an energy density of 5 J/cm^2, to a 3 mm defocused spot. The pulse is very short, well under 1 ms. This vaporizes tissue so rapidly and completely that little heated tissue is left to transmit heat to non-target tissues.

The second desirable characteristic of a high-energy, short pulsed CO_2 laser system is that the power applied to the skin is determined solely by the number of pulses per second which can be varied. With this system, each pulse is an individual event that applies a certain amount of energy to the skin; the energy density per unit area (fluence) determines the effect on tissue. The laser is passed over the skin at a speed that allows each area to be treated by a single pulse. Further passes may be necessary to achieve the desired depth of tissue ablation. For maximum surgical control (e.g., removing small lesions), minimum power or number of pulses per second is used.

A major advance is the collimated handpiece, a lens which keeps the beam always defocused, allowing the distance from the target tissue to be varied without varying the spot size or power density. This ensures even vaporization of tissue.

Recently, a scanning device (computerized pattern generator) has become available for this laser and has reduced the effect of hand speed variation. It places pulses in patterns of a different size, shape and area of overlap, enabling uniform application of laser energy to the skin and precise reproducibility between operators. The device also collimates the beam, enabling the operator to work at a distance from the skin.

(ii)   Short-dwell-time Scanning CO_2 Lasers

These produce char-free ablation by sharply focusing the beam, allowing high energy to be applied from a comparatively low energy laser system. The scanner rapidly moves a continuous beam in a spiral , keeping the dwell time at any particular point below 1 ms.

Both these systems achieve superficial ablation by delivering their energy within the thermal relaxation time of skin (less than 1 ms), thus achieving selective photothermolysis. The characteristic brown char caused by earlier CO_2 lasers, which correlates with slow boiling of tissue and indicates heat transmission outside the intended target, is replaced by a clean, white appearance, resulting in faster healing with fewer complications [18].

Uses of these lasers for treating abnormalities of surface topography or texture are shown in Table 2. For solar-induced epidermal damage and facial wrinkling, these laser systems have largely replaced dermabrasion and stronger chemical peeling as the treatment of choice. Areas that were previously untreatable (such as the eyelids) are now able to be treated.

Char-free carbon dioxide lasers are being used to treat facial wrinkles [19].   Results have been positive, although side effects have included transient erythema and pigmentation changes [20]. More recently, long pulsed ($\sim$ 10 ms) near-infrared (2940 nm) erbium-YAG lasers have been introduced. They have a very high degree of water absorption ($\sim$ 10 times that of CO_2 lasers) and a very short ($\sim$ 1μm) extinction coefficient. The effect of pulsed CO_2 lasers have been compared with long pulsed erbium:YAG lasers in the treatment of periocular and perioral wrinkles [21], assessing efficacy both clinically and histologically. The study suggested that the primary mechanism in the reduction of wrinkles may be a thermally induced collagen shortening and coagulation. The results were satisfactory with both systems.

For the difficult problem of acne scarring, modern CO_2 lasers are probably the best available treatment. However, in some cases they are still best supplemented with other methods, such as punch and dermal grafting, collagen implantation and fat transfer. Treatment of acne scars is always difficult, as results rarely meet patient expectations.

8.3.1.2   Keloids, Scars and Warts

The first lasers used to treat keloids and scars were continuous wave lasers. Results were disappointing, however, with a high rate of recurrence [22-23]. More recently, the pulsed dye laser (PDL) was successfully employed to treat hypertrophic scars [24]: scars flattened and skin markings reappeared. Keloid therapy may be improved by combining laser therapy with intralesional steroids and/or partially compressing the site. As with other therapies, it is keloids of the ear lobe that do best, and published results on keloid management should note the proportion of cases treated from this site in any series.

Table 2. Uses and effectiveness of the CO_2 laser

Problems	Effectiveness	Treatment of choice
Wrinkles (Perioral, periorbital, facial)	Excellent	Yes
Scars (Facial acne, traumatic, chickenpox)	Good	Often
Sun damage (Facial solar keratoses, actinic cheilitis, blotchy hypo-and hyperpigmentation)	Excellent	Often
Benign skin appendage tumours and infiltrates (Facial syringomas, trichoepitheliomas, adenoma sebaceum, xanthelasmas)	Good	Yes
Rhinophyma	Good	Yes
Warts (any region)	Fair	Rarely
Seborrhoeic keratoses (any region)	Fair	Rarely

A controlled study [25] on post-cardiac surgery mediastinal sternotomy scars evaluated 16 adults with hypertrophic or keloidal scars and compared laser-treated (pulsed dye, 585 nm, 450 µs) with untreated portions of the scars clinically and histologically. Color, texture, height, and symptoms improved significantly in all cases. Histology specimens of laser-treated areas contained normal numbers of fibroblasts compared with an increased number of fibroblasts found in untreated scars. Additionally, dermal collagen after PDL treatment was less dense than that of the untreated scars and an increased number of mast cells was also seen after laser treatment. Scars from surgeries as diverse as facelift, breast reconstruction, liposuction and trauma can be minimized with excellent patient satisfaction [26]. Red facial acne scars also improved with PDL treatment [27].

The carbon dioxide laser was the mainstay for the treatment of recalcitrant warts for many years. Warts responded variably to this modality, however, and a variety of side effects including scarring and painful healing accompanied treatment [28,29].

More recently investigators employed the PDL to treat 39 patients with recalcitrant warts. Excellent response rates and few side effects were seen [30]. A subsequent study examined the safety and efficacy of using the PDL to treat 721 recalcitrant and 25 untreated warts [31]. Warts were pared prior to treatment and sequential pulses (3-10) were delivered to the wart. Energy fluences varied with body site from 7 to 9.5 J/cm^2, and subjects were treated up to five times at 2 to 4 weeks intervals. PDL therapy was shown to be a highly effective and safe method to selectively destroy warts without damaging the surrounding skin. Response rates varied (84% - 99%) depending on location, and complications included transient hypopigmentation and scarring in one individual.

8.3.1.3   Skin Lesions

(i)   Vascular lesions

Laser therapy of vascular lesions uses wavelengths that match the absorption wavelengths of the target and short illumination times, around the thermal relaxation time of the target vessel (1-10 ms for diameters of 50 - 100 μm). All vascular lesions contain the endogenous chromophores hemoglobin and deoxyhemoglobin, which provide a convenient laser target. The pulsed dye laser (585 nm, 450 μs: several kW power output) is the treatment of choice for most vascular lesions. Vascular blemishes can be divided into those with clearly visible individual vessels and essentially normal-colored background skin (e.g. some telangiectasia) and those with diffuse erythema (e.g. port wine stains, surgical erythema, rosacea etc).

For telangiectasia with normal background skin, achieving selective photothermolysis is relatively unimportant, as focusing the laser beam to damage the precise area of the vessel is sufficient to spare adjacent tissue. Almost all laser systems that deliver wavelengths in the blue-green visible light range of 500-600 nm are acceptable, if used with a focused handpiece approximating the size of the vessel. Examples include the argon , argon dye-tunable, krypton, copper vapor and copper bromide lasers. The laser   is applied by slowly tracing the lesions with either a continuous beam or electronically shuttered 30 -100 ms flashes.

Diffuse erythema requires treatment of the entire area rather than tracing of individual vessels. This can be achieved with a "large footprint" laser, which treats an area 5-10 mm in diameter at a fixed distance in a single pulse. Usually this is done at eight-week intervals and several treatments are required. The optimal effect of the argon laser, especially for deeper lesions, may not be realized for twelve months.

Currently the treatment of choice for pediatric port wine stains and some pediatric hemangiomas is the pulsed dye laser, which has dramatically increased our capacity to treat pale port wine stains [32]. It produces selective short impact damage to vessels, resulting in purpura rather than the pallor, scabbing and blistering produced by older non-pulsed lasers. It has minimal complications but multiple treatment sessions are needed. Lighter port wine stains respond better than those that are dark or hypertrophic. It is usual to avoid overlap, and therefore initial results give a reticulate appearance which is improved by subsequent treatment.

Unfortunately port wine stains tend to darken in color and may thicken or develop nodules as the lesions age, thereby making treatment difficult in adult patients since they may require several laser sessions producing unpredictable results. A new technique using a combination of wavelengths and pulse durations (590-600 nm at 1.5 ms, and 585 nm at 450 µs) has shown complete removal of thick and nodular adult port wine stains in just a few sessions [33].

The flashlamp-pumped pulsed dye laser is expensive to operate and post-treatment purpura is inconvenient for cosmetic applications. It has been suggested that lengthening the pulses to 1-10 ms could prevent this side effect, while being short enough not to damage adjacent tissue. This has been achieved both with scanning systems and with high energy, large area, single pulse treatment with 532 nm, frequency-doubled Nd:YAG lasers. The Neodymium:Yttrium/Aluminum/Garnet laser is absorbed by tissue proteins rather than water, and is capable of penetration to a depth of 6 mm and able to coagulate vessels 4 mm in diameter. These lasers also achieve selective photothermolysis. Dynamic rapidly delivered refrigerant can be applied to the skin to protect the epidermis while energy is delivered to dermal chromophores, further increasing the safety margin.

With the pulsed dye laser, it is possible to treat, with a very low risk of side effects, most superficial (1-2 mm in depth) vascular lesions (Table 3), especially port wine stains and telangiectasia such as spider nevi (Figure 1), venous lakes and senile angiomas. In deeply pigmented skin, absorption by melanin diminishes its effectiveness. Scarring occurs in less than 1% of patients and it is not as effective as sclerotherapy for ectatic leg veins. Temporary hyperpigmentation occurs in about 10% of patients. It is the treatment of choice for pediatric port wine stains. Treatment of pediatric hemangiomas can also be effective, but only if started very early, when the lesion is flat. The short penetration of the laser (1.2 mm) limits its effectiveness to lesions in the upper dermis; it has no role in treating subcutaneous hemangiomas. Surprisingly, however, it can be very effective in aiding healing of ulcerated hemangiomas.

Other large-footprint and scanning vascular lasers (copper vapor, argon-pumped, continuous-wave, tunable dye) are proving effective in treating diverse erythema, telangiectasia and some adult port wine stains. This is a therapy for which large fees may be charged, and it should not be forgotten that lesions such as spider nevi can be treated cheaply and effectively by older technology such as cautery and electrolysis. The aim of producing

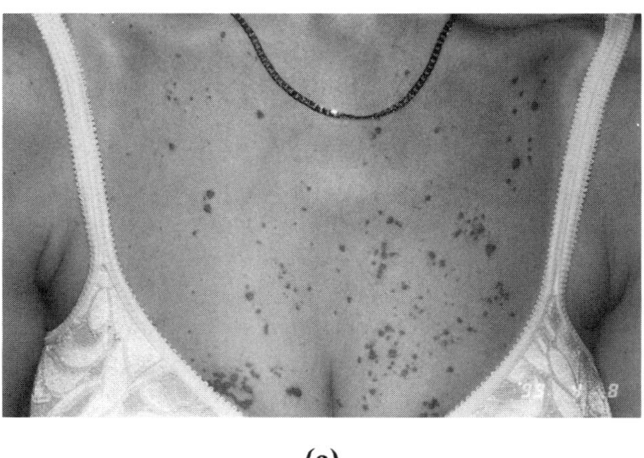

(a)

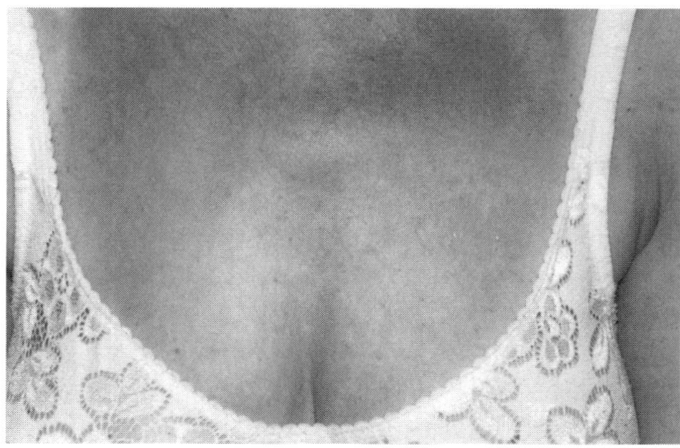

(b)

Figure 1. The use of a pulsed dye laser to remove a vascular nevus of the anterior of the chest, a site which quite frequently produces scarring: (a) The nevus before treatment; (b) The nevus after a subsequent therapy, showing satisfactory clearance without any evidence of scarring. The patient was satisfied with this improvement, the residual nevus being easy to camouflage, and no further therapy was planned. (Courtesy of Dr. Neil Walker, Oxford).

Table 3. Effectiveness of flashlamp-pumped dye laser treatment of vascular lesions.

Problems	Effectiveness	Treatment of choice
Port wine stains, hemangiomas	Good to excellent	Yes
Telangiectasia	Excellent	Yes
Rosacea flushing	Good	Often
Spider nevi, angiofibromas	Good to excellent	Yes
Cherry angiomas	Excellent	Often
Venous lakes	Good	Often
Postsurgical erythema	Good	Often

maximum improvements requires patience, since it usually takes several sessions and up to a year for repair processes and reorganization of the damaged tissue to completely heal. The scarring, for instance, which occurs in only 10% of lesions may resolve during that time and vascular and pigmented lesions may recur. Not to be forgotten is that paling of the lesion allows more effective use of camouflage creams.

(ii) *Pigmented lesions*

Cutaneous pigment may be endogenous (usually melanin) or exogenous (tattoo). Q-switched lasers, which allow ultrashort high intensity pulses, are effective for treating most tattoos and some benign pigmented lesions.

Tattoo pigment exists as tiny particles, about the same size as melanosomes, within macrophages, perivascular fibroblasts and mast cells in the dermis [34]. These particles are too large to be effectively removed by the reticuloendothelial system.

Treatment of tattoos before Q-switched lasers were available was unsatisfactory. Because of the small size of tattoo pigment granules and melanosomes, their thermal relaxation time is only about 1 µs. Pulses as short as this, to allow selective photothermolysis of the pigments, were impossible with conventional lasers. Some epidermal pigmented lesions were able to be treated with older, non-pulsed lasers, but there was a significant incidence of textural change and hypopigmentation. Conventional surgery, dermabrasion and lasers, such as argon, argon dye-tunable, and CO_2 lasers, were unsatisfactory in the treatment of deeper melanin or tattoos, producing significant scarring as damage was not confined to the target pigment granules. Q-switched lasers were able to deliver pulses of laser light with high peak power and ultrashort duration (in the nanosecond range). As this is shorter than the thermal relaxation time of pigment granules, heat damage to adjacent tissues is avoided.

Melanin absorbs light well across the visible spectrum and slightly less well in the near-infrared range, thus allowing different wavelengths to be used. In general, shorter, less penetrating wavelengths are used for epidermal pigment and longer, more penetrating wavelengths (red to infrared) for deeper pigment. The short impact of the laser breaks up the ink granules and may induce death of the surrounding cell. The granule fragments are to beremoved by the macrophage system. Melanosomes are also small enough to be susceptible to selective photothermolysis with these laser systems. However, the precise mechanism by which melanin pigmentation is lightened is not completely understood; it is not known whether the melanocyte is injured or the melanosomes are simply destroyed.

It is now possible to remove or significantly lighten most tattoos with only a small risk of scarring (less than 5%). After each treatment, fading occurs slowly for up to three months or more. Amateur tattoos are easier to remove than professional tattoos, since they usually have a single color at a less concentrated level in the skin. A degree of scarring is often preferred to incomplete removal, especially for pornographic tattoos. Confetti-like hypopigmentation is a common side effect lasting a year or more. The uses of Q-switched lasers are summarized in Table 4.

Table 4. Effectiveness of Q-switched laser treatment of pigmented lesions

Problem	Effectiveness
Tattoo, pigments	Excellent
Nevus of Ota	excellent
Cafe au lait macules	Fair
Lentigines, freckles	Excellent
Benign junctional and compound nevi	Unpredictable
Hemosiderin (postinflammatory pigmentation)	Unpredictable
Chloasma	Unpredictable

All the Q-switched lasers are efficient at treating black pigment, but the YAG laser is more efficient for red and the alexandrite and ruby lasers for green, blue and black. Neither is effective for aqua. The YAG laser uses a near-infrared wavelength, which is less absorbed by melanin, and is therefore probably the laser of choice for treating tattoos in darker skin types [8].

An interesting new use for these lasers is the modification or removal of cosmetic facial tattoos (eyeliner and lip liner). This form of tattooing seems to be increasing in popularity, but problems can occur. If lower-lid eyeliner is implanted too deeply, pigment may migrate, producing a smeared appearance. Poor color choice and placement may also lead the patient to seek removal.

In general, results of laser treatment of black or blue-black cosmetic pigments are uniformly excellent. However, treatment may drastically blacken red, flesh-colored and white pigments by changing the oxidation state of their iron base [35]. This sometimes, but not always, responds to further treatment. Therefore, test treatments are mandatory before treating such colors.

Q-switched lasers are at their best in treating the rare nevus of Ota [36] and the more common freckles [37] (Figure 2), examples of benign pigmented lesions. *Cafe au lait* spots are less predictable in response and will require long term maintenance treatment as they tend to recur.

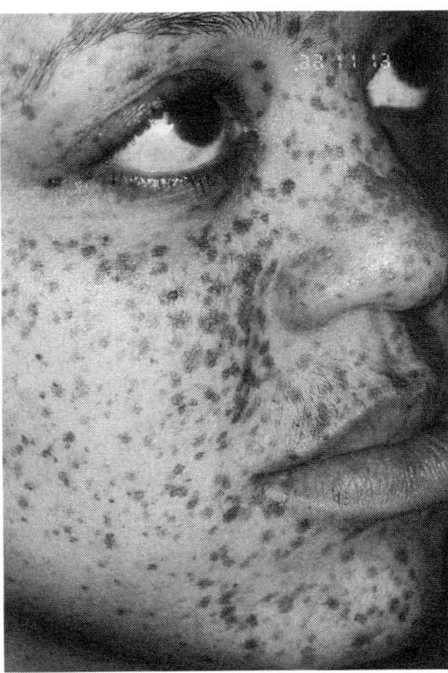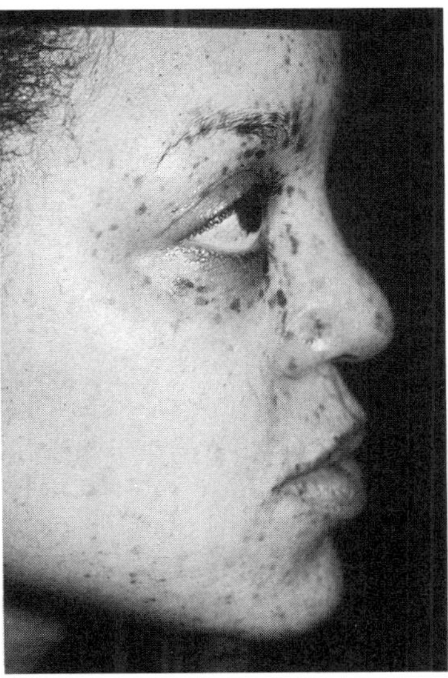

Figure 2. Before and after pictures of successful partial reduction of pigmented freckles (lentigenes) without scarring. The histology shows the localized nature of the destruction of the melanocytes with epidermal cells largely intact and the dermis unaffected.

8.3.1.4   Hair Removal

Laser removal of unwanted hair resulting from hirsutism or other causes has recently emerged as a viable modality [38]. Although various lasers had been used for hair removal in ophthalmology as well as surgery, specific laser applications using the principles of selective photothermolysis were not used for hair removal until recently. The problems are numerous, since there is great variability in response: patients with darker hair and lighter skin respond best. Melanin in the hair shaft or follicles, or both, is the target chromophore. It is reported (*Cosmetic Surgery Times*, July 1998) that the ruby laser has the greatest treatment effect, but also the greatest risk of adverse events. The Nd:YAG laser is the least efficacious, but has the most favorable safety profile. At three months after the third laser treatment, the long-pulse ruby laser was associated with 100% reduction in hair, compared with a 90% reduction for the long-pulse alexandrite and only 40% for the Q-switched Nd:YAG. The hair that grows between the three- and six-months period is finer and lighter.

A ruby laser (694 nm, 270 μs) was used in normal volunteers: six sites were treated at varying fluences (30-60 J/cm^2) and compared with untreated sites [39]. Clinical evaluation after 1, 3, and 6 months showed a statistically significant growth delay. Histology showed follicular damage with minimal surrounding collagen damage. Side effects included transient pigmentary changes in some subjects without scarring. A long-pulse (~ ms) increases follicular damage [40].

A Nd:YAG laser used in combination with a carbon-suspension solution was also reported to produce a hair growth delay in treated areas. The carbon suspension is believed to collect in the follicle and serve as a chromophore for the laser light. Preliminary results showed a growth delay of 3 months [41].

Patients should be warned that pigmentary changes are common, and that immediate blistering also occurs. Since the hair follicle often contains bacteria, episodes of infection are not rare, particularly in the groin or around the mouth and nose. Selective photothermolysis with a ruby laser has been used for hair follicle destruction [42] in black-haired dog skin with follow-up histology, and the results applied to humans. At six months, there was significant hair loss only in areas shaved before treatment at the highest fluence. Four subjects had less than 50% regrowth, even though two of these subjects had shown no change between three and six months. Obviously, therefore, a program for hair removal should be planned over a prolonged period of perhaps one to two years.

A promising new laser for hair removal is the long pulse (10 -20 ms) alexandrite laser [43,44] (Figure 3), whose wavelength (755 nm) is between that of the ruby laser (694 nm) and the Nd: YAG (1064 nm). It is safe and effective, and carries a lower risk of pigmentary alterations.

8.3.1.5 Darker Skin Types

In black skin, the epidermal melanosomes are large, numerous, and spread uniformly throughout the entire epidermis: whereas in white skin, the melanosomes are small, sparse, clumped together in aggregates, and located primarily in the lower portion of the epidermis. Black skin shows little to no overt solar elastosis with aging, whereas white skin develops moderate to extensive elastosis. These unique features of black skin protect it against actinic damage, making resurfacing for rhytides a non-issue.

Ethnic skin, however, has other challenges. Blacks are more susceptible to keloid development, and they have a higher incidence of pseudofolliculitis barbae. The higher numbers of melanocytes in ethnic skin, plus their labile nature, mean that trauma - including that caused by dermatologic treatment - more easily causes pigmentation disturbances. In spite of these concerns and in spite of black skin absorbing laser light differently from white skin, many lasers can effectively treat and improve the appearance of ethnic patients.

Pre-Treatment

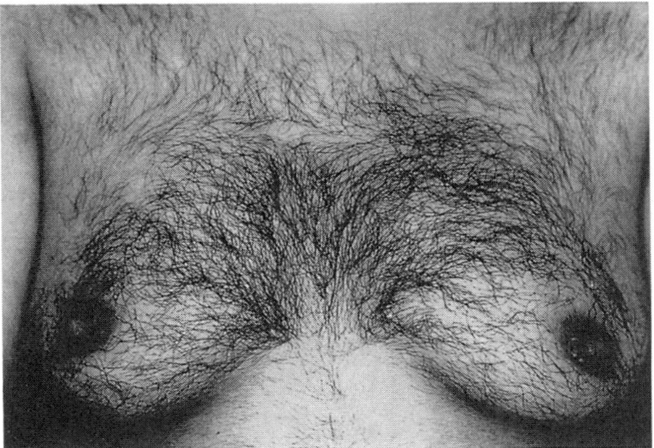

Post-Five Months

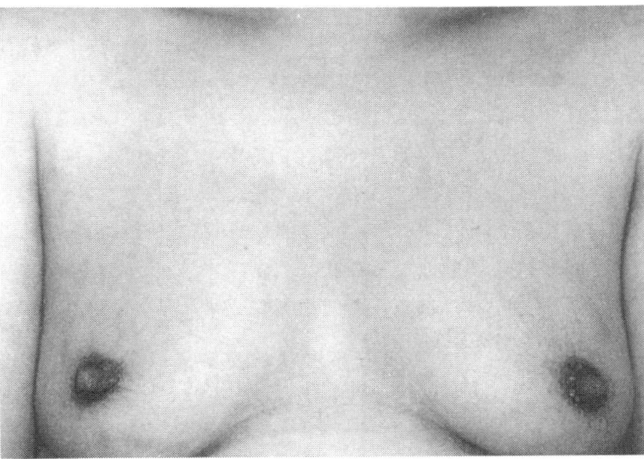

Figure 3. Before treatment and after two treatments using a long pulse (20 ms) alexandrite laser with 10 nm spot size. (Photos courtesy of Dr. Med. Christian Raulin).

Treating black patients for vascular lesions is more difficult than treating white patients because black skin has more melanin, and melanin has a fairly wide absorption spectrum. Melanin competes for absorption with laser energy intended for the hemoglobin in the blood vessels. Nevertheless, lasers can be used to treat port wine stains, telangiectases, verrucae, hypertrophic scars, striae, and some keloids. Lasers for pigmented lesions must generate a wavelength more highly absorbed by melanin than by hemoglobin or water. These are the green-light, continuous-wave lasers and the Q-switched lasers.

Although black patients do not have such a problem with photoaging, they often request resurfacing for acne scarring and dermal lesions such as syringomas and dermatosis papulosa nigra. Resurfacing is safe in ethnic skin as long as patients adhere to pre-treatment and post-treatment regimens regarding bleaching and sun avoidance.

Hirsutism and hypertrichosis, including lesions of pseudofolliculitis barbae and acne keloid, both of which are caused by ingrown hairs, are extremely common in many ethnic groups. Because side effects are more likely in pigmented skin, prospective patients should avoid acquiring a tan. It appears that longer pulse duration is more appropriate for use in darker skin. Ruby lasers, used in normal (long-pulse) mode rather than the Q-switched mode used for tattoo removal, and long-pulse alexandrite lasers are most effective.

8.3.1.6 Photodynamic Therapy

Photodynamic therapy avoids thermal damage and induces toxic metabolites. Photodynamic agents are given intravenously and irradiated one or two days later. The therapy is used mostly for malignant tumors, and it should not be forgotten that tumors such as basal cell epitheoliomata can be treated very effectively with less expensive lower technology. Porphyrin, and porphyrin derivatives, which absorb light at 630 nm have a selective affinity for tumour cells, making them photosensitive and targets for laser light irradiation. Tunable dye laser irradiation excites photosensitizer molecules to their triplet state, whereupon energy is transferred to endogenous oxygen-producing singlet oxygen which is cytotoxic and destroys the tumor cells [45]. Photodynamic therapy has been successfully used in the treatment of non-melanoma skin cancers [46,47].

The major side effect is the prolonged cutaneous photosensitivity that may continue for up to 8 weeks. Phototoxic reactions may also occur months after administration of these photosensitizing drugs [48]. The future of photodynamic therapy lies in the synthesis of new photosensitizing drugs that are less toxic, have shorter periods of photosensitivity, are cleared more rapidly by normal cells, or can be applied topically. Newer investigational photosensitizing drugs include benzoporphyrin-derivative monoacid ring A (BPD-MA) and 5-aminolevulinic acid (5-ALA), a precursor of porphyrin IX and various phthalocyanines. BPD-MA has the advantage of being cleared from normal cells faster than DHE [49]. 5-ALA can be applied topically and is absorbed through abnormal stratum corneum into epidermal and appendageal tumors, sparing normal skin and the dermis [50]. In the future, monoclonal antibodies specific for the tumor may act as carriers of the photosensitizer.

8.3.1.7 Low Energy Laser Systems: helium-neon and gallium-arsenide lasers

Low-energy lasers are a controversial area of laser application in dermatology. These devices produce little or no temperature elevation following exposure. Since the generation of heat does not occur, it is felt that any effects seen are due directly to the laser radiation. Studies in the laboratory and clinical studies have suggested that cells absorb low energy doses of laser energy which may modify cell membranes and influence such processes as wound healing [51-53] or immunological reactions. Laboratory techniques have shown that low energy laser radiation increases the rate of DNA and RNA synthesis [54], fibroblast proliferation [55] and collagen synthesis [56]. Although the mechanism for these effects remains unclear, it may be due to photoactivation of a porphyrin-containing enzyme, which stimulates the mitochondrial synthesis of ATP [57]. The concept was developed particularly in Eastern Europe but the effects that have been widely reported are not consistently reproduced by other centers.

8.3.1.8 Robotized Scanners

There are two types of robotized laser scanners: fully automated scanning devices and automated scanning handpieces [58]. The fully automated scanning devices have no contact with the skin and can be used with continuous-wave lasers [59]. These scanners map out a predetermined treatment area, which is then treated by passing the beam in parallel lines over the lesion. The patients need to be completely immobilized, usually by general anesthesia, during the procedure. This allows large areas to be treated quickly. A disadvantage is the potential appearance of post-treatment stripes that can be cosmetically unappealing.

The automated handpieces are microprocessor-controlled to deliver quickly small, nonadjacent spots in a predetermined geometric area. These handpieces are light-weight and easy to use. They move the beam over the skin quickly so that the patient does not need to be immobilized and may not even require anesthesia. Automated handpieces may be used with continuous or "pseudo-continuous"-wave lasers such as the argon, argon-pumped dye, and copper lasers [60].

The most studied automated hand piece is the Hexascan^{TM} (Prein & Partners, Ferney-Voltaire, France). It delivers nonadjacent 1 mm circular spots until a predetermined size of hexagon has been filled. Delivering these spots 2 mm apart at intervals of 50 ms allows dissipation of undesired thermal energy between pulses [61]. The pulse durations can be adjusted from 30 to 990 ms by varying the energy fluence. The diameter of the hexagonal grid can be preset from 1 to 13 mm. With a pulse duration of 30 ms, a hexagonal grid 13 mm in diameter can be treated in 20 s. Therefore relatively large areas can be irradiated in a controlled, uniform manner. The Autolase^{TM} scanner (Innovative Health Concepts, Inc., Pleasanton, Calif.) has the option of spot sizes smaller than 1 mm allowing shorter pulse durations with lower output lasers.

Automated scanners have produced good results in the treatment of port wine stains, spider angiomas, telangiectases, and a variety of benign pigmented lesions (benign lentigines, *café au lait* macules, nevus spilus, Becker's nevus, and ephelides [62-64]).

8.3.1.9 Anesthesia

Cutaneous laser therapy with the pulsed lasers is relatively painless. The discomfort has been described as like a rubber band being snapped against the skin or like a drop of hot grease on the skin. However, if large areas are being treated, the patient may request anesthesia. Anesthesia may consist of topical anesthetics, local intradermal injection, localized nerve block, iontophoresis, oral and intravenous sedation, or general anesthesia [58]. The topical anesthetic cream EMLA (Astra Pharmaceuticals, Sodertalje, Sweden) is a eutectic mixture of local anesthetics, lidocaine 2.5% and prilocaine 2.5%, suspended within an oil-in-water emulsion. When used for pulsed dye laser treatment of port wine stains in children, EMLA is applied at least 60 minutes before treatment for maximum effect and should not be used in children younger than 1 month of age or in patients with methemoglobinemia [65,66]. Other topical preparations such as tetracaine hydrochloride 0.5% and lidocaine 40% in acid mantle base under occlusion for 90 minutes can also be used. Supraorbital and infraorbital nerve blocks with lidocaine 1% have also been used in the treatment of facial port wine stains [67]. Iontophoresis of lidocaine with or without epinephrine has been used to provide anesthesia in the treatment of port wine stains with the pulsed dye laser [68]. Mild sedation with oral agents such as chloral hydrate alone or in combination with promethazine (Phenergan) and chlorpromazine

(Thorazine) is frequently used. Anxious patients may benefit from oral diazepam (2 mg) or halcinonide (0.2 mg). Sedation with intramuscular meperadine (2 mg/ml) and promethazine (1 mg/ml) allows communication with the patient during the procedure, but an extended recovery period is needed until the patient is alert [67]. Side effects are uncommon with this type of anesthesia but may include vomiting and respiratory depression; monitoring with a pulse oximeter is necessary. General anesthesia is seldom warranted but can be used in children who require an extended treatment session or who are combative. General anesthesia induction and maintenance may be attained with a combination of halothane, nitrous oxide, and oxygen. Today, a commonly preferred general anesthetic is propofol (Deprivan).

8.3.1.10 Dynamic Cooling

There is a long tradition in medicine of using cooling as an analgesic procedure. Theoretically, cooling the epidermis during laser treatment may enhance the ability to clear resistant port wine stains by allowing increased delivery of energy to the lesion, without damaging the epidermis. A recent study examined the use of a cryogen pulse in combination with the pulsed dye laser (585 nm, 450 µs) to keep the epidermis cool without cooling the dermal vessels. Preliminary results suggest that this technique may be useful [69].

A clinical study was performed in which ten patients with port- wine stains were treated with high fluence (9.0 - 10.5 J/cm^2) pulses from the pulsed dye laser 25 to 30 s after the application of ice. Resistant port wine stains lightened at these high fluences with an absence of scarring [70].

A cold air device is now available as a handpiece (Smartcool^{TM}, Cynosure, Chelmsford, MA) to deliver a continuous flow of chilled air to the treatment area.

8.3.2 Diagnostic

8.3.2.1 Laser Doppler Flowmetry

Laser Doppler flowmetry (LDF) is a useful diagnostic technique for monitoring microvascular blood flow [71-74]. The technique is non-invasive, relying on the detection of laser light backscattered from the skin surface. Low power laser light (usually < 2 mW) is directed towards the tissue using an optical fiber, and is scattered both by moving red blood cells (RBCs) and static tissue structures. Those photons scattered by moving RBCs undergo a shift in frequency that is proportional to the velocity of the RBCs: typically this is several kHz for light of wavelength around 780 nm.

Thus the backscattered light contains both frequency shifted and non-shifted photons. A portion of the backscattered light is collected by a second optical fiber which directs the light on to the surface of a sensitive photodetector. The resulting photocurrent is processed electronically to produce several parameters related to blood flow within the measured volume. The blood flux parameter, for example, is proportional to the product of the mean RBC velocity and the mean RBC concentration.

Conventional LDF cannot distinguish between blood flow in the superficial (papillary) vessels and bulk flows in the deeper dermal regions. Such information would be of significant use in the study of pathophysiological changes in human tissue, particularly in the area of inflammatory skin diseases such as psoriasis, dermatitis, and eczema and in evaluating burn injury depth. Its value is for simultaneous comparison of two sites or the measurement of changes in flow affected by therapy. Absolute measurement is not possible.

Blood flow can be investigated at different depths within the skin by varying the coherence length of a diode laser source [75]. The coherence length is varied by regulating its input drive current. This results in a reproducible means of controlling the mean optical pathlength in tissue over which laser Doppler signals can be remitted. If a short coherence length is selected, coherent interference with the reference beam will be obtained only for backscattered light from the superficial dermal plexus: light from the deeper dermis will no longer be coherent with the reference beam and will not produce a Doppler signal. Conversely, as the coherence length is increased Doppler signals will be obtained over depths commensurate with the penetration of that light in the tissue. Because the technique relies on the ability to control the efficiency of heterodyne mixing, it is largely independent of the actual penetrability of the particular wavelength of laser light chosen: and the circumvention of the wavelength dependence of the Doppler effect itself greatly simplifies the interpretation of experimental results.

Scanning LDF systems have been developed to move the beam slowly over a large area of the skin, recording small pinpoint variations in fast or slow blood flow [76]. Normal vasomotion is very variable, and ideally several repeat readings must be taken after a prolonged period of room temperature and patient stabilization. The resulting scattered light contains the Doppler -shifted component, which is detected and processed to form an image of the flow in the scanned region. In practice, a 2 mW He-Ne laser is directed at a mirror, driven by a motor, so that the reflected beam scans over the patient's skin, the mirror-patient distance being above 1.5 m. Areas of 500 to 700 mm^2 can be imaged with 2 mm spatial resolution. Laser light, scattered from the skin and travelling back to the mirror, is directed to lenses which focus the light on photodetectors. The component of signal from the detectors representing the Doppler-shifted light can then be compared, by analogue signal processing, with the signal from the unscattered laser light to obtain the difference frequency. The data is processed to generate an image with colors representing the blood flow values. The mean depth at which blood flow sampling takes place within the instrument is 390 µm, so the surface microcirculation is imaged.

Various applications have been examined, including dermatology, burns, vascular assessment and plastic surgery. A case of particular interest is psoriasis, a condition causing large red patches to appear on the patient's skin. These patches are characterized by increased blood flow, which can vary markedly from region to region within a patch and from patch to patch. Treatment is not always efficacious and although it may reduce the size of a patch, laser Doppler has shown that in some patches, not affected by medication, the high blood flow remains. Scanning LDF is also useful in the examination and assessment of burn wounds [77,78], since it reveals where blood is flowing well, with good prognosis for repair, and those areas with reduced or zero flow, which may not recover and need a skin graft. A scanning LDF imaging system has been developed that can accurately image and analyze three-dimensional (3-D) surfaces in healing wound tissue [79]. The laser beam diameter is 1 x 2 mm and can measure distances as small as 8 µm. The system produces a 3-D image that can be used to calculate the volume of the wound.

There are compelling clinical advantages in being able to monitor, simultaneously and continuously, blood oxygen saturation and tissue perfusion from the same volume of tissue. Laser Doppler flowmetry and reflection pulse oximetry are essentially complementary techniques, which use changes in the frequency and amplitude of backscattered light to monitor blood supply to the tissues and its oxygenation status. In reflection pulse oximetry differences in collected red and infrared light resulting from arterial blood pulsation in a vascular bed can be used to measure arterial hemoglobin oxygen saturation [80], S_aO_2. Absolute calibration of reflection pulse oximeters is notoriously difficult [81,82]. Backscattered light from living skin depends not only on the optical absorption of the blood but also on the complex physiology of the sampled tissue volume. In practice, both the derived Doppler and oximetry signals are often complicated by the effects of multiple scattering from the RBCs [83]. An instrument capable of combining both functions has been designed [84]. It uses a laser diode at 805 nm to give a blood flow index and oxygenation information at that wavelength, and a pulsed LED at 660 nm to complete the estimation of oxygen saturation. By using a compensating photodetector these readings can be made relatively insensitive to sampling site. It provides a unique means for the assessment and clinical management of a whole range of ischemic-related tissue disorders, and has important applications in dermatology, plastic surgery, anesthesiology and critical-care monitoring. It could also be used to provide an effective method of assessing the viability of skin during clinical procedures such as amputation and free-flap transfer surgery. The ability to measure flow and oxygen independently (instead of simply using the oxygenation as a guide to perfusion) is a major advance. Considering that the most common cause of anesthesia-related preventable deaths is hypoxia [85], the use of such an instrument is likely to prove of significant benefit. Further applications include its use in monitoring treatment of, for example, port wine stains [86] and in investigating vascular responses at tumor and normal tissue sites induced by porphyrin-mediated photodynamic therapy [87].

8.3.2.2 Microscopy

Skin imagery and especially subsurface imagery are at the forefront of laser diagnostics [88]. The skin surface has been studied with everything from the simple ancient magnifier to the most sophisticated scanning electron microscope [89].

Currently, common instruments used for magnified surface and subsurface imagery of living skin include: (i) the new dermatoscopes with all their accessories (ii) the coaxial polarizing microscope (iii) the infra-red microscope (iv) the ultrasonic biomedical microscope (v) the confocal scanning microscope for microscopy of living skin and (vi) the new holographic optical phase conjugation microscope [90]. As a result of this exciting renaissance in optical technology, *in vivo* study of the normal and pathologic skin is e.g., the details of the topography of living skin, particularly pigment distribution on the surface and below the surface of the skin is becoming a fertile area of future research. Although transillumination and the recent use of the dermatoscope have provided some information for help in diagnosis, additional developments of technology are necessary. Some of these factors are monochromatic versus polychromatic light sources, polarized versus unpolarized light with vertical versus oblique direction of polarization, vertical versus angulated direction of illumination, phase conjugation versus other nonlinear types of optics, and direct transillumination versus subsurface fiberoptic transillumination. All of these many factors are used in an attempt to recognize the earliest pathologic changes in skin, especially the living skin.

A laser scanning confocal microscope has been recently used to image skin *in vivo* [91]. Normal skin from subjects of varying types was imaged. Epidermal cells of each layer were easily visualized and distinguishable.

Additionally blood flow could be seen in the dermis. Images obtained with the confocal microscope were compared with stained skin specimens. A compound nevus was also visualized with this technique and dermal nevus cells were seen.

8.3.3 Research and Recent Advances

It is still early days and clinical experience is important. Some physicians get much better results than others, and the reasons for this are not always apparent. There is a great deal of enthusiasm, and many practitioners can make a great deal of money by advertising their high technology. Careful controlled trials are still in their infancy. The major advances in the field of dermatologic surgery are in the areas of the diagnosis and management of cutaneous melanoma, advances in laser surgery, tumescent liposuction, and tumorigenesis [92]. Advances in the current therapy for cutaneous melanoma include clear guidelines in its surgical management, new staging of the disease, and an improvement in the evaluation and therapy of advanced disease. Advances in laser surgery include the use of pulsed due laser for the treatment of telangiectases, poikiloderma of Civatte, red noses, flushing, recalcitrant warts, hypertrophic scars, and striae distensae, apart from its successfully proven use in the treatment of port wine stains and hemangiomas. With the application of new technology to new laser development, a multi-wavelength, flashlamp-pumped light source has been used for the treatment of leg veins [93] though Goldman (personal communication) still finds that in his hands sclerotherapy is a reliable technique. A long pulsed alexandrite laser has been shown to be effective in treating leg telangiectasias, especially when used alongside sclerotherapy [94]. The 755 nm wavelength was intended to take advantage of the increased penetration of the dermis for deeper vessels, while simultaneously benefiting from the second absorption peak of hemoglobin and decreased interference by melanin. Also, high peak power short-pulse carbon dioxide lasers are being used for tissue resurfacing in the removal of rhytides of the face, acne scars, and actinic damage. Advances in photodynamic therapy as treatment for cutaneous malignancies might expand the treatment options for patients with multiple nonmelanoma skin cancers. With the development of the tumescent technique the procedure of liposuction has become safer and less painful, and general anesthesia is no longer needed, permitting the use of microcannulas with which a more complete removal of fatty tissue has been accomplished. In the field of tumorigenesis there is no a better understanding of the role of accumulations of specific mutations in tumor suppressor genes and oncogenes in the development of cutaneous malignancies.

In addition to use in skin resurfacing, new generation carbon dioxide lasers are also being studied to facilitate hair transplantation. Hair growth in subjects was examined using a pulsed carbon dioxide laser to make the slits in which hair grafts were placed [95,96]. Decreased bleeding, absence of graft compression, and increased hair density in laser-treated areas have been reported [97]. Disadvantages included the need for operator experience, an increase in time required to produce laser slits, potential laser plume toxicities, increased postoperative thermal damage [98] and crusting, and hair regrowth delay.

High-powered semiconductor diode lasers have recently been developed that emit energy at a wavelength of 805 nm in continuous or pulsed fashion [99]. Light from this laser can be transmitted by fiber optics and delivered using synthetic sapphire tips in a contact mode to incise or vaporize soft tissue.

Another phase of laser development is the attempt to offer multiple frequencies and multiple laser instruments in one or two systems in one area. There are several examples of these multiple wavelength units currently available, such as the tunable dye lasers pumped by argon lasers. Titanium sapphire units offer another example. Another, more versatile approach is the use of interchangeable metal vapor lasers to drive interchangeable solid-state modules. These lasers deliver nanosecond pulse widths without Q-switching [88]. Barring the development of a continuously variable tunable wavelength, continuously variable tunable pulse width and frequency, and continuous variable tunable pulse power, these metal vapor lasers may offer a satisfactory and rather economical approach to a variety of clinical problems in dermatology.

REFERENCES

1. Anderson RR, Levins PC, Grevelink JM. Lasers in dermatology. In: Fitzpatrick TB, Eisen AZ, Wolff K. et al, eds. Dermatology in general medicine. 4th ed. New York: McGraw-Hill. 1993: 1755-66
2. Dixon JA, Huether S, Rotering R. Hypertrophic scarring in argon laser treatment of port wine stains. Plast Reconstr Surg 1984; **73**: 771-9
3. McBurney EI, Rosen DA. Carbon dioxide laser treatment of verrucae vulgares. J Dermatol Surg Oncol 1984; **10**: 45-8
4. Fairhurst MV, Roenigk RK, Brodland DG. Carbon dioxide laser surgery for skin disease. Mayo Clin Proc 1992; **67**: 49-58
5. Goldberg DJ. Benign pigmented lesions of the skin: treatment with the Q-switched ruby laser. J Dermatol Surg Oncol 1993; **19**: 376-9
6. Anderson RR, Parrish RR. Selective photothermolysis: precise microsurgery by selective absorption of pulsed radiation. Science 1983; **220**: 524-7
7. Goodman GJ, Bekhor PS, Richards SW. Update in lasers in dermatology. Med J Aust 1996; **164**: 681-6

8. Hruza GJ , Geronemus RG, Dover JS, Arndt JA. Lasers in dermatology. Arch Dermatol 1993; **129**: 1026-35

9. Spicer MS, Goldberg DJ. Lasers in dermatology. J Am Acad Dermatol 1996; **34**: 1-25

10. Sawchuk WS, Weber PJ, Lowy DR, et al. Infectious papillomavirus in the vapor of warts treated with carbon dioxide laser or electrocoagulation: detection and protection. J Am Acad Dermatol 1989; **21**: 41-9

11. Baggish MS, Poiesz BJ, Joret D, et al. Presence of human immunodeficiency virus DNA in laser smoke. Lasers Surg Med 1991; **11**: 197-203

12. David LM. Laser vermilion ablation for actinic cheilitis. J Dermatol Surg Oncol 1985; **11**: 605-8

13. Wheeland RG, Bailin PL, Reynolds OD, Ratz JL. CO_2 laser vaporisation of multiple facial syringomas.. J Dermatol Surg Oncol 1986; **12**: 225 - 8

14. Whitaker DC. Microscopically proven cure of actinic cheilitis by CO_2 laser. Lasers Surg Med 1987; **7**: 520 - 3

15. Apfelberg DB, Master MR, Lash H, et al. Superpulse CO_2 laser treatment of facial syringomata. Lasers Surg Med 1987; **4**: 533-8

16. Apfelberg DB, Druker D, Maser MR, et al. Benefits of the CO_2 laser for verruca resistant to other modalities of treatment. J Dermatol Surg Oncol 1989; **15**: 371-5

17. Albricht SM, Stern RS, Tang SV, et al. Complications of cutaneous laser surgery. Arch Dermatol 1987; **123**: 345-9

18. Kauvar AN, Geronemus RG, Waldorf HA. Char free tissue ablation: a comparative histopathological analysis of new carbon dioxide (CO_2) laser systems. Lasers Surg Med 1995; **15** (Suppl 7):50

19. Fitzpatrick RE, Goldman MP, Satur NM, et al. Pulsed CO_2 laser resurfacing of photoaged facial skin. Arch Dermatol 1996; **132**: 395-402

20. Ross EV, Glatter RD, Duke D, Grevelink JM. Effects of pulse and scan stacking in CO_2 laser skin resurfacing: a study of residual thermal damage, cell death, and woud healing. Lasers Surg Med 1997; **17** (Suppl 9):42

21. Adrian RM. Pulsed carbon dioxide and long pulse 10-ms erbium-YAG laser resurfacing: a comparative and histologic study. J Cutan Laser Ther 1999; **1**: 197-202

22. Hulsbergen-Henning JP, Roskam Y, Van Gemert MJ. Treatment of keloids and hypertrophic scars with an argon laser. Laser Surg Med 1986; **6**: 72-5

23. Apfelberg DB, Maser MR, While D, et al. Failure of carbon dioxide laser excision of keloids. Lasers Surg Med 1989; **9**: 382-8

24. Alster TS, Kurban SK, Grove GL. Alteration of argon laser induced scarring by the pulsed dye laser. Lasers Surg Med 1993; **13**: 368-78

25. Alster TS. Improvement of erythematous and hypertrophic scars by 585 nm flash lamp pumped pulsed dye laser. Ann Plast Surg 1994; **32**: 186-90

26. McCraw JB et al. Prevention of unfavourable scars using early pulsed dye laser treatments: a preliminary report. Annals of Plastic Surgery 1999; **42**: 7-14

27. Alster TS, McMeekin TO. Improvement of facial acne scars by the 585 nm flash lamp-pumped pulsed dye laser. J Am Acad Dermatol 1996; **35**: 79-81

28. Logan RA, Zachary CB. Outcome of carbon dioxide laser therapy for persistent cutaneous viral warts. Br J Dermatol 1989; **121**: 99-105

29. Lim JT, Goh CL. Carbon dioxide laser treatment of periungual and subungual viral warts. Aust J Dermatol 1992; **33**: 87-91

30. Tan OT, Hurwitz RM, Stafford TJ. Pulsed dye laser treatment of recalcitrant verrucae: a preliminary report. Lasers Surg Med 1993; **13**: 127-9

31. Kauvar ANB, McDaniel DH, Geronemus RG. Pulsed dye laser treatment of warts. Arch Fam Med 1995; **4**: 1035-40

32. Reyes BA, Geronemus RG. Treatment of port wine stains during childhood with the flashlamp pumped pulsed dye laser. J Am Acad Dermatol 1990; **23**: 1142-8

33. Bencini PL. The multilayer technique: a new and fast approach for flashlamp-pumped pulse (PLPP) dye laser treatment of port wine stains (preliminary reports). Dermatol Surg 1999; **25**: 786-9

34. Taylor CR, Anderson RR, et al. Light and electron microscopic analysis of tattoos treated by Q-switched ruby laser. J Invest Dermatol 1991; **97**: 131-6

35. Anderson RR, Geronemus R, Kilmer SC, et al. Cosmetic tattoo ink darkening; a complication of Q-switched and pulsed laser treatment. Arch Dermal 1993; **129**: 1010-4

36. Geronemus RG. Q-switched ruby laser therapy of nevus of Ota. Arch Dermatol 1992; **128**: 1618-22

37. Tse Y, Levine VJ, McClain SA, Ashinoff R. The removal of cutaneous pigmented lesions with the Q-switched ruby laser and the Q-switched neodymium:yttrium-aluminum-garnet laser: a comparative study. J Dermatol Surg Oncol 1994; **20**: 795-800

38. Grossman MC. What is new in cutaneous laser research. Adv Clin Res 1997; **15**: 1-8

39. Grossman MC, Ferinelli W, Flotte T, et al. Laser targeted at hair follicles. Laser Surg 1995; **5** ; 47

40. Dierickx C, Grossman M, Farinelli W, Manuskiatte W, Anderson RR. Long-pulsed ruby laser hair removal. Lasers Surg Med 1997; **17** (Suppl 9): 36-7

41. Goldberg D. Topical solution assisted laser hair removal. Lasers Surg Med 1995; **5**:45

42. Grossman MC, Dierickx C, Farinelli W, Flotte T, Anderson RR. Damage to hair follicles normal-mode ruby laser pulses. J Amer Acad Dermatol 1996; **35**: 889-94

43. Connolly CS and Paolini LP. Study reveals successful removal of unwanted hair with LPIR laser. Cosmetic Dermatol 1997; **10**: 38-40

44. McDaniel DH, Lord J, Ash K, Newman J, Zukowski M. Laser hair removal: a review and report on the use of the long-pulsed alexandrite laser for hair reduction of the upper lip, leg, back and bikini region. Dermatol Surg 1999a; **25**: 425-30

45. Weishaupt KR, Gomer CJ, Dougherty TJ. Identification of singlet oxygen as the cytotoxic agent in photo-inactivation of a murine tumor. Cancer Res 1979; **36**: 2326-9

46. Keller GS, Razum NJ, Dorion DR. Photodynamic therapy for nonmelanoma skin cancer. Facial Plast Surg 1989; **6**: 180 - 4

47. Svanberg K, Andersson T, Killander D, et al. Photodynamic therapy of non-melanoma malignant tumours of the skin using topical δ-amino levulinic acid sensitization and laser irradiation. Br J Dermatol 1994; **130**: 743-51

48. Dougherty TJ, Cooper MT, Mang TS. Cutaneous photo-toxic occurrences in patients receiving Photofrin[R]. Lasers Surg Med 1990; **10**: 485-8

49. Richter AM, Yip S, Waterfield E, et al. Mouse skin photosensitization with benzoporphyrin derivatives and photofrin[R]: macroscopic and microscopic evaluation. Photochem Photobiol 1991; **53**: 281-6

50. Goff BA, Bachor R, Kollias N, et al. Effects of photodynamic therapy with topical application of 5-aminolevulinic acid on normal skin of hairless guinea pigs. Photochem Photobiol 1992; **55**: 239-51

51. Abergel RP, Meeker CA, Lam TS, et al. Control of connective tissue metabolism by lasers:Recent developments and future prospects. J Am Acad Dermatol 1984; **11**:1142-50

52. Longo L, Evangelista S, Tinacci G, Sesti AG. Effect of diodes-laser silver arsenide aluminium (Ga-Al-As) 904 nm on healing of experimental wounds. Lasers Surg Med 1987; **7**: 444-7

53. Braverman B, McCarthy RJ, Ivankovich AD, et al. Effect of helium-neon and infrared laser irradiation on wound healing in rabbits. Lasers Surg Med 1989; **9**: 50-8

54. Fava G, Marchesini R, Melloni E, et al. Effect of low energy irradiation by He-Ne laser on mitosis rate of HT-29 tumor cells in culture. Lasers Life Sci 1986; **1**: 135-41

55. Boulton M, Marshall J. He-Ne laser stimulation of human fibroblast proliferation and attachment in vitro. Lasers Life Sci 1986; **1**: 125-34

56. Lam TS, Abergel RP, Meeker CA, et al. Laser stimulation of collagen synthesis in

human skin fibroblast cultures. Lasers Life Sci 1986; **1**: 61-77

57. Pasarella S, Dechecchi MS, Quagliariello E, et al. Optical and biochemical properties of NADH irradiated by high peak power Q-switched ruby laser or by low power CW He-Ne laser. Bioelectrochem Bioenerg 1981; **8**: 315-9

58. Spicer MS and Goldberg DJ. Lasers in dermatology. J Amer Acad Dermatol 1996; **34**: 1-25

59. Smithies DJ, Butler PH, Pickering JW, et al. A computer controlled scanner for the laser treatment of vascular lesions and hyperpigmentation. Clin Phys Physiol Meas 1991; **12**: 261-7

60. Mordon S, Rotteleur G, Brunetaud JM, et al. Rationale for automatic scanners in laser treatment of port wine stains. Lasers Surg Med 1993; **13**: 113-23

61. Apfelberg DB, Smoller B. Preliminary analysis of histological results of Hexascan^{TM} device with continuous tunable due laser at 514 (argon) and 577 nm (yellow). Lasers Surg Med 1993; **13**: 106-12

62. Rotteleur G, Mordon S, Buys B, et al. Robotized scanning laser handpiece for the treatment of port wine stains and other angiodysplasias. Lasers Surg Med 1988; **8**: 283-7

63. Apfelberg DB. Atlas of cutaneous laser surgery. New York: Raven Press, 1991: 404-27

64. McDaniel DH. Clinical usefulness of the Hexascan: Treatment of cutaneous vascular and melanocytic disorders. J Dermatol Surg Oncol 1993; **19**: 312-9

65. Tan OT, Stafford TJ. EMLA for laser treatment of port wine stains in children. Lasers Surg Med 1992; **12**: 543-8

66. Sherwood KA. The use of topical anesthesia in removal of port wine stains in children. J Pediatr 1993; **122** (suppl):S36-S40

67. Rabinowitz LG, Esterly NB. Anesthesia and/or sedation for pulsed dye laser therapy. Pediatr Dermatol 1992; **9**:132-53

68. Kennard CD, Whitaker DC. Iontophoresis of lidocaine for anesthesia during pulsed dye laser treatment of port wine stains. J Dermatol Surg Oncol 1992: **18**: 287-94

69. Nelson JS, Milner TE, Anvari B, et al. Dynamic epidermal cooling during pulsed laser treatment of port wine stain: A new methodology with preliminary clinical evaluation. Arch Dermatol 1995; **131**: 695-700

70. Adrian RM. Cutaneous cooling facilitated high fluence pulsed dye laser therapy of port wine stains. Lasers Surg Med 1995; **5**: 57

71. Nilsson GE, Tenland T, Oberg PA. A new instrument for continuous measurements of tissue blood flow by light beating spectroscopy. IEEE Trans Biomed Eng 1980 ; **BME-27**:12-9

72. Belcaro G, Vasdekis S, Rulo A, Nicolaides AN. Evaluation of skin blood flow and venoarterial response in patients with diabetes and peripheral vascular disease by laser Doppler flowmetry. Angiology 1989: 953-7

73. Hirkaler GM, Rosenberger LB. Simultaneous two-probe laser Doppler velocimetric assessment of topically applied drugs in rats J Pharmocol Methods 1989; **21**: 123-7

74. Dougherty G. Spectral analysis of laser Doppler signals in real time using digital processing. Med Eng Phys 1994; **16**: 35-8

75. Dougherty G. A laser Doppler flowmeter using variable coherence to effect depth discrimination. Rev Sci Instrum 1992; **63**: 3220-1

76. Niazi ZBM, et al. New laser Doppler scanner, a valuable adjunct in burn assessment. Burns 1993; **19**: 485-9

77. Yeong EK, Mann R, Goldberg M, Engrav L, Heimbach D. Improved accuracy of burn wound assessment using laser Doppler. J Trauma 1996; **40**: 856-61

78. Park DH, Hwang JW, Jang KS, Han DG, Ahn KY, Baik BS. Use of laser Doppler flowmetry for estimation of the depth of burns. Plast Reconstr Surg 1998; **101**: 1516-23

79. Patete PV, Bulgrin JP, Shabani MM, Smith DJ. A non-invasive, three-dimensional, diagnostic laser imaging system for accurate wound analysis.Physiol Meas 1996; **17**:71-9

80. Yoshiya I, Shimada Y, Tanaka K. Spectrophotometric monitoring of arterial oxygen saturation in the fingertip. Med Biol Eng Comp 1980; **18**: 27-32

81. Mendelson Y, Kent J.C, Yocum BL, Birle MJ. Design and evaluation of a new reflectance pulse oximeter sensor. Medical Instrumentation 1988; **22**: 167-73

82. Shimada Y, Nakashima K, Fujiwara Y, Komatsu T, Kawanishi M, Takezawa J, Takatani S. Evaluation of a new reflectance pulse oximeter for clinical applications. Med Biol Eng Comp 1991; **29**: 557-61

83. Shimada Y, Yoshiya I, Oka N, Hamaguri K. Effects of multiple scattering and peripheral circulation on arterial oxygen saturation measured with a pulse-type oximeter. Med Biol Eng Comp 1984; **22**: 475-8.

84. Dougherty G, Lowry J. Design and evaluation of an instrument to measure microcirculatory blood flow and oxygen saturation simultaneously. J Med Eng Tech 1992;**16**:123-8

85. Tremper KK, Barker SJ. Pulse oximetry. Anesthesiology 1989; **70**: 98-108

86. Troilius AM, Ljunggren B. Evaluation of port wine stains by laser Doppler perfusion imaging and reflectance photometry before and after pulsed dye laser treatment. Acta Derm Venereol 1996; **76**: 291-4

87. Feather JW, Driver I, Leslie G, Hajizadehsaffar M, Gilson D, King PR, Dixon B. Reflectance spectrophotometric investigation of tissue response in photodynamic therapy of cancer. SPIE Optical Fibres in Medicine III 1988; **906**: 162-8

88. Goldman L. Future of laser dermatology. Lasers Surg Med 1998; **22**: 3-8

89. Kenet RO, Sewon K, Barney J, Kenet TB, Fitzpatrick AJ, Sober RL, Barahill PH. Dermatology 1993; **129**:157

90. Goldman L. Direct skin microscopy of the skin in vitro as a diagnostic aid and as a research tool. J Dermatol Surg Oncol 1980; **6**:9

91. Rajadyaksha M, Grossman MC, Easerowitz D, et al. In vivo confocal scanning laser microscopy of human skin: melanin provides strong contrast. J Invest Dermatol 1995; **104**: 946-52

92. Perez M. Advances in dermatologic surgery. Adv Clin Res 1997; **15**: 9 - 16

93. Goldman MP, Eckhouse S. Photothermal sclerosis of leg veins. Derm Surg 1996; **22**: 323-30

94. McDaniel DH, Ash K, Lord J, Newman J, Adrian RM, Zukowski M. Laser therapy of spider leg veins: clinical evaluation of a new long pulsed alexandrite laser. Dermatol Surg 1999; **25**: 52-8

95. Unger WP, David LD. Laser hair transplantation. J Dermatol Surg Oncol 1994;**20**:515-21

96. Unger WP. Laser hair transplantation II. J Dermatol Surg 1995; **21**: 759-65

97. Grevelink JM. Laser hair transplantation. Dermatol Clin 1997; **15**: 479-86

98. Smithdeal CD. Carbon dioxide laser assisted hair transplantation. The effect of laser parameters on scalp tissue - a histology study. Dermatol Surg 1997; **23**: 835-40

99. Wyman A, Duffy S, Sweetland HM et al. Preliminary evaluation of a new high power diode laser. Lasers Surg Med 1992; **12**: 506-9

Chapter 9

LASER DENTISTRY

Markolf H. Niemz
Mannheim Biomedical Engineering Laboratories, University of Heidelberg, GERMANY

9.1 INTRODUCTION

Although dentistry was the second medical discipline where lasers were applied, it basically remained a field of research. Especially in caries therapy - the most frequent dental surgery (conventional mechanical drills are still superior compared to most types of lasers, particularly CW or long-pulse lasers). Only laser systems capable of providing ultrashort pulses might be an alternative to mechanical drills according to Niemz [1]. However, many clinical studies and an extensive engineering effort still remain to be done in order to achieve satisfactory results. We should keep in mind that mechanical drills have improved over several decades until the present stage was reached, and that the development of suitable application units for laser radiation also takes time. Other topics of interest in dentistry include laser treatment of soft tissue as well as laser-welding of dental bridges and dentures. In some of these areas, research has been very successful. In this chapter, laser treatment of hard tooth substances, soft dental tissues, and filling materials will be addressed.

9.2 THE HUMAN TOOTH

Before going into the details of laser dentistry, a brief summary of the anatomy of the human tooth as well as its physiology and pathology shall be given. In principle, the human tooth consists of mainly three distinct segments called enamel, dentin, and pulp. A schematic cross-section of a human tooth is shown in Figure 1.

The *enamel* is the hardest substance of the human body. It is made of approximately 95% (by weight) hydroxyapatite, 4% water, and 1% organic

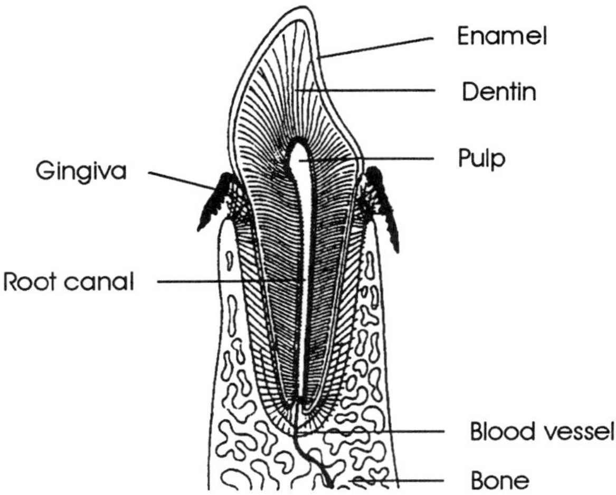

Figure 1. Cross-section of a human tooth.

matter. Hydroxyapatite is a mineralized compound with the chemical formula $Ca_{10}(PO_4)_6 (OH)_2$. Its substructure consists of tiny crystallites which form so-called *enamel prisms* with diameters ranging from 4 μm to 6 μm. The crystal lattice itself is intruded by several impurities, especially Cl^-, F^-, Na^+, K^+, and Mg^{2+}.

The *dentin*, on the other hand, is much softer. Only 70% of its volume consists of hydroxyapatite, whereas 20% is organic matter - mainly collagen fibers - and 10% is water. The internal structure of dentin is characterized by small tubuli which measure up to a few millimeters in length, and between 100 nm and 3 μm in diameter. These tubuli are essential for the growth of the tooth.

The *pulp*, finally, is not mineralized at all. It contains the supplying blood vessels, nerve fibers, and different types of cells, particularly odontoblasts and fibroblasts. Odontoblasts are in charge of producing the dentin, whereas fibroblasts contribute to both stability and regulation mechanisms. The pulp is connected to peripheral blood vessels by a small channel called the *root canal*. The tooth itself is embedded into soft tissue called the *gingiva* which keeps the tooth in place and prevents bacteria from attacking the root.

The most frequent pathologic condition of teeth is called *decay* or *caries*. Its origin lies in both cariogeneous nourishment and insufficient oral hygiene. Microorganisms multiply at the tooth surface and form a layer of *plaque*. These microorganisms produce lactic and acetic acid, thereby reducing the pH down to values of approximately 3.5. The pH and the solubility of hydroxy-apatite are strongly related by

$$Ca_{10}(PO_4)_6(OH)_2 + 8\,H^+ \longleftrightarrow 10\,Ca^{2+} + 6\,HPO_4^{2-} + 2\,H_2O$$

By means of this reaction, the enamel can be demineralized within a few days only. Calcium bound to the hydroxyapatite is ionized and washed out by saliva. This process turns the hard enamel into a very porous and permeable structure as shown in Figure 2. Usually, this kind of decay is associated with a darkening in color. Sometimes, however, carious lesions appear bright at the surface and are thus difficult to detect. At an advanced stage, the dentin is demineralized, as well. In this case, microorganisms can even infect the pulp and its interior which often induces severe pain. Then, at the latest, the dentist must remove all infected substance and refill the tooth with suitable alloys, gold, ceramics, or composites. Among alloys, amalgam has been a very popular choice of the past. Recently, though, a new controversy has arisen concerning the toxicity of this filling material, since it contains a significant amount of mercury.

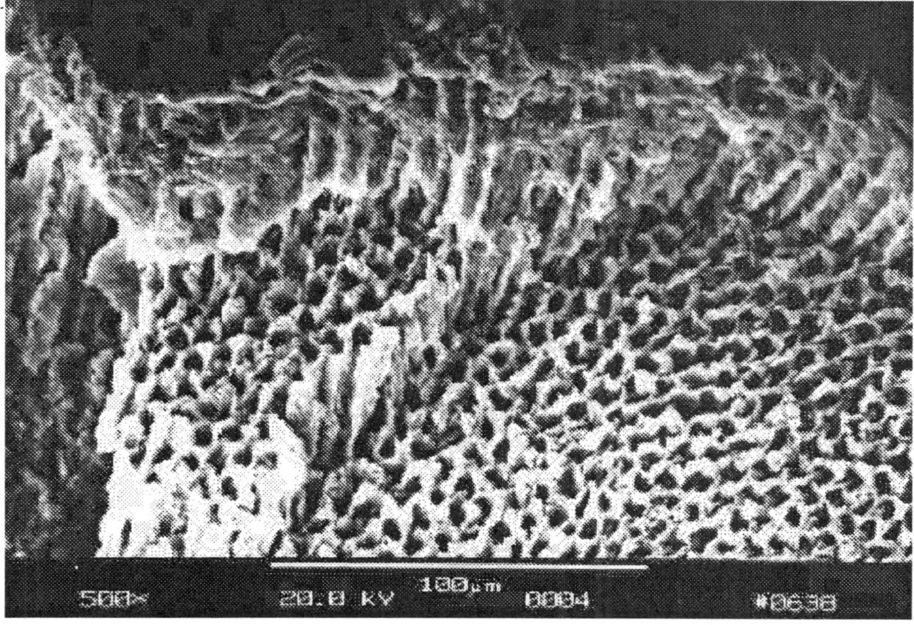

Figure 2. High magnification photograph of caries taken with a scanning electron microscope. Reproduced from [2].

The removal of infected substance is usually accomplished with conventional mechanical drills. These drills do evoke additional pain because of two reasons. First, tooth nerves are very sensitive to the induced vibrations. Second, tooth nerves also detect sudden increases in temperature which are induced by friction during the drilling process. Pain relief without injection of anaesthetic was the basic ulterior motive when looking for laser applications in caries therapy. However, it turned out that not all types of lasers fulfill this task. Although vibrations are avoided due to the contactless technique, thermal side effects are not always eliminated when using lasers. CW and long-pulse lasers, in particular, induce extremely high temperatures in the pulp as shown in Figure 3 . Even air cooling does not reduce this temperature to a tolerable value. Thermal damage is negligible only when using ultrashort pulses in the picosecond or femtosecond range.

Meanwhile, other advantages are being discussed which could even be more significant than just pain relief. Very important among these are the so-called conditioning of dental substance and a possibly more precise procedure of caries removal. Conditioning provides additional protection of the tooth by means of sealing its surface. Thereby, the occurrence of caries can be significantly delayed. Improved control of caries removal, e.g. by a spectroscopic analysis of laser-induced plasmas, as shown in Figures 4, could minimize the amount of healthy substance to be removed. The information is derived from specific calcium transitions and the process of demineralization associated with caries, since carious teeth contain far less calcium than healthy teeth. It is emphasized, though, that this method is not suitable for a complete screening of all teeth. It shall only assist the dentist in regulating the laser power during the treatment of a specific tooth and in determining the best moment for finishing this treatment. Then, indications for expensive dental crowns or bridges are effectively reduced.

9.3   LASER TREATMENT OF HARD TOOTH SUBSTANCE

First experiments with teeth using the laser as a surgical tool were performed by Goldman *et al.* [4] and Stern and Sognnaes [5]. Both of these groups used a pulsed ruby laser at a wavelength of 694 μm. This laser induced severe thermal side effects such as irreversible injury of nerve fibers and tooth cracking. Thus, it is not very surprising that these initial studies never gained clinical relevance. A few years later, a CO_2 laser system was investigated by Stern *et al.* [6]. However, the results did not improve very much compared with the ruby laser. These observations are due to the fact that both ruby and CO_2 lasers are typical representatives of thermally acting lasers. Thus, it was straightforward to conclude that without being able to eliminate these thermal effects, lasers would never turn into a suitable tool for the preparation of teeth [7].

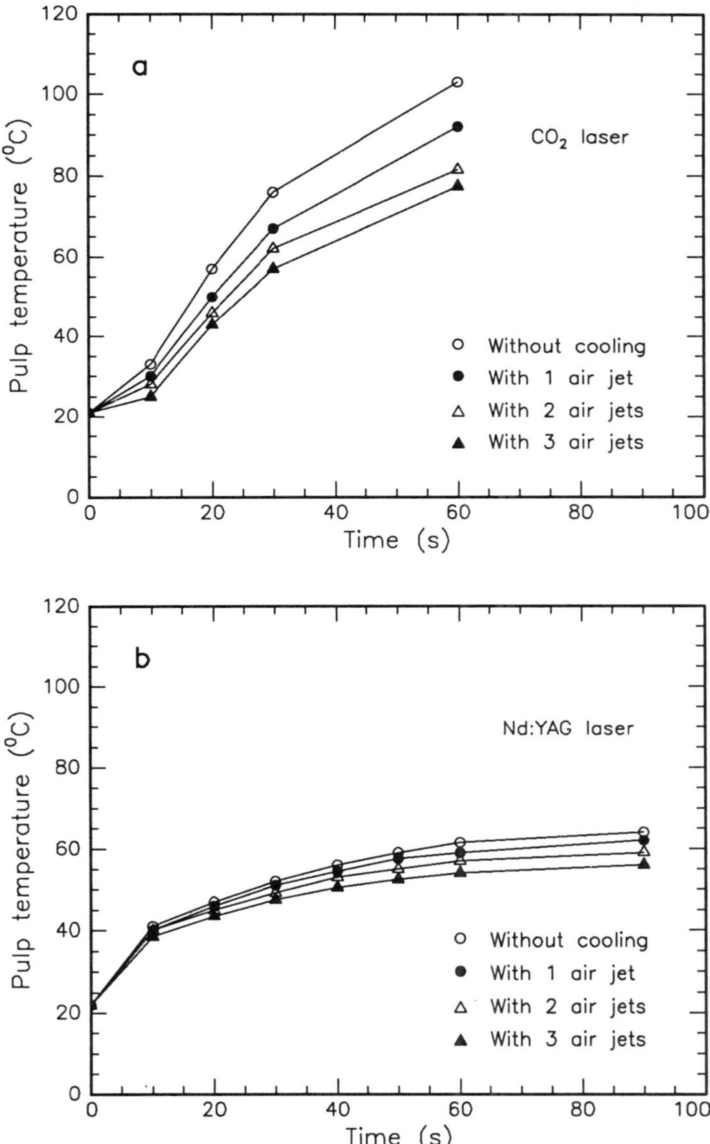

Figure 3. (a) Mean temperatures in the pulp during exposure to a CW CO2 laser (power: 5W) without and with air cooling, respectively, (b) Mean temperatures in the pulp during exposure to a CW Nd:YAG laser (power: 4W) without and with air cooling, respectively [3].

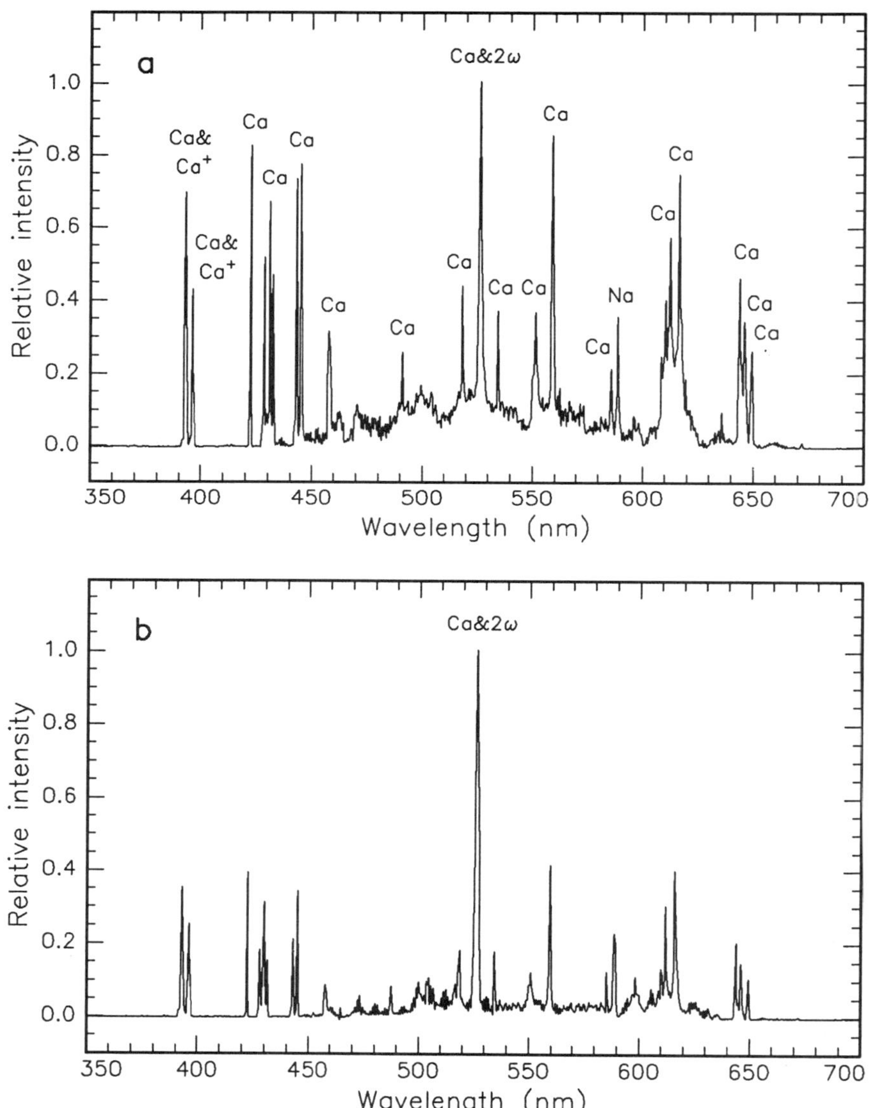

Figure 4. (a) Spectrum of a laser-induced plasma on healthy tooth substance (laser type: Nd:YLF, pulse duration: 30 ps, pulse energy: 500 μJ). Lines of neutral calcium (Ca), singly ionized calcium (Ca⁺), and neutral sodium (Na) are seen. The signal at 526.5 nm partly originates from calcium and from second harmonic generation (SHG) of the laser beam, (b) Spectrum of a laser-induced plasma on carious tooth substance (same laser parameters as above). Due to the process of demineralization, the intensity of all mineral lines is reduced [2].

Meanwhile, several experiments have been conducted using alternative laser systems. At the end of the 1980s, the Er:YAG laser was introduced to dental applications by Hibst and Keller [8,9], and Kayano *et al.* [10]. The wavelength of the Er:YAG laser at 2.94 µm matches the resonance frequency of the vibrational oscillations of water molecules contained in the teeth. Thereby, the absorption of the Er:YAG radiation is strongly enhanced, resulting in a high efficiency. However, the sudden vaporization of water is associated with a pressure gradient. Small microexplosions are responsible for the break-up of the hydroxyapatite structure. A high magnification photograph of a human tooth after Er:YAG laser exposure is shown in Figure 5. The coincidence of thermal (e.g. vaporization)and mechanical (e.g. pressure gradient) ablation effects has led to the term "thermomechanical interaction".

Initially, Er:YAG lasers seemed to be very promising because of their high efficiency in ablating dental substances. Meanwhile, though, some indication has been given that microcracks can be induced by Er:YAG laser radiation. It was found by Niemz *et al.* [11] and Frentzen *et al.* [8], using scanning electron microscopy and dye penetration tests, that these fissures can extend up to 300 µm in depth. They could thus easily serve as an origin for the development of a new decay. External cooling of the tooth might help to reduce the occurrence of cracking but further research needs to be performed prior to clinical applications.

Even worse results were found with the Ho:YAG laser at a wavelength of 2.12 µm as reported by Niemz *et al.* [11]. A high magnification photograph of a human tooth after Ho:YAG laser exposure is shown in Figure 6. Severe thermal effects including melting of tooth substance were observed. Moreover, cracks up to 3 mm in depth were measured when performing dye penetration tests.

Dye penetration tests are suitable experiments for the detection of laser-induced tooth fissures. After laser exposure, the tooth is stained with a dye, e.g. neofuchsine solution, for several hours. Afterwards, the tooth is sliced using a microtome, and the maximum penetration depth of the dye is determined. The results of some representative measurements are summarized in Figure 7. Obviously, tooth fissures induced by Ho:YAG and Er:YAG lasers must be considered as a severe side effect.

Another laser type - the ArF excimer laser - was investigated by Frentzen *et al.* [13] and Liesenhoff *et al.* [14] regarding its usefulness in dentistry. Indeed, initial experiments proved that only very little thermal effects were induced which was attributed to the shorter pulse duration of approximately 15 ns and the gentle interaction mechanism of photoablation. However, the ablation rate achieved with this laser, i.e. the ablated volume per unit time, is too low for clinical applications. Although very successful in refractive

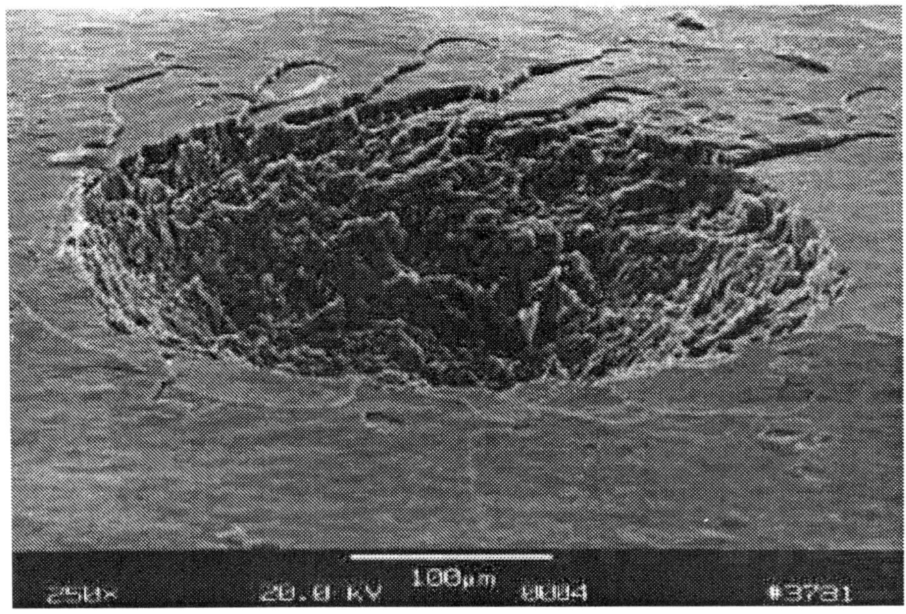

Figure 5. Human tooth exposed to 20 pulses from an Er:YAG laser (pulse duration: 90 µs, pulse energy: 100 mJ, repetition rate: 1 Hz).

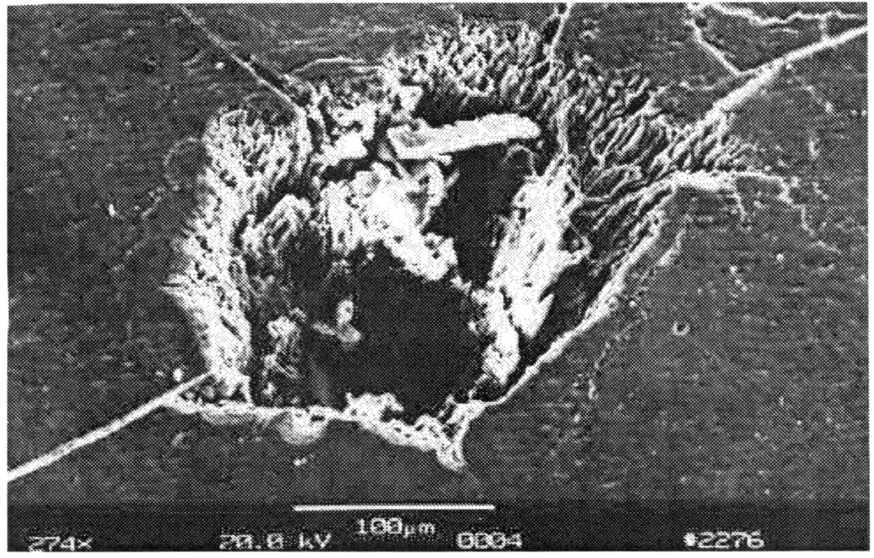

Figure 6. Human tooth exposed to 100 pulses from a Ho:YAG laser (pulse duration: 3.8 µs, pulse energy: 18 mJ, repetition rate: 1 Hz

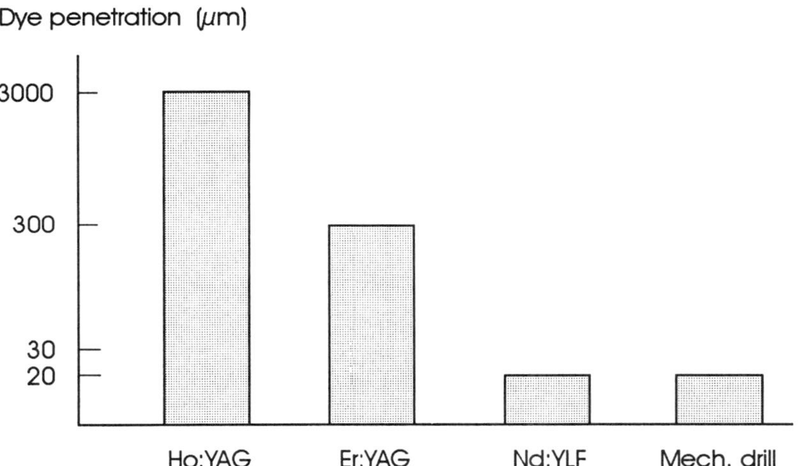

Figure 7. Results of dye penetration tests for three different solid-state lasers and the mechanical drill. Listed are the maximum penetration depths inside the enamel of human teeth. Pulse durations: 250 μs (Ho:YAG), 90 μs (Er:YAG), and 30 ps (Nd:YLF) [11].

corneal surgery because of its high precision, it is exactly this accuracy with ablation depths less than 1 μm per pulse and the rather moderate repetition rates which pull the ablation rate down. This ineffectiveness and the general risks of UV radiation are the major disadvantages concerning the use of the ArF laser in dentistry.

A second UV laser, the frequency-doubled Alexandrite laser at 377 nm, was studied by Steiger *et al.* [15] and Rechmann *et al.* [16]. It was observed that this laser offers a better selectivity for carious dentin than the Er:YAG laser, i.e. the required fluence at the ablation threshold of healthy dentin is higher when using the Alexandrite laser, whereas the thresholds for carious dentin are about the same.

A novel approach to laser caries therapy has been made by Niemz *et al.* [11], Pioch *et al.* [17] and Niemz [18] when using ultrashort laser pulses. Although, at the early stage of experiments, uncertainty predominated concerning potential shock wave effects, it has meanwhile been verified by five independent tests that mechanical impacts are negligible. These consist of *scanning electron microscopy, dye penetration tests, hardness tests, histology, and polarized microscopy.* Detailed results have been published by Niemz [19].

9.3.1 Scanning Electron Microscopy (SEM)

In Figures 8 and 9, two SEM are shown demonstrating the ability of ultrashort laser pulses to produce extremely precise tetragonal cavities in human enamel. The cavities were achieved by scanning the laser focus of a picosecond Nd:YLF laser at a wavelength of 1053 nm and of a femtosecond Ti:Sapphire laser at a wavelength of 780 nm respectively. In either case, the cavity walls are very steep and are characterized by a sealed glass-like structure. This is of great significance for the prevention of further decay. The roughness of the cavity bottom is of the order of 10-20 μm and thus facilitates the adhesion of most filling materials.

9.3.2 Dye Penetration Tests

The results of dye penetration tests after exposure to a picosecond Nd:YLF laser have already been presented in Figure 7. Laser-induced fissures typically remained below 20 μm. This value is of the same order as fissure depths obtained with the mechanical drill.

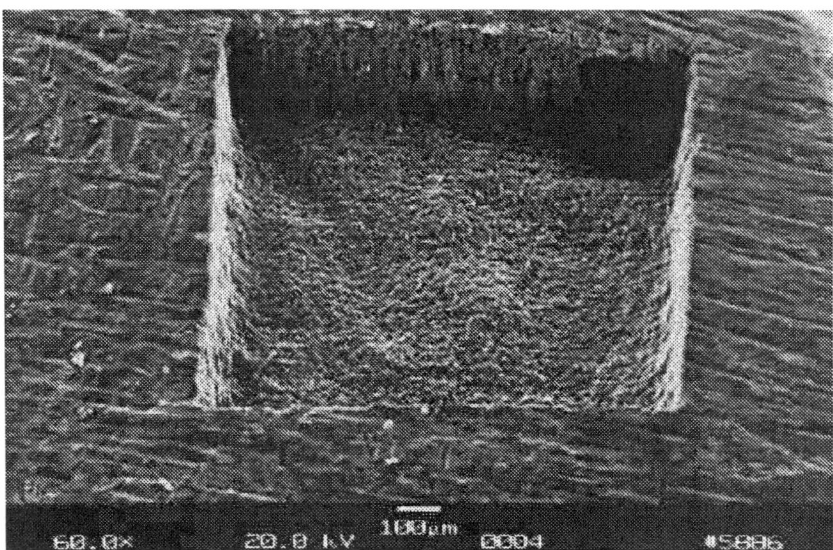

Figure 8. Human tooth exposed to a picosecond Nd:YLF laser (pulse duration: 30 ps, pulse energy: mJ).

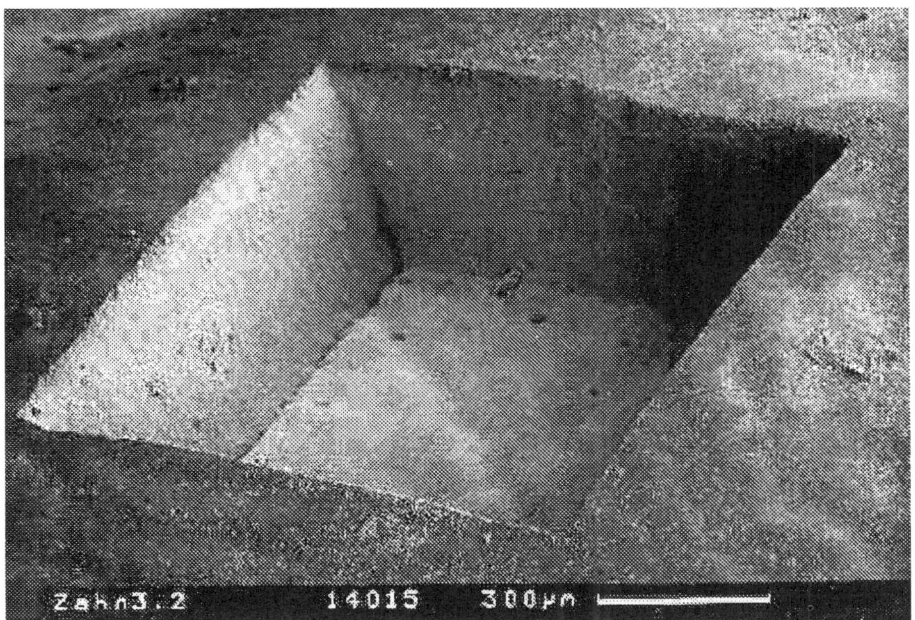

Figure 9. Human tooth exposed to a femtosecond Ti:Sapphire laser (pulse duration: 130 fs, pulse energy: 50 µJ).

9.3.3 Hardness Tests

One obvious test for the potential influence of shock waves is the measurement of hardness of a tooth before and after laser exposure. In hardness tests according to Vickers, the impact of a diamond tip into a tooth surface is determined. Softer material is characterized by a deeper impact of the diamond tip - and thus a larger impact diameter. The hardness itself is defined as:

$$H_V = 1.8544 \ K/D^2$$

where $K = 5.0 \times 10^4$ N, and **D** is the impact of a diamond tip cut at an angle of 136° and expressed in millimeters. The results of hardness tests after exposure to picosecond Nd:YLF pulses are presented in Table 1. According to Niemz [1], no significant alteration in hardness is observed in exposed and unexposed enamel. As expected, though, dentin appears much softer due to its lower content of hydroxyapatite.

Table 1. Mean hardness values of teeth before and after exposure to a Nd:YLF laser (pulse duration: 30 ps, pulse energy: 1 mJ).}

	D (mm)	H_V (N/mm^2)
Exposed enamel	5.9	2660
Unexposed enamel	5.8	2760
Unexposed dentin	11.5	700

9.3.4 Histology

The most important touchstone for the introduction of a new therapeutic technique is the biological response of the tissue, i.e., the survival of cells. Histologic sections enable specific statements concerning the condition of cells due to highly sophisticated staining techniques. Odontoblasts do not intrude into the dentin after exposure to ultrashort laser pulses as shown by Niemz [19]. Moreover, they do have a similar appearance as in unexposed teeth. Thus, potential shock waves do not have a detectable impact on the pulp - not even on a cellular level.

9.3.5 Polarized Microscopy

Polarized microscopy is an efficient tool for detecting alterations in optical density which might arise from the exposure to shock waves. If these shock waves are reflected, e.g., at the enamel-dentin junction, such alterations might even be enhanced and should thus become evident. For polarized microscopy, exposed teeth are dehydrated in an upgraded series of ethanol. Afterwards, they are kept in fluid methacrylate for at least three days. Within the following period of seven days, polymerization takes place in a heat chamber set to 43° C. Then, the embedded samples are cut into 100 µm thick slices using a saw microtome. Finally, the slices are polished and examined with a polarized light microscope. According to Niemz [19], no evidence for laser-induced shock waves is given when applying ultrashort laser pulses.

In Figure 10, the ablation curves of healthy enamel, healthy dentin, and carious enamel are given, respectively. In healthy enamel, plasma sparking was already visible at approximately 0.2 mJ. Taking the corresponding focal spot size of 30 µm into account, the ablation threshold is determined to be about 30 J/cm^2. For carious enamel, plasma generation started at roughly 0.1

mJ, i.e., at a threshold density of 15 J/cm^2. In the range of pulse energies investigated, all three ablation curves are mainly linear. Linear regression analysis yields that the corresponding slopes in Figure 10 are 1 μm /0.2 mJ, 3 μm /0.2 mJ, and 8 μm /0.2 mJ, respectively. Thus, the ablation efficiency increases from healthy enamel and healthy dentin to carious enamel. From the ablation volumes, we derive that, at the given laser parameters, approximately 1.5 mm^3 of carious enamel can be ablated per minute. To cope with conventional mechanical drills, a ten times higher ablation efficiency would be desirable. It can be achieved by increasing both the pulse energy and repetition rate. The Nd:YLF picosecond laser might represent a considerable alternative in the preparation of hard tooth substances. The potential realization of such a clinical laser system is currently being evaluated.

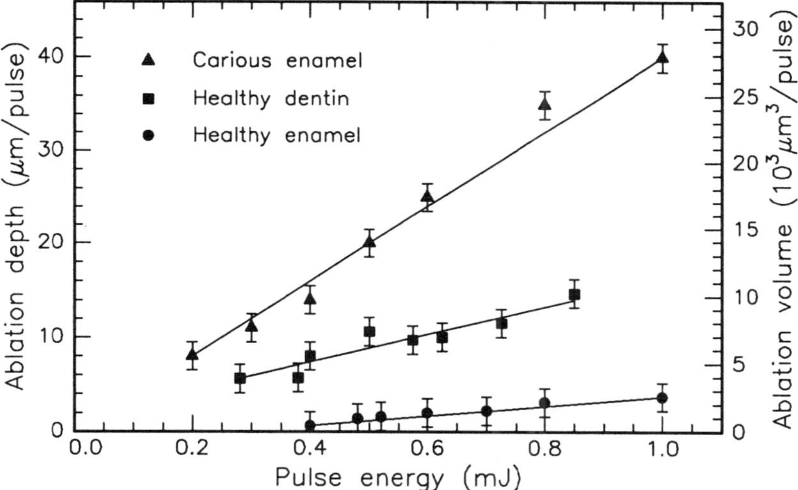

Figure 10. Ablation curves of carious enamel, healthy dentin, and healthy enamel, respectively, obtained with a Nd:YLF laser (pulse duration: 30 ps, focal spot size: 30 μm) [1].

One very important issue associated with dental laser systems is the temperature increase inside the pulp where odontoblasts, blood vessels, and tooth nerves are located. Only increments below 5° C are tolerable, otherwise thermal side effects might occur. Moreover, the feeling of pain is induced at pulp temperatures which exceed approximately 45°C. It is thus very important to remain below these temperatures when striving for clinical applicability. In Figure 11, the temperature increments induced by a picosecond Nd:YLF laser at a repetition rate of 1 kHz are summarized. For this experiment, human teeth were cut into 1 mm thick slices. On one surface of these slices, the laser beam was scanned over a 1 × 1 mm^2 area, while the temperature was measured at the opposite surface by means of a thermocoupler. The observed temperature increments depend on the number of consecutive pulses as well as on the total duration of exposure. A higher temperature is obtained when applying 30 instead of only 10 consecutive pulses before moving the focal spot to the next position. The total duration of exposure also affects the final temperature, although the increase during the first minute is most significant. From these results, we can conclude that up to approximately 10 consecutive pulses may be applied to a tooth at a repetition rate of 1 kHz if the temperature in the pulp shall not increase by more than 5 °C.

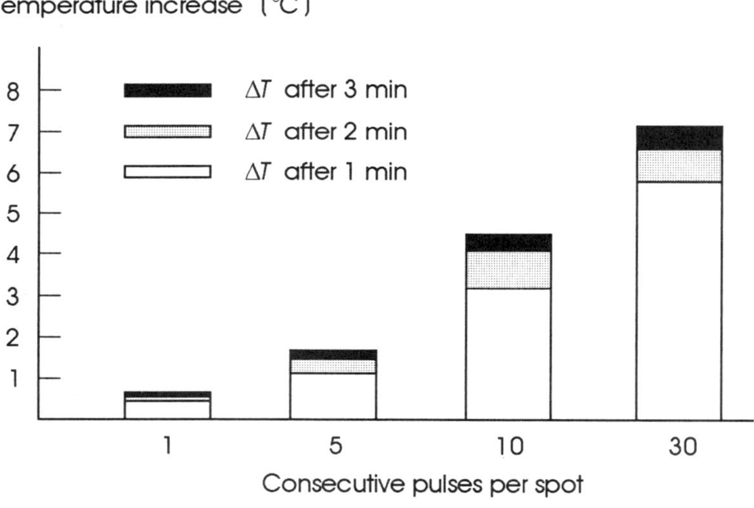

Figure 11. Increase in temperature in a distance of 1 mm from cavities achieved with a Nd:YLF laser (pulse duration: 30 ps, pulse energy: 1mJ, repetition rate: 1 kHz) [1].

9.4 LASER TREATMENT OF SOFT DENTAL TISSUE

Several studies have been reported on the use of a CO_2 laser in the management of malignant, pre-malignant, and benign lesions of the oral mucosa, e.g., by Strong *et al.* [20], Horch and Gerlach [21], Frame *et al.* [22], and Frame [23]. Since the oral environment is very moist, radiation from the CO_2 laser is predestined for such purposes because of its high absorption. When treating a soft tissue lesion inside the mouth, the surgeon has a choice of two techniques - either excision or vaporization. It is usually preferable to excise the lesion because this provides histologic evidence of its complete removal and confirmation of the preceding diagnosis.

During vaporization, a risk always remains that not all altered tissue is eliminated. Hence, if a pathologic lesion is vaporized, a biopsy should be obtained from the adjacent tissue after the treatment.

The CO_2 laser is particularly useful for small mucosal lesions. Most of them can be vaporized at a power of 5-10 W in pulsed or CW mode. After laser treatment, the wound is sterile and only minimal inflammatory reactions of the surrounding tissue occur. One major advantage is that there is no need to suture the wound, since small blood vessels are coagulated and bleeding is thus stopped. The wound edges can even be smoothed with a defocused beam. Wound healing usually occurs within a period of two weeks, and the process of reepithelialization is complete after about 4-6 weeks. Frame [23] states that patients tolerate the procedure well and initially complain of little pain only. However, the treated area may become uncomfortable for approximately 2-3 weeks.

Cases of leukoplakia are difficult to treat by conventional surgery, since they are frequently widespread inside the mouth. The lesion is usually outlined with a focused CO_2 laser beam for easy visualization. Afterwards, it is vaporized with a defocused beam at a power of about 15-20 W. According to Horch [24], laser-treated leukoplakias heal very well, and there is only little evidence of recurrence. Even leukoplakias on tongue and lips can be treated without losses in performance of these organs.

Malignant lesions require a higher laser power of approximately 20-30 W to deal with the bulk of the tumor. Lanzafame *et al.* [25] state that the recurrence of local tumors is reduced when using the CO_2 laser rather than a mechanical scalpel. The thermal effect of the radiation is made responsible for this observation. However, it is questionable whether laser treatments of malignant oral tumors are successful during a longer follow-up period, since metastases have often already spread to other parts of the body. In these cases, laser application is restricted to a palliative treatment. Specimen for biopsy can also be excised with a CO_2 laser as one would do with a conventional scalpel. Patel [26] reported on the application of a Nd:YAG laser in the treatment of oral cancer. However, in the treatment of soft dental tissues, this laser has not gained clinical relevance so far.

Wound healing and pain relief are sometimes attributed to laser irradiation, as well. They belong to the group of biostimulative effects. However, biostimulation is still a research field with a lot of speculation involved. Detailed investigations in this area and reproducible experimental results are badly needed.

9.5 LASERS IN ENDODONTICS

Endodontics is concerned with the treatment of infections of the root canal. These arise from either a breakthrough of decay into the pulp or from plaque accumulation beneath the gingiva and subsequent bacterial attacks of the root. In either case, once the pulp or the root canal are infected by bacteria, the only treatment is to sterilize both pulp and root, thereby taking into account the associated death of the tooth. However, even a dead tooth may reside in place for years.

The mechanical removal of bacteria, plaque, infected root cementum, and inflammated soft tissues is regarded as an essential part of a systematic periodontal treatment. The excavation of the root itself is a very complicated and time-consuming procedure, since roots are very thin and special tools are required. The procedure can be supported by antimicrobial chemicals to ensure sterility which is a mandatory condition for success of the treatment. Along with the rapid development of medical laser systems, it has been discussed whether lasers could improve conventional techniques of endodontics, especially in removal of plaques and sterilization. First experimental results using CO_2 and Nd:YAG lasers in endodontics were published by Weichmann and Johnson [27,28]. By means of melting the dentin next to the root, the canal wall appears to be sealed and thus less permeable for bacteria. Indeed, Melcer *et al.* [29] and Frentzen and Koort [30] stated that lasers may have a sterilizing effect. Sievers *et al.* [31] observed very clean surfaces of the root canal after application of an ArF excimer laser. However, both the CO_2 laser and the ArF laser will not gain clinical relevance in endodontics, since their radiation cannot be applied through flexible fibers. Even other laser systems will not be applicable exclusively, since suitable fiber diameters of 400 μm are still too large for unprepared roots. Thinner fibers are very likely to break inside the root causing severe complications and additional mechanical operation.

9.6 LASER TREATMENT OF FILLING MATERIALS

In dental practice, not only tooth substance needs to be ablated but also old fillings have to be removed, e.g., when a secondary decay is located underneath. For the removal of metallic fillings, infrared lasers cannot be used, since the reflectivity of these materials is too high in that spectral range.

Amalgam should never be ablated with lasers at all. During irradiation, the amalgam is melted and a significant amount of mercury is released which is extremely toxic for both patient and dentist. For other filling materials, e.g., composites, few data are available only. Hibst and Keller [32] have shown that the Er:YAG laser removes certain kinds of composites very efficiently. However, it is quite uncertain whether lasers will ever be clinically used for such purposes.

Another very interesting topic in dental technology is laser-welding of dental bridges and dentures. It can be regarded as an alternative to conventional soldering. During soldering, the parts to be joined are not melted themselves but are attached by melting an additional substance which, in general, is meant to form an alloy between them. Laser-welding, on the other hand, attaches two parts to each other by means of transferring them to a plastic or fluid state. This is achieved with high power densities ranging from 10^2 - 10^9 W/cm^2. According to Benthem [33], CO_2 lasers and Nd:YAG lasers are preferably used. Since the reflectivity of metals is very high in the infrared spectrum, it must be assured that either a laser plasma is induced at the surface of the target or that the target is coated with a highly absorbing layer prior to laser exposure. Dobberstein *et al.* [34] state that some laser-welded alloys are characterized by a higher tear threshold than soldered samples as shown in Figure 12.

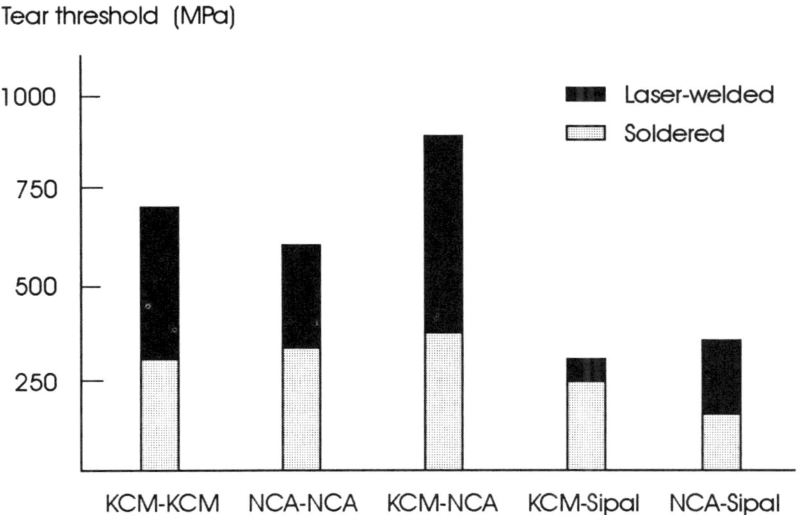

Figure 12. Tear thresholds of laser-welded and soldered dental alloys (KCM: cobalt-based alloy, NCA: nickel-based alloy, Sipal: silver-palladium-based alloy) [34].

However, Benthem [33] argues that such a behavior cannot be observed in all alloys, but tear thresholds in laser-welded alloys can definitely reach the same values as the original cast. According to his studies, the major advantages of laser-welding are: higher resistency against corrosion, ability to weld different metals, ability to weld coated alloys, and lower heat load. Moreover, the reproducibility of laser-welded alloys is significantly higher than during soldering. For further results, the interested reader should consult the excellent review given by Benthem [33].

REFERENCES

1. Niemz, M.H. (1996). *Laser-Tissue Interactions:Fundamentals and Applications*. Springer-Verlag, Berlin, Heidelberg, New York.
2. Niemz, M.H. (1994*). Investigation and Spectral Analysis of the Plasma-Induced Ablation Mechanism of Dental Hydroxyapatite*. Appl. Phys. **B 58**, 273-281.
3. Frentzen, M., Koort, H.-J. (1992). *Excimer Laser - Grundlagen und Mogliche Anwendungen in der Zahnheilkunde*. In: Laser in der Zahnmedizin (Eds.: Vahl, J., van Benthem, H.). Quintessenz-Verlag, Berlin, Chicago, London.
4. Goldman, L., Hornby, P., Mayer, R., Goldman, B. (1964*). Impact of the Laser on Dental Caries*. Nature **203**, 417.
5. Stern,, R.H., Sognnaes, R.F. (1964). *Laser Beam Effect on Dental Hard Tissues*. J. Dent. Res. **43**, 873.
6. Stern, R.H., Vahl, J., Sognnaes R. (1972). *Lased Enamel: Ultrastructural Observations of Pulsed Carbon Dioxide Laser Effects*. J. Dent. Res. **51**, 455-460.
7. Stern, R.H. (1974). *Dentistry and the Laser*. In: Laser Applications in Medicine and Biology (Ed.: Wolbarsht, M.L.). Plenum Press, New York.
8. Hibst, R., Keller, U. (1989). *Experimental Studies of the Application of the Er:YAG Laser on Dental Hard Substances: I. Measurement of the Ablation Rate*. Lasers Surg. Med. **9**, 338-344.
9. Keller, U., Hibst, R. (1989). *Experimental Studies of the Application of the Er:YAG Laser on Dental Hard Substances: II. Light Microscopic and SEM Investigations*. Lasers Surg. Med. **9**, 345-351.
10. Kayano, T., Ochiai, S., Kiyono, K., Yamamoto, H., Nakajima, S., Mochizuki, T. (1989). *Effects of Er:YAG Laser Irradiation on Human Extracted Teeth*. J. Stomat. Soc. Jap. **56**, 381-392.
11. Niemz, M.H., Eisenmann, L., Pioch, T. (1993). *Vergleich von drei Lasersystemen zur Abtragung von Zahnschmelz*. Schweiz. Monatsschr. Zahnmed. **103**, 1252--1256.
12. Frentzen, M., Winkelstrater, C., van Benthem, H., Koort, H.-J. (1994). *Bearbeitung der Schmelzoberfachen mit gepulster Laserstrahlung*. Dtsch. Zahnarztl. Z. **49**, 166--168.
13. Frentzen, M., Koort, H.-J., Kermani, O., Dardenne, M.U. (1989). *Bearbeitung von Zahnhartgeweben mit einem Excimer-Laser--eine in- vitro Studie*. Dtsch. Zahnarztl. Z. **44**, 431-435.
14. Liesenhoff, T., Bende, T., Lenz, H., Seiler, T. (1989). *Abtragen von Zahnhartsubstanzen mit Excimer-Laserstrahlen*. Dtsch. Zahnarztl. Z. **44**, 426--430.
15. Steiger, E., Maurer, N., Geisel, G. (1993). *The Frequency-Doubled Alexandrite Laser: an Alternative Dental Device*. Proc. SPIE **1880**, 149-152.
16. Rechmann, P., Hennig, T., von den Hoff, U., Kaufmann, R. (1993). *Caries Selective Ablation: Wavelength 377 nm versus 2.9 μm}*. Proc. SPIE **1880**, 235-239.

17. Pioch, T., Niemz, M., Mindermann, A., Staehle, H.J. (1994). *Schmelzablationen durch Laserimpulse im Pikosekundenbereich.* Dtsch. Zahnarztl. Z. **49**, 163-165.

18. Niemz, M.H. (1998*). Ultrashort Laser Pulses in Dentistry -- Advantages and Limitations.* Proc. SPIE **3255**, 84-91.

19. Niemz, M.H. (1995). *Cavity Preparation with the Nd:YLF Picosecond Laser.* J. Dent. Res. **74**, 1194-1199.

20. Strong, M.S., Vaughan, C.W., Healy, G.B., Shapshay,~S.M., Jako, G.J. (1979). *Transoral Management of Localised Carcinoma of the Oral Cavity Using the CO_2 Laser* Laryngoscope **89**, 897-905.

21. Horch, H.-H., Gerlach, K.L. (1982). *CO_2 Laser Treatment of Oral Dysplastic Precancerous Lesions: a Preliminary Report.* Lasers Surg. Med. **2**, 179-185.

22. Frame, J.W., Das Gupta, A.R., Dalton, G.A., Rhys Evans, P.H. (1984). *Use of the Carbon Dioxide Laser in the Management of Premalignant Lesions of the Oral Mucosa.* J. Laryngol. Otol. **98**, 1251-1260.

23. Frame, J.W. (1985). *Carbon Dioxide Laser Surgery for Benign Oral Lesions.* Br. Dent. J. **158**, 125-128.

24. Horch,H.-H. (1992). *Laser in der Mund-Kiefer-Gesichts-Chirurgie.* In: Laser in der Zahnmedizin (Eds.: Vahl, J., van Benthem, H.). Quintessenz-Verlag, Berlin, Chicago, London.

25. Lanzafame, R.J., Rogers, D.W., Naim, J.O., De France, C.A., Ochej, H., Hinshaw, J.R. (1986). Reduction of Local Tumor Recurrence by Excision with the CO_2 Laser}. Lasers Surg. Med. **6**, 439-441.

26. Patel, D.D. (1988). *Nd:YAG Laser in Oral Cavity Cancer Report of 200 Cases - Minimum Follow Up of One Year.* In: Laser-Optoelectronics in Medicine (Ed.: Waidelich, W.). Springer-Verlag, Berlin, Heidelberg, New York.

27. Weichmann, G., Johnson, J. (1971). *Laser Use in Endodontics. A Preliminary Investigation.* Oral Surg. **31**, 416-420.

28. Weichmann, G., Johnson, J., Nitta, L. (1972*). Laser Use in Endodontics. Part II.* Oral Surg. **34**, 828-830.

29. Melcer, J., Chaumette, M.T., Melcer, F. (1987). Dental Pulp Exposed to CO_2 Laser Beam}. Lasers Surg. Med. **7**, 347-352.

30. Frentzen, M., Koort, H.-J. (1990*). Lasers in Dentistry.* Int. Dent. J. **40**, 323-332.

31. Sievers, M., Frentzen, M., Kosina, A., Koort, H.-J. (1993). *Scaling of Root Surfaces with Laser - an in vitro Study.* Proc. SPIE **2080**, 82-87.

32. Hibst, R., Keller, U. (1991*). Removal of Dental Filling Materials by Er:YAG Laser Radiation.* Proc. SPIE **1200**, 120-126.

33. van Benthem, H. (1992). *Laseranwendung in der zahnarztlichen Prothetik und der dentalen Technologie.* In: Laser in der Zahnmedizin (Eds.: Vahl, J., van Benthem, H.). Quintessenz-Verlag, Berlin.

34. Dobberstein, H., Dobberstein, H., Zuhrt, R., Thierfelder, C., Ertl, T. (1991). *Laserbearbeitung von Dentalkeramik und Dentallegierungen.* In: Angewandte Lasermedizin (Eds.: Berlien, H.-P., Muller, G.). Ecomed-Verlag, Landsberg.

Chapter 10

LASERS IN GYNAECOLOGY

D. Takkar and Alka Sinha
Department of Obstetrics and Gynaecology
All India Institute of Medical Sciences, New Delhi, INDIA

10.1 INTRODUCTION

Lasers have come a long way since Schawlow and Townes explained how the process of stimulated emission of radiation could be used to amplify visible light [1]. Subsequently, Maiman produced the first working laser [2]. Lasers have since then found wide and varied applications in many specialties in the medical field including that of gynecology. Gynecologists, all over the world, are becoming increasingly aware of the potential applications of lasers in both conventional surgeries and newer endoscopic and microsurgical procedures. The types of lasers now used are as diverse as the diseases they are used to treat.

The most useful lasers in gynaecology are the CO_2, Nd:YAG and the argon and KTP lasers. A comparison of the physical properties of these lasers regarding their use in gynaecology is given here.

CO_2 laser is most commonly used by gynaecologists for colposcopic procedures and during laparotomy. It is safe with minimal depth of thermal injury. However it has several limitations. Its coagulating power is less and it is a non-contact laser. It cannot be transmitted down a fibre, so it cannot be used for operative hysteroscopy. During laparoscopy, it necessitates the use of a direct or indirect laser coupler or a special laser laparoscope. Recently waveguide delivery systems have been introduced for CO_2 laser laparoscopy using standard laparoscopes. These are slender cannula through which the beam is transmitted. This eliminates the problem of alignment associated with the couplers.

The Nd:YAG (neodymium:yttrium aluminium garnett) laser is the primary endoscopic instrument. Nd is the active lasing medium while YAG is a solid with good crystalline strength. It is used for deep coagulation. Nd:YAG laser can be used through the bare fibre or in association with a variety of contact saphire tips which increases its precision. A helium-neon beam for aiming is needed as the light of the Nd:YAG laser is in the infrared spectrum.

The properties of the Argon and the KTP (potassium titanyl phosphate) lasers are like Nd:YAG and they can be used similarly. However these lasers are best used as colour selective photocoagulators.

A comparison of the properties of the CO_2 and the Nd:YAG lasers is presented in Table 1.

Table 1 : Comparison of properties of lasers commonly used in gynaecology

	CO_2	Nd:YAG	Argon	KTP
Coagulation	Less	Good	Good	Good
Depth of coagulation	0.1mm	7-8 mm	4mm	4mm
H_2O absorption	Absorbed	No	No	No
Spectrum	Infrared, needs He-Ne for aiming	Infrared, need He-Ne for aiming	Blue/ Green	Green
Excision	Good	Average	Average	Average
Transmission down fibers	No	Yes	Yes	Yes

Applications of lasers in gynaecology can be classified as follows:

I.   Laparotomy / laparoscopy

    1.   Endometriosis
- Excision of endometriomas
- Ovarian cystectomy
- Vaporization of endometrial implants
- Uterosacral nerve ablation and presacral neurectomy

    2.   Fibroids and other conditions of uterus
- Myomectomy
- Myolysis
- Hysterectomy
- Metroplasty

3.   Tubal surgery
   - Tubal surgery for infertility
       i.   Neosalpingostomy
       ii.   Cuff salpingostomy
       iii.   End to end anastomosis
       iv.   Cornual implantation
   - Ectopic pregnancy
4.   Ovarian cysts
   - Cystectomy
   - Oophorectomy
   - Ovarian drilling for polycystic ovarian disease
5.   Adhesions
   - Adhesiolysis

II.   Hysteroscopy
1.   Endometrial laser ablation
2.   Resection of submucous myoma
3.   Myolysis
4.   Resection of uterine septum
5.   Division of uterine synechiae

III.   Colposcopy
1.   Cervical intraepithelial neoplasia
2.   Vaginal intraepithelial neoplasia
3.   Vulvar intraepithelial neoplasia
4.   Non-neoplastic vulvar lesions

IV.   Assisted reproductive techniques

10.2 LAPAROSCOPY/ LAPAROTOMY WITH LASERS

10.2.1 Endometriosis

Endometriosis is a common condition affecting women in the reproductive age group leading to infertility, pain and dysmenorrhoea. Lasers are particularly effective in the treatment of endometriosis because of their precision and coagulating capacity. Endometriotic implants in moderate to severe endometriosis may be treated laparoscopically by laser vaporization and/or resection. In a few comparative studies, CO_2 laser therapy was found to be more effective than non-laser therapy [3]. Advanced laparoscopic surgery with the CO_2 laser may also be more efficient than other modalities in treating infertile women with minimal to mild endometriosis in terms of pregnancy rates [4]. The pregnancy rates seem to be related to the severity of the disease e.g., 62% for mild, 52% for moderate and 42% for severe disease [5].

It is important to ensure complete vaporization of the endometriotic implants as evidenced by the appearance of 'bubbling of water' created by vaporization of the intraperitoneal fat. A margin of 2mm around each lesion should be vaporized. Flimsy periovarian and peritubal adhesions may be vaporised at the same time.

Small ovarian endometriomas may be vaporized completely. Longer endometriomas, may be drained and then started on GnRH therapy followed by vaporization of the inner wall of the endometrioma. A cumulative pregnancy rate of 5.1% after 1 year was achieved with a recurrence rate of 8% in a follow up of 2-11 years [6]. Improvement or resolution of pain was reported in 74% [7].

The Nd:YAG laser [8] and the KTP laser [7] have been used similarly. The argon laser may have a benefit because of its colour spectrum. The CO_2 laser, though most commonly used, has the disadvantage that it is absorbed by water.

Patients with severe dysmenorrhoea may benefit from presacral neurectomy in combination with other treatment for endometriosis. The performance of presacral neurectomy with the standard laparoscopic approach utilising a contact tip Nd:YAG laser with a sapphire tip is feasible, effective and safe [9].

The pain impulses from the uterus, travelling through the inferior hypogastric plexus into the intermediate and superior hypogastric plexus, can be interrupted by this procedure. The intermediate hypogastric plexus lying on the body of L5 vertebra is the most appropriate site for resection and it results in significant relief of midline pain. Laparoscopic uterosacral nerve ablation (LUNA) is another procedure used for pain relief in these patients [5,10].

10.2.2 Fibroids and Other Conditions of Uterus

10.2.2.1 Myomectomy

Subserous and interstitial fibroids are amenable to laparoscopic removal. Laparoscopic myomectomy is specially suited for fibroid size less than 8-10cms and numbering 4 or less. In a report of 43 cases by Dubuisson *et al.*, no complications were observed [11]. Lasers can be used both for laparopscopic myomectomy as well as for conventional open myomectomy [12]. The procedure for myomectomy remains essentially the same except that the incision is made with laser.

10.2.2.2 Laparoscopic Myolysis

Myolysis involves multiple punctures of the fibroid with the laser fibre (bare fibre of Nd:YAG) so that the vasculature is dessicated and a reduction in fibroid size is achieved (Figure 1). Concentric puncture are made 5mm apart at 30-50 watts power. Subserous and interstitial fibroids, 3-10 cm in size and less than 4 in number are ideal for this procedure. Reduction in myoma size of upto 30-40% have been reported, with no regrowth over 2 years [13]. This procedure has been successfully performed in Indian setting [14].

Interstital hyperthermia is a variant of this procedure in which delayed necrosis of the myoma is achieved secondary to hyperthermia [15]. Laser induced thermotherapy has been described with the YAG, KTP and the diode laser [16].

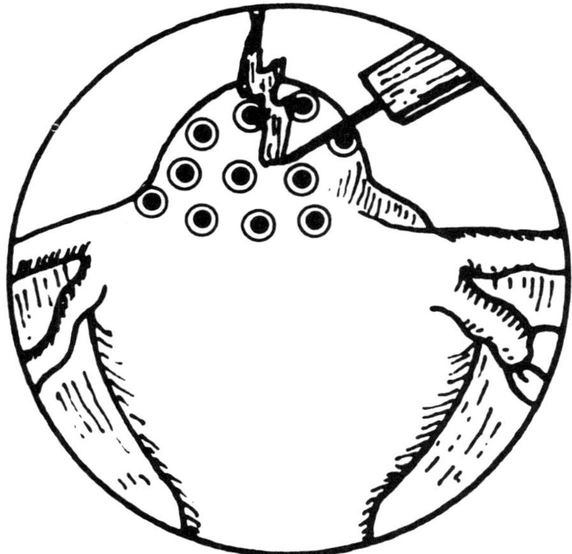

Figuer1. Nd:YAG laser laparoscopic myolysis

10.2.2.3 Hysterectomy

Lasers may be used as a cutting and coagulating tool during laparoscopic assisted vaginal hysterectomy (LAVH). Here lasers act as an alternative to electrocautery as a source of energy. Nd:YAG lasers have been used successfully for LAVH by Saye *et al.* [17] in 167 women, Howard and Sanchez [18] in 15 women, Hur *et al.* [19] in 176 women and Takkar *et al.* [20] in 21 women without increased morbidity.

10.2.2.4 Metroplasty

Lasers may be used during metroplasty for bicornuate uterus. Incision of the uterus is less prone to bleed with the use of laser. Uterine septa may also be dealt with by metroplasty procedures. However now-a-days, hysteroscopic septal resection is the preferred method of treatment for uterine septa where laser application is very useful.

10.2.3 Tubal Disease

Tubal disease is one of the most frequent cause of female infertility accounting for 40% of cases. Tubal surgery with lasers may be performed for these tubes as well as reversal of sterilization.

10.2.3.1 Proximal Tubal Disease

These tubes are dealt with by tubal anastomosis or uncommonly tubal (cornual) implantation. Laser incision of the tube in preparation for anastomosis in isthmic and ampullary disease has been suggested to require less time and facilitate better hemostasis. The CO_2 laser has been generally used for this purpose [21].

The serosal and muscular layers of the tube can be incised with the laser and then the mucosa is divided with a knife or iris scissors. Alternatively, the full thickness of the tube can be divided with the laser and then the mucosa freshened. The anastomosis is then performed with fine sutures. CO_2 /Nd:YAG laser tissue welding may be an alternative to the use of sutures in the future [22].

The laser is most useful in cornual or interstitial anastomosis where it may be used to outline the tube at the serosal area and to incise down through the interstitial portion of the tube. The CO_2 laser has also been used for tubal desterilization through laparoscopic route [23].

Although anastomosis is the preferred technique for interstitial block, in some cases, tubal implantation into the uterus may be needed for a completely damaged or destroyed cornual and/or interstital segment. In such cases the laser may be used to drill a hole into the endometrial cavity in preparation for implantation of the tube. Alternatively the laser may be used to incise the fundus of the uterus and then the tubes are implanted there. The latter technique is preferred by the author.

10.2.3.2 Distal Tubal Disease

When the fimbria are agglutinated, fimbrioplasty may be performed. The laser may be used to vaporize the adhesions between the fimbria to create normal fimbrial architecture. On the other hand, when the fimbrial end is completely closed, a neosalpingostomy is required. The point of puckering, corresponding to the fimbrial opening is noted and then incisions are made radiating outward from the point to create four flaps. Following the creation of flaps a flowering technique is adopted.

The peritoneal surface of the flap is coagulated lightly which results in retraction of the peritoneum and thus eversion of the edges of the flaps. Terminal tuboplasties by CO_2 laser laparoscopy have been reported to yield intrauterine pregnancy rates of 25.8% and 29.4% after fimbrioplasty and neosalpingostomy respectively [24]. The Nd:YAG laser has also been used for the purpose [25].

Fertility outcome after tubal surgery is influenced by the tubal mucosal appearance which is an indicator of the extent of tubal damage [26]. Use of salpingoscopy for studying the mucosal pattern in association with argon laser laparoscopy has been described [27].

10.2.3.3 Ectopic Pregnancy

The recent reported increase in the rate of ectopic pregnancy is in a major part due to better tools available for increasing accuracy in diagnosis. Unrupruted ectopic pregnancies are now diagnosed at an early gestational age and conservative surgery may be more appropriate for management of such cases.

Laparoscopic linear salpingostomy is ideal for an unruptured ectopic pregnancy in the distal tube (Figure 2). The laser provides haemostases as it cuts along the length of the tube. After incising the tube, the products of conception are removed and the incison left to heal by itself. The CO_2 laser [28] Nd:YAG laser [29] and the argon laser [30] have all been used for this purpose. Use of the diode laser has also been reported [31]. Segmental resection and anastomosis is more appropriate for the isthmic area. Anastomosis can be undertaken at the same time or later as an elective procedure.

The laser has the advantage that both precise cutting and haemostasis can be achieved by the same instrument. The fibre optic lasers may be preferred because of their convenience of use during operative laparoscopy. The CO_2 laser is also used, but its absorption by water is a disadvantage.

Salpingectomy is indicated with large, ruptured ectopic pregnancies or when conservation of the tube is not a priority. However, one study assessed the feasibility of CO_2 laser laparoscopic treatment for large and/or ruptured ectopic pregnancies [32]. The study concluded that endoscopic treatment was feasible in such cases and resulted in a shorter hospital stay, and in nulliparous women with history of pelvic infection or infertility, in higher cumulative pregnancy rates. However, laparoscopy cannot be a procedure of choice for haemodynamically unstable patients.

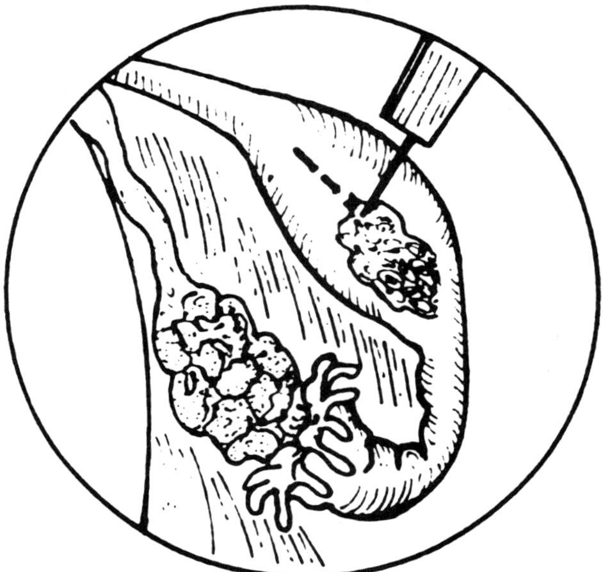

Figure 2. Laser salpingostomy for ectopic pregnancy

10.2.4 Ovarian Cysts

10.2.4.1 Ovarian Cystectomy

The treatment of ovarian endometriomas with lasers has already been discussed. Other benign ovarian cysts amenable to laparoscopic cystectomy may also be treated with lasers. However the exact role of laser laparoscopy in the management of such cysts is yet to be established [27].

10.2.4.2 Ovarian Drilling

Polycystic ovarian disease is a common cause of anovulatory infertility. Induction of ovulation with clomiphene may not be successful. Such patients may be treated by drilling multiple holes in the ovarian stroma to decrease androgen production by destruction of ovarian cysts. Either cautery or laser (CO_2, Nd:YAG, Argon) may be used for this purpose (Figure 3). This procedure yields good results with reported pregnancy rates of 42% to 68% with laser [33,34]. However, whether laser caries any advantage over cautery, in terms of pregnancy rates is again debatable [35]. This technique as now preferred over wedge resection of the ovaries which was advocated in the past. The CO_2/Nd:YAG lasers were used for this procedure. The major disadvantage was the significant incidence of postoperative adhesions.

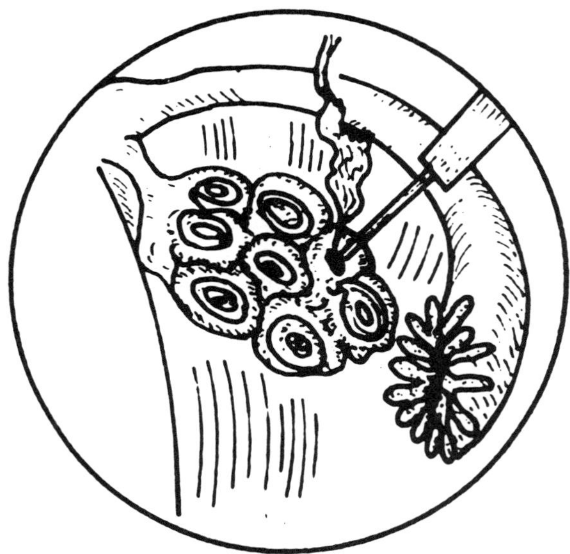

Figure 3. Laser laparoscopic drilling for polycystic ovary

10.2.5 Adhesions and Adhesiolysis

Adhesions within the abdominal cavity are relatively common and generally innocuous. However, in certain locations they can lead to significant problems, e.g., bowel obstruction, dyspareunia and infertility. Chronic abdominal and pelvic pain may also be attributed to adhesions, though the association is less certain. Gross pelvic adhesions, leading to distorted anatomy, are a definite cause for infertility. Such adhesions may result from previous surgery or pelvic inflammatory disease. Adhesiolysis may be performed laparoscopically or during laparotomy. Adhesiolysis by CO_2 lasers has been reported to have good results in patients with thin peritubal or periovarian adhesions [36]. However, with thick and vascular adhesions laparotomy may be more effective. The visible light lasers may be used, but the greater depth of damage associated with these may be a disadvantage.

10.3 HYSTEROSCOPIC PROCEDURES WITH LASER

10.3.1 Endometrial Laser Ablation

Endometrial laser ablation (ELA) is a comparatively newer technique for treatment of dysfunctional uterine bleeding (DUB) as well as for menorrhagia associated with fibroids. Either a contact or a non-contact technique can be used for endometrial ablation with the Nd:YAG laser [37]. In a study, using the Nd:YAG laser by Lomano, 68% of patients with normal sized uterus and 91% of patients with uterine fibroids became amenorrhoeic or had lighter flow [38]. Hysterectomy rates following ELA vary in different series depending on many factors, including the duration of follow up and the underlying pathology. In one series it has been reported to be 13.3% in a mean follow up of 32 months while another projected an overall hysterectomy rate of 21% over a follow up period of 6.5 years [39,40]. Thus ELA is a safe and effective procedure with the potential to reduce the rate of hysterectomy for fibroids and DUB. In comparison with TCRE (transcervical resection of endometrium), ELA has been found to be equally effective but associated with more fluid absorption, and more time consuming [41,42].

10.3.2 Hysteroscopic Resection of Myoma

This is a conservative procedure suitable for patients with one or two submucous fibroids, less than 6 cm in diameter with their major portions protruding in the uterine cavity, with an uterocervical length less than 12 cm. The limitation of fibroid size is, however, not absolute. More important is the operating time which usually should not exceed 60 minutes. Satisfactory results have been achieved with the Nd:YAG laser [43]. This procedure, performed either with the resectoscope or laser, is ideally suited for patients desirous of future pregnancies. Whether the use of laser offers any significant advantages over cautery for hysteroscopic resection will only be determined by large comparative studies. The risks of the procedure include uterine perforation, fluid absorption and haemodilution and haemorrhage from the resected surface. In subsequent pregnancies, there are chances of placenta accreta and intrauterine growth restriction.

10.3.3 Hysteroscopic Myolysis

This procedure is suited for large submucous fibroids with their largest portion inside the myometrium which cannot be dealt with by hysteroscopic resection alone. Donnez *et al* [44] has described a two step procedure in which preoperative GnRH treatment is followed by hysteroscopic resection of the submucous part of the myoma, along with myolysis of the remaining intramural portion. After a further 8 weeks treatment with GnRH agonist, hysteroscopic myomectomy of the remaining part of the fibroid is easily performed as the fibroid now protrudes into the uterine cavity and is less vascular. The principle and procedure of hysteroscopic myolysis is similar to that of laparoscopic myolysis (Figure 4).

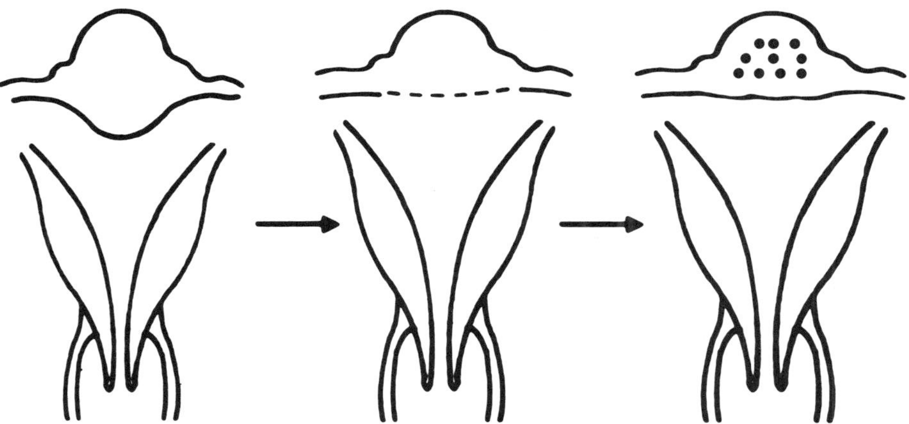

Figure 4. Hysteroscopic laser myolysis

10.3.4 Hysteroscopic Resection of Septum

Choe and Baggish [45] reported the use of Nd:YAG laser in the hysteroscopic resection of septate uterus in 19 patients. Of the 14 patients who wanted to conceive, 13 succeeded. Recently a multicenter retrospective study reported good pregnancy rates with hysteroscopic treatment of septate uterus [46]. However in this study the resectoscope was most commonly used followed by scissors and laser. Whether laser confers any advantage over scissors or cautery is not yet clear, with most studies showing no definite advantages [47].

10.3.5 Hysteroscopic Division of Intra-uterine Synechia

Hysteroscopic treatment of Asherman's syndrome has dramatically improved the prognosis of this disease. Scissors, diathermy and laser have all been used to divide the synechiae. Nd:YAG laser [48] and the KTP laser [49] have been reported to have good results with return of normal menstrual cycles and subsequent uncomplicated pregnancy. In severe disease a two step procedure may be opted for [49]. The KTP laser with a lesser depth of thermal damage may be the preferred choice of laser for the procedure [49].

10.4 COLPOSCOPY WITH LASERS

10.4.1 Cervical Intraepithelial Neoplasia (CIN)

Laser vaporization or laser excision may be used to treat CIN. Another novel approach is photodynamic therapy.

10.4.1.1 Laser Vaporization

Before opting for this therapy, invasive cancer has to be ruled out. The entire lesion should be colposcopically seen and endocervical curettage should be negative for malignancy. The tissue should be ablated to a depth of 7mm which is the location of the deepest endocervical gland. Laser vaporization is particularly effective for large lesions, lesions with extensive glandular involvement, cases of vaginal involvement and associated irregularity of the cervix. CO_2 laser vaporization has been quoted to give clearance rates of 96% [50]. An advantage of laser vaporization is that the outcome of subsequent pregnancies is not influenced adversely [51].

10.4.1.2 Laser Conization

Laser may be used in the cutting mode to perform conization in patients with CIN whose lesions extend into the endocervical canal and who require excisional biopsy to rule out invasive cancer. The clearance rates with laser conization has been reported to be similar to laser vaporization [50]. These figures compare favourably with those reported for electrocautery and cryosurgery [52,53]. The advantage of laser conization is high efficacy with low complication rates [54]. Complications are mainly in the form of bleeding or occurrence of cervical stenosis. However, bleeding is much less compared to cold knife conization [55].

In a study comparing laser conization with LEEP (Loop electrosurgical excision procedure), LEEP proved to be faster, less costly and required less expertise [56].

Combination of laser vaporization of the ectocervix and excisional cone of endocervix is useful in patients with positive endocervical curettage, with a very wide exocervical abnormality. In order to achieve good results with laser, it is important to realize that the entire transformation zone has to be treated and not just the individual lesions.

10.4.1.3 Photodynamic Therapy (PDT)

This is a novel treatment modality that produces local tissue necrosis with laser light after prior administration of a photosensitizing agent. Topically administered 5-aminolevulinic acid and dihematoporphyrin ether have been used as photosensitizing agents. They are applied using a cervical cap, and a cylindrical applicator for the endocervix, three to 24 hrs prior to exposure to argon pumped dye laser. This procedure has been proved to be safe but its efficacy is not yet established [57]. However it has been found to be effective in phase I trials in some studies [58].

10.4.2 Vaginal Intraepithelial Neoplasia (VAIN)

Conservative management of VAIN is indicated in young patients in order to preserve sexual function. Carbon dioxide laser ablation therapy has been found to be safe and effective treatment for VAIN, though repeat procedures may be required [59,60]. As VAIN 3 lesions are likely to harbour an early invasive lesion, they have to be adequately sampled to rule out invasive disease before they can be treated with laser. Lasers can also be used for treatment of non-neoplastic lesions like condylomas.

10.4.3 Vulvar Intraepithelial Neoplasia (VIN)

CO_2 laser excision of the lesion is an effective treatment for VIN. In additional to the cosmetic and consequent psychological benefits, it also allows evaluation of the operative specimen and detection of occult early invasion with good preservation of vulvar morphology [61]. Laser vaporization is less effective than laser excision (cure rates of 75% vs 87%) and it also destroys the specimen [62]. Therefore, excisional treatment is preferred to ablative treatment.

Photodynamic therapy using aminolevulinic acid has been tried and found to have the advantages of minimal tissue destruction, excellent cosmetic results and low side effects with good results [63]. However, multifocal VIN disease with pigmented and hyperkaratinic lesions are difficult to treat by this modality.

10.5 ASSISTED REPRODUCTIVE TECHNIQUE (ART)

Lasers with their unique precision, have found several uses in ART. It works without actually physically touching the cell in most cases and does not have any traceable toxic effects. It has been used for the immobilization of sperms prior to intracytoplasmic sperm injection (ICSI) [64]. Zona drilling with the diode laser or 'non-contact' UV laser has been used for 'assisted hatching' with improved implantation and pregnancy rates [65,66]. Zona thinning has also been performed with laser for the same purpose [67].

Preimplantation diagnosis is another field in which lasers have proved to be useful. Blastocyst or polar body biopsy using the diode or Erbium YAG (Er:YAG) laser to open the zona pellucida have been found to be safe and reliable for pre-implantation diagnosis [68,69,70].

10.6 FUTURE TRENDS OF LASERS IN GYNAECOLOGY

The last three decades have witnessed the evolution of lasers from a novelty to a common modality of treatment for a variety of diseases. And in the foreseably near future, the use of lasers may become much simpler, enabling us to use it for many other purposes as well. For a start newer lasers with better delivery systems may become available. The free electron laser (FEL) which is not being used clinically at present, has the potential to deliver several hundred watts of average power. Other wave lengths, apart from the commonly used lasers, are being explored for their possible roles in gynaecological laser surgery. Newer delivery systems have enabled us to use the CO_2 laser in laparoscopic surgeries [71].

Photodynamic therapy is one area where a lot of research is going on with the application of lasers. If successfully used, this therapy would be the ideal example of tissue specific therapy. In addition photodynamic therapy is being studied for nor-neoplastic disease also, e.g. photodynamic therapy of the endometrium for patients with menorrhagia. Assisted reproductive techniques provide yet another field for extensive use of lasers. At present we are just touching on the fringes of the vast and unexplored potential of lasers in this field.

Apart from therapy lasers could also prove to be useful diagnostic aids e.g. endoscopic holography. This is a procedure by which a three dimensional endoscopic picture of the tissue is taken with the aid of laser. The photograph yields detail similar to that of a microscopic picture.

There may be may other applications which we cannot even envisage at the moment. However it is of the utmost importance to realise the lasers are just a source of energy which can be supplemented and complimented by other energy delivery systems like electrocautery. Most of the procedures described with the use of lasers can also be done quite satisfactorily without laser also. Lasers only help in making the procedure simpler and faster in experienced hands. But the health hazards of lasers and the possible complications in untrained hands cannot be overlooked. Lasers are just tools and the surgeon should use the tool with which he or she is most familiar with and which is best suited for the patient and the procedure.

REFERENCES

1. Schawlow AL, Townes CH. Infrared and optical masers. Physiol Rev 1958; 112 : 1940.
2. Maiman T. Stimulated optical radiation in ruby. Nature. 1960; **187** : 493.
3. Soong YK, Chang FH, Chou HH, Chang MY, Lee CL, Lai YM, Chang SY. Life table analysis of pregnancy rates in women with moderate or severe endometriosis comparing danazol therapy after carbon dioxide laser laparoscopy plus electrocoagulation or laparotomy plus electrocoagulation versus danazol therapy only. J Am Assoc Gynecol Laparosc 1997; **4**(2) : 225-30.
4. Chang FH, Chou HH, Soong YK, Chang MY, Lee CL, Lai YM. Efficacy of isotopic 13CO$_2$ laser laparoscopic vaporization in the treatment of infertile patients with minimal and mild endometriosis : A life table cumulative pregnancy rates study. J Am Assoc Gynecol Laparosc 1997; **4**(2) : 219-23.
5. Donnez J. CO$_2$ laser laparoscopy in infertile women with endometriosis and women with adnexal adhesions. Fertil Steril 1987; **48**(3) : 390-4.
6. Donnez J, Nisolle M, Gillet N, Smets M, Bassil S, Casanas Roux F. Large ovarian endometriomas. Hum Reprod 1996; **11**(3) : 641-6.
7. Sutton CJ, Ewen SP, Jacobs SA, Whitelaw NL. Laser laparoscopic surgery in the treatment of ovarian endometriomas. J Am Assoc Gynecol Laparosc 1997; **4**(3) : 319-23.
8. Kojima E, Morita M, Otaka K, Yano Y. Nd:YAG laser laparoscopy for ovarian endometrioma. J Reprod Med 1990; **35**(6) : 592-6.
9. Carter JE. Laparoscopic presacral neurectomy utilizing contact tip Nd:YAG laser. Keio J Med 1996; **45**(4) : 332-5.
10. Donnez J, Nisolle M, CO$_2$ laser laparoscopic surgery. Adhesiolysis, salpingostomy, laser uterine nerve ablation and tubal pregnancy. Baillieres Clin Obstet Gynecol 1989;3:525-43.
11. Dubuisson JB, Lecuru F, Foulot H, Mandelbrot L, Aubriot FX, Mouly M. Myomectomy by laparoscopy : a preliminary report of 43 cases. Fertil Steril 1991; **56**(5) : 827-30.
12. McLaughlin DS. Micro-laser myomectomy technique to enhance reproductive potential : a preliminary report. Lasers Surg Med 1982; **2**(2) : 107-27.
13. Goldfarb HA. Laparoscopic coagulation of myoma (myolysis). Obstet Gynecol Clin North Am 1995; *22*(4) : 807-19.
14. Takkar D, Roy KK, Sinha A, Kriplani A, Maya. Myolysis in parous women with application of Nd:YAG lasers (Abstract). Int J Obstet & Gynecol 2000; **70** (Supp I): 105-6
15. Jourdain O, Roux D, Cambon D, Dallay D. A new method for the treatment of fibromas : interstitial laser hyperthermia using the Nd:YAG laser. Preliminary study Eur J Obstet Gynecol Reprod Biol 1996; **64**(1) : 73-8.
16. Chapman R. New therapeutic technique for treatment of uterine leiomyomas using laser-induced interstitial thermotherapy (LITT) by a minimally invasive method. Lasers Surg Mod 1998; **22**(3) : 171-8.
17. Saye WB, Espy GB, Bishop MR, Slinkard P, Miller W, Hertzmann P. Laparoscopic Doderlein Hysterectomy : A rational alternative to traditional abdominal hysterectomy. Surg Lap and Endoscopy 1993; **3** : 88-94.
18. Howard FM, Sanchez R. A comparison of laparoscopically assisted vaginal hysterectomy and abdominal hysterectomy. J Gynecol Surg 1993; **9** : 83-87.
19. Hur M, Kim JH, Moon JS, Lee JC, Seo DW. Laparoscopically assisted vaginal hysterectomy.J Reprod Med 1995; **40** : 820-833.

20. Takkar D, Roy KK, Kriplani A, Chaudhary M, Jayalaxmi TS. Laparoscopic assisted vaginal hysterectomy with application of Nd:YAG lasers (Abstract). Int J Obstet & Gynaecol 2000; **70** Supp I : 26.

21. Kelley RW, Roberts DK. Experience with carbon dioxide laser in gynecologic microsurgery. Am J Obstet Gynecol 1983; **146**(5) : 585-8.

22. Wallwiener D, Meyer A, Bastert G. Carbon dioxide laser tissue welding : an alternative technique for tubal anastomosis? J Clin Laser Med Surg 1997; **15**(4) : 163-9.

23. Sedbon E, Delajolinieres JB, Boudouris O, Madelenat P. Tubal desterilization through exclusive laparoscopy. Hum Reprod 1989; **4**(2) : 158-9.

24. Dubuisson JB, Bouquet-de-Joliniere J, Aubriot FX, Darai E, Foulot H, Mandelbrot L. Terminal tuboplasties by laparoscopy: 65 consecutive cases. Fertil Steril 1990; **54**(3) : 401-3.

25. Yanagibori A, Kojima E, Ontaka K, Morita M, Hirakawa S. Nd:YAG laser therapy for infertility with a contact type probe. J Reprod Med 1989; **34**(7) : 456-60.

26. Dubuisson JB, Chapron C, Morice P, Aubriot FX, Foulot H, Bouquet-de-Joliniere J. Laparoscopic salpingostomy : fertility results according to the tubal mucosal appearance. Hum Reprod 1994; **9**(2) : 334-9.

27. Brosens IA, Puttemans PJ. Double-optic laparoscopy. Salpingoscopy, ovarian cystoscopy and endovarian surgery with the argon laser. Baillieres Clin Obstet Gynecol 1989; **3**(3) : 595-608.

28. Paulson JD. The use of carbon dioxide laser laparoscopy in the treatment of tubal ectopic pregnancies. Am J Obstet Gynecol 1992; **167**(2) : 382-5.

29. Keckstein J, Hepp S, Schneider V, Sasse V, Steiner R. The contact Nd:YAG laser : a new technique for conservation of the fallopian tube in unruptured ectopic pregnancy. Br J Obstet Gynecol 1990; 97(4) : 352-6.

30. Kekstein J, Kekstein S, Wolf AS, Shneider V, Steiner R. Argon laser laparoscopy : an effective technique for conservative treatment of unruptured ectopic pregnancy. Int J Fertil 1992; **37**(2) : 82-5.

31. Abrao MS, Ikeda F, Podgaec S, Pereira PP. Microlaparoscopy for an intact ectopic pregnancy and endometriosis with the use of a diode laser : Case report. Hum Reprod 2000; **15**(6) : 1369-71.

32. Koninickx PR, Witters K, Brosens J, Stemers N, Oosterlynck D, Meuleman C. Conservative laparoscopic treatment of ectopic pregnancy using the CO_2 laser. Br. J Obstet Gynecol 1991; **98**(12) : 1254-9.

33. Heylen SM, Puttemans PJ, Brosens IA. Polycystic ovarian disease treated by laparoscopic argon laser capsule drilling : Comparison of vaporization versus perforation technique. Hum Reprod 1994; **9** (6) : 1038-42.

34. Kekstein G, Rossmanith W, Spatzier K, Schneider V, Borchers K, Steiner R. The effect of laparoscopic treatment of polycystic ovarian disease by CO_2 laser or Nd:YAG laser. Surg Endosc 19990; **4** : 103-7.

35. Li TC, Saravelos H, Chow MS, Chisabingo R, Cooke ID. Factors affecting the outcome of laparoscopic ovarian drilling for polycystic ovarian syndrome in women with anovulatory infertility. Br J Obstet Gynecol 1998; **105** : 338-44.

36. Donnez J. CO_2 laser laparoscopy in infertile women with adnexal adhesions and women with tubal occlusion. J Gynecol Surg 1989; **5** : 47-53.

37. Indman PD. High power Nd:YAG laser ablation of the endometrium. J Reprod Med 1991; **36** (7) : 501-4.

38. Lomano J. Endometrial ablation for the treatment of menorrhagia : a comparison of patients with normal, enlarged and fibroid uteri. Lasers Surg Med 1991; **11**(1) : 8-12.

39. Jourdain O, Joyeux P, Lajus C, Sfaxi I, Harli T, Roux D, Dallay D. Endometrial Nd:YAG laser ablation by hysterofibroscopy : long term results of 137 cases. Eur J Obstet Gynecol Reprod Biol 1996; **69**(2) : 103-7.

40. Phillips G, Chien PF, Garry R. Risk of hysterectomy after 1000 consecutive endometrial laser ablations. Br J Obstet Gynecol 1998; **105**(8) : 897-903.

41. Bhattacharya S, Cameron IM, Parkin DE et al. A pragmatic randomised comparison of transcervical resection of the endometrium with endometrial laser ablation for the treatment of menorrhagia. Br J Obstet Gynecol 1997; **104**(5) : 601-7.

42. Parkin DE. Laser ablation or endometrial resection ? In. Progress in Obstetrics and Gynaecology. Eds. Studd J. Volume 12, Churchill Livingstone : New York. 1996; pp. 345-54.

43. Baggish MS, Sze EHM, Morgan G. Hysteroscopic treatment of symptomatic myomata uteri with the Nd:YAG laser. J Gynecol Surg 1989; **5** : 27-36.

44. Donnez J, Gillerot S, Bourgonjon D, Clerekx F, Nisolle M. Nd:YAG laser hysteroscopy in large submucous fibroids. Fertil Steril 1990; **54**(6) : 999-1003.

45. Choe JK, Baggish MS. Hysteroscopic treatment of septotic uterus with Neodymium YAG laser. Fertil Steril 1992; **57**(1) : 81-4.

46. Colacurci N, DePlacido G, Peririo A, Mencaglia L, Gubbini G. Hypoteroscopic metroplasty. J Am Assoc Gynecol Laparosc 1998; **5**(2) : 171-4.

47. Candiani GB, Vercellini P, Fedele L, Garsia S, Brioschi D, Villa L. Argon laser versus microscissors for hysteroscopic incision of uterine septa. Am J Obstet Gynecol 1991; **164**(1) : 87-90.

48. Newton JR, MacKenzie WE, Emens MJ, Jordan JA. Division of uterine adhesions (Asherman's syndrome) with the Nd:YAG laser. Br J Obstet Gynaecol 1989; **96**(1) : 102-4.

49. Chapman R, Chapman K. The value of two stage laser treatment for severe Asherman's syndrome. Br J Obstet Gynecol 1996; **103**(12) : 1256-8.

50. Stentella P, Pace S, Villani C, Palazzetti PL, Di-Renzi F, Stolfi G, Frega A. Cervical intraepithelial neoplasia : carbon dioxide laser vaporization and conization. Our experience. Eur J Gynecol Oncol 1995; **16**(4) : 282-9.

51. Van-Rooijen M, Persson E. Pregnancy outcome after laser vaporization of the cervix. Acta Obstet Gynecol Scand 1999; **78**(4) : 346-8.

52. Chanen W, Rome RM. Electrocoagulation diathermy for cervical dysplasia and carcinoma in situ : a 15 year survey. Obstet Gynecol 1983; **61** (6) : 673-9.

53. Townsend DE, Richart RM. Cryotherapy and carbon dioxide laser management of cervical intraepithelial neoplasia : a controlled comparison. Obstet Gynecol 1983; **61**(1) : 75-8.

54. Hagen B, Skjeldestad FE, Bratt H, Tingulstad S, Lie AK. CO_2 laser conization for cervical intraepithelial neoplasia grade II-III : complications and efficacy. Acta Obstet Gynecol Scand 1998; **77**(5) : 558-63.

55. Bostofte E, Berget A, Falk-Larsen J, Hjortkjaer Pederson P, Rank F. Conization by carbon dioxide laser or cold knife in the treatment of cervical intrapiehtelial neoplasia. Acta Obstet Gynecol Scand 1986; **65** (3) :192-202.

56. Santos C, Galdos R, Alvarez M et al One session management of cervical intraepithelial neoplasia : a solution for developing countries. Gynecol Oncol 1996; **61**(1) : 11-5.

57. Hillemanns P, Korell M, Schmitt-Sody M, et al. Photodynamic therapy in women with cervical intraepithelial neoplasia using topically applied 5-amino levulinic acid. Int J Cancer 1999; **81**(1) : 34-8.

58. Monk BJ, Brewer C, Van Nostrand K, Berns MW, McCullough JL, Tadir Y, Manetta A. Photodynamic therapy using topically applied dihematoporphyrin ether in the treatment of cervical intra-epithelial neoplasia. Gynecol Oncol 1997; **64**(1) : 70-5.

59. Campugnutta E, Parin A, De-Piero G, Giorda G, Gallo A, Scarabelli C. Treatment of vaginal intraepithelial neoplasia (VAIN) with the carbon dioxide laser. Clin Exp Obstet Gynecol 1999; **26**(2) : 127-30.

60. Diakomanolis E, Rodolakis A, Sakellaropoulos G, Kalpaktsoglou K, Aravantinos D. Conservative management of vaginal intra-epithelial neoplasia (VAIN) by laser CO_2. Eur J Gynecol Oncol 1996; **17**(5) : 389-92.

61. Sideri M, Spinaci L, Spolti N, Schettino F. Evaluation of CO_2 laser excision or vaporization for the treatment of vulvar intraepithelial neoplasia. Gynecol Oncol 1999; **75**(2) : 277-81.

62. Herod JJ, Shaji MI, Rollason TP, Jordon JA, Luesley DM. Vulvar intraepithelial neoplasia : long-term follow up of treated and untreated women. Br J Obstet Gynecol 1996; **103**(5) : 446-52.

63. Hillemanns P, Untch M, Dannecker C et al. Photodynamic therapy of vulvar intraepithelial neoplasia using 5-aminolevulinic acid. Int J Cancer 2000; **85**(5) : 649-53.

64. Schopper B, Ludwig M, Edenfield J, Al-Hasani S, Diedrich K. Possible applications of lasers in assisted reproductive technologies. Hum Reprod 1999; **14** Suppl. 1 : 186-93.

65. Antinori S, Selman HA, Caffa B, Panci C, Dani GL, Versaci C. Zona opening of human embryos using a non-contact UV laser for assisted hatching in patients with poor prognosis of pregnancy. Hum Reprod 1996; **11**(11) : 2488-92.

66. Montag M, van-der ver H. Laser-assisted hatching in assisted reproduction. Croat Med J 1999; **40**(3) : 398-403.

67. Antinori S, Panci C, Selman HA, Caffa B, Dani G, Versaci C. Zona thinning with the use of laser: a new approach to assisted hatching in humans. Hum Reprod 1996; **11**(3) : 590-4.

68. Veiga A, Sandalinas M, Benkhalifa M et a. Laser blastocyst biopsy for pre-implantation diagnosis in the human. Zygote 1997; **5**(4) : 351-4.

69. Obruca A, Strohmer H, Blaschitz A, Schonickle E, Dohr G, Feichtinger W. Ultrastructural observations in human oocyte and pre-implantation embryos after zona opening using an erbium-yttrium aluminium-garnett (Er:YAG) laser. Hum Reprod 1997; **12** (10): 2242-5.

70. Montag M, van-der ven K, Delacretaz G, Rinki K, vander ven H. Laser assisted microdissection of the zona pellicida facilitates polar body biopsy. Fertil Steril 1998; **69**(3) : 539-42.

71. Adamson GD, DeNatale ML, Harman S. A new wave guide for use with a CO_2 delivery system for laparoscopic surgery. J Reprod Med 1993; **389** (11) : 875-8.

Chapter 11

LASER SAFETY IN MEDICINE

Ken Barat
Lawrence Berkeley National Laboratory, Berkeley, U.S.A.

11.1   INTODUCTION

There is no doubt that the laser technology is being applied to a vast number of procedures, many of which have clear advantages over the other methods. Regardless of the kind of medical applications; lasers safety to the patient and administering staff against any harmful exposure or effects that may arise in the use and handling of lasers is an important consideration. The goal of this chapter is to present information that will assist all parties involved to work in a safe manner. Throughout the chapter, and particularly at the end of this chapter, a number of laser accidents in the medical field will be presented. It is hoped that the reader will see a comparison to one's own experiences and take corrective steps.

11.2   CLASSIFICATION OF LASER HAZARDS

Central to any review of laser safety is an understanding of the laser hazard classification system. This system was made popular with the first American National Standard Institute Laser Safety Standard in 1970. In order to inform the user of the potential hazard of a laser system or laser product, a laser hazard classification system was developed. Let us, first, define the terms laser system and laser product. A laser system is a laser cavity and a power supply. A laser product or device is generally something a laser system has been incorporated into. A common example would be the laser printer. The internal laser diode is the laser system, but the printer, as a whole, is the laser product. Lasers are broken up into four broad hazard classifications. These classifications are followed by all the users and manufacturers of laser equipment. They also serve as a basis for defining appropriate control measures and medical surveillance. Lasers and laser systems received from manufacturers should be classified and appropriately labeled by the manufacturer.

The classification may, however, change whenever the laser or laser system is modified to accomplish a given task. Also, the Laser Safety Officer (LSO) shall effect the classification in cases where the laser or laser system classification is not provided or where the class level may change because of alterations to the laser or laser system. It should be mentioned that the U.S. Federal Government does not "approve" laser systems. The manufacturer of the laser system first classifies the laser and then certifies that it meets all performance requirements of the Federal Laser Product Performance Standard (FLPPS). Therefore, all lasers and laser systems that are manufactured or purchased by a company and relabeled or incorporated into a system and placed into commerce, shall be classified in accordance with the FLPPS. The classification shall be confirmed by the LSO at the laser installation site.

CLASS I: Cannot emit laser radiation at known hazard levels (typically CW: 0.4 μW at visible wavelengths). Users of Class I laser products are generally exempt from radiation hazard controls during operation and maintenance (but not necessarily during service).

CLASS II: Low power visible lasers, with radiant power above Class I levels but not above 1 mW. The concept is that the human aversion reaction to bright light will protect a person.

CLASS IIIA: Intermediate power lasers (CW: 1-5 mW). These are hazardous for beam viewing, but can be considered safe for momentary viewing except by focussing or directing optics. Some limited controls are usually recommended.

> NOTE: There are different labeling requirements for Class IIIA lasers with a beam irradiance that does not exceed 2.5 mW/cm^2 (Caution logotype) and those where the beam irradiance does exceed 2.5 mW/cm^2 (Danger logotype).

CLASS IIIB: Moderate power lasers (CW: 5-500 mW, pulsed: 10 J/cm^2). In general, Class IIIB lasers will not be a fire hazard and generally are not capable of producing a hazardous diffuse reflection, except under situations of intentional staring at distances close to the diffuser.

CLASS IV: High power lasers (CW: 500 mW) are hazardous to view under any condition (directly or diffusely scattered) and are a potential fire hazard and a skin hazard. Significant controls are required for Class IV laser facilities.

EMBEDDED LASER: A Class II, Class III, or Class IV laser or laser system contained in a protective housing and operated in a lower classification (Class I, Class II or Class III). Specific control measures may be required to maintain the lower classification.

Now that the laser hazard classification system has been defined, it is easy to see why safety concerns and controls of laser use tends to gravitate toward class IIIB and class IV lasers. Under the correct circumstances, these systems do present a hazard to the user and those around them.

11.3   COMMON WAVELENGTHS

Medical laser applications are not confined to just one or two wavelengths of laser radiation. Wavelengths and types of lasers, earlier thought to be inaccessible or too complex, are common today. The excimer laser is a good example of this. A laser product using toxic halogen gases, at one time, was seen as too complex to be used in a medical setting outside of the research institution. Today, the use of excimer lasers in corneal surgery is common. Table 1 gives a list of typical wavelengths that are available to the medical community.

Table 1. Typical wavelengths and penetration depths of various types of lasers

Type of Laser	Wavelengths (nm)	Penetration depth mm
Argon Ion	488 & 515	1-1.5
Nd:YAG	1064	3-4
Carbon Dioxide	10, 6000	0.1-0.2
Nd:YAG doubled	532	833 microns
Krypton Ion	335-800	
Excimer	180-350	
ArF	193	<25 microns
XeCl	308	50 "
XeFl	351	250 "
Erbium:YAG	2940	1.0 "
Erbium:YLF	1730	667 microns
Holmium:YAG	2100	
Copper Vapor	511 & 578	
Gold Vapor	628	
Diodes	600-1600	
HeNe	633	2.5 microns
HFL	2730	10 microns

11.4 FIBER OPTICS

The use of fiber optics has allowed a wider range of laser medical applications that would be impossible with lasers alone. A laser fiber optic is similar to the catheter used in many established diagnostic and invasive procedures. The fiber comprises a center core of an optically transmissive material (the most commonly used material is Silica). The core is covered by a cladding that has a lower refractive index than the core, effectively trapping the laser radiation within the core. Internal reflections bounce the beam down the fiber to an end where it can escape, or transfer heat to a specially designed tip. At the right angle bend, total internal reflection can occur. Medical fiber optics are made to have a certain degree of bend, after which they can be broken. The bend performance of fiber optics is determined by numerical aperture, cladding material, wavelength and core size. For medical applications, fiber can come as single-use devices or re-useable. Avoid the temptation to cut the edge of a single-use fiber, and then re-use. While this is technically possible, this action will void any guarantees by the manufacturer and could place the patient at risk.

Hazards associated with fiber optic work include silica slithers on one's fingers which can go unnoticed and get in touch with eyes or mouth, flammable chemicals that are used to clean fibers, and the beam escaping from a broken fiber. The greatest problem with fiber optic use is the false sense of security it creates (the business end of the fiber is within the patient, all is safe and no eyewear needs to be worn). In addition, the divergence is so large that the beam would not present a hazard even if it comes out. Remember; fibers can break, tips come loose and break off. Also, the laser can be activated while the fiber is outside the body; either before or after the procedure. Following are the three examples of accident/equipment malfunctions due to optical fiber failures.

Laser Accident Case # 1 Event description: during a laparoscopic procedure a tip broke off the laser that was to be utilized. The scrub nurse connected the fiber delivery system and probe and handed off the connector to the circulator to attach to the laser. The delivery system was inserted into the abdomen. An attempt to turn on the laser was made. However, the laser lamp would not activate. After two attempts, the laser fiber was removed. Upon examination, it was noted that the probe was missing. The metal connector was intact. The surgeon irrigated and suctioned the abdominal cavity. The suction container was strained and examined. The probe tip was not visible. This event could have been avoided if the laser had been turned on and the fiber calibrated prior to insertion of the delivery system into the abdominal cavity via the laparoscope. This sequence would have identified the laser lamp problem, which would not allow the laser to be used.

Laser Accident Case # 2 Nd:YAG surgical laser event description: the nurse saw there was no laser output and checked the connector of the Yttrium Aluminum Garnert fiber to ensure it was tightly secured on the laser. The connector was hot and burned her thumb and forefinger. The connector was removed from the laser and another fiber and connector were installed and the system performed okay. The nurse was treated for second degree burns. The user installed a fiber manufactured by another company onto the company's laser. There was little laser output and the nurse touched the connector portion of the fiber. The connector was hot and burned her thumb and forefinger. The other company's fiber was the cause of the injury. This type of event would not have occurred with company's own fiber.

Laser Accident Case # 3 Event description: during urological procedure, which was being performed on a 73 year old male out-patient, the distal tip of a lateral fire laser fiber detached after the surgeon activated the laser beam. (Lateral fire laser fiber was not manufactured by this firm. However, it was distributed by it). Just prior to occurrence of event, the user indicated that it appeared that the laser beam traveled in a retrograde manner through laser fiber. The tip was retrieved from the patient's bladder without adverse consequence, and the procedure was successfully completed with a second lateral fire laser fiber. During the investigation into the circumstances leading up to the event, the user facility did not provide details whether or not there was a constant irrigation flow around the fiber in order to provide an adequate coolant effect, or if the reflective aperture had been fouled with either tissue or debris that could have presented an obstacle to transmission of the laser beam.

11.4.1 Surgical Fiber Optical Density Hazard Analysis

A hazard analysis of a typical Nd:YAG surgical laser with a fiber optic hand-piece attachment could be based upon the following parameters:
Laser power: 100 Watts (maximum/CW); beam divergence: 210 milliradian (12 degrees from fiber tip); exposure time: 10 seconds (maximum); wavelength: 1.06 μm. Using these parameters, a mathematical hazard analysis can be done to estimate the general region around the surgical site where hazardous exposures may be possible. Although, the following analysis is based upon one specific unit, it is representative of Nd:YAG surgical lasers. This analysis is based upon the maximum permissible exposure (MPE) criteria of the ANSI Z-136.1 standard.

The "worst case" MPE value for a direct intrabeam Nd:YAG laser exposure of 10 seconds is 50.6 mj/cm^2. The MPE for a 10-second diffuse reflection of this laser is 10(8) J/cm^2 sr. contained within an apparent visual angle (alpha min) which is not smaller than 24 milliradians. The 10 second MPE value for skin exposure is 10.5 J/cm^2.

To estimate a diffuse reflection from the site, one can estimate, using the inverse square law, an approximate scattering distance of 40 cm from the beam (on the tissues) to the eye. Using the ANSI Z-136.1 point source criteria (because the focused beam acts as a point source), the irradiance at the eye will be 19.9 mW/cm^2. This produces a radiant exposure of nearly 200 mJ/cm^2 during a ten second exposure.

The optical density required for safe viewing of the diffuse reflection off tissues is substantially reduced from the 100-watt intrabeam case. Using a 40 cm "viewing distance", and assuming a "point source condition", the required optical density at 1.06 μm would be OD = 0.6 for a 10 second exposure and OD = 1.1 for an 8 hour (occupational) exposure. The "worst case" conditions suggest than an optical density ranging from 0.6 to 5.2 depending upon viewing time and conditions.

11.5 LASER TISSUE INTERACTION

The interaction of laser radiation with tissue is epresented by a number of mathematical and physical laws and theories. This section will state the interaction of different bands of laser radiation with the eye and skin, in an absolute way. We need to remember that any photon of laser radiation, which strikes tissue, has the ability to be absorbed, reflected, or scattered. The scattering can occur at the surface or while it is traveling through the tissue. For tissue coagulation, scattering also strongly affects the dosimetery of laser radiation during therapeutic procedures that depend on absorption. From this point of view, we can consider blood to have the same properties of absorption, reflection or scattering. Understanding laser tissue interaction helps one to understand why so many lasers are used in medicine today. Different lasers will be used to obtain different effects and absorption by different targets. An example would be the CO_2 laser, which is highly absorbed by water, and is extremely useful where the rapid removal of tissue is desired.

Thermal effects are the major cause of tissue damage by lasers. Energy from the laser is absorbed by the tissue in the form of heat, which can cause localized and intense heating of sensitive tissues. In other words, the tissue proteins are denatured due to the rapid temperature rise; egg on a frying pan, are an example. The amount of thermal damage that can be caused to tissue varies depending on the thermal sensitivity of the type of tissue. Thermal effects can range from erythema (reddening of the skin) to burning of the tissue.

Laser beams are capable of causing a localized vaporization of tissue that in turn can create a mechanical shockwave to be propagated through the tissue (acoustic effects). Shockwaves can cause tearing of tissue. Laser radiation can also cause changes to the chemistry of cells, which can result in changes to tissue (photochemical effects). The thermal damage process (burns) is generally associated with lasers operating at exposure times greater than 10 microseconds and in the wavelength region of the near ultraviolet to the far infrared (0.315 μm-103 μm). Tissue damage may also come from thermally induced acoustic waves following exposures to sub-microsecond laser exposures. Basic biological effects of light are summarized in Table 2.

Table 2. Summary of basic biological effects of light in photobiological spectral domain.

Eye Effects	Skin Effects
Ultraviolet C (0.200-0.280 μm) Photokeratitis	Erythema (sunburn) Skin cancer
Ultraviolet B (0.280-315 μm) Photokeratitis	Accelerated skin aging Increased pigmentation
Ultraviolet A (0.315-0.400 μm) Photochemical UV cataract	Pigment darkening Skin burn
Visible (0.400-0.780 μm) Photochemical and thermal Retinal injury	Photosensitive reactions Skin burn
Infrared A (0.780-1.400 μm) Cataract, retinal burns	Skin burn
Infrared B (1.400-3.00 μm) Corneal burn Aqueous flare IR cataract	Skin burn
Infrared C (3.00-1000 μm) Corneal burn only	Skin burn

With regard to repetitively pulsed or scanning lasers, the major mechanism involved in laser-induced biological damage is a thermal process wherein the effects of the pulses are additive. Factors that affect thermal damage to tissue are:

- size of the area irradiated
- wavelength of laser radiation
- energy of the beam (Irradiance)
- length of time that the tissue is irradiated and pulse repetition factors
- the absorption and scattering coefficients of the tissues at the laser wavelength
- extent of the local vascular flow

Photochemical reactions are the principal cause of threshold level tissue damage following exposures to either actinic ultraviolet radiation (0.200 μm-0.315 μm) for any exposure time or "blue light" visible radiation (0.400 μm-0.550 μm) when exposures are greater than 10 seconds.

Visible and IR-A wavelengths of light are transmitted through the cornea and lens of the eye and are absorbed mostly by the retina. The visible and IR-A portions of the spectrum (400-1200 nm) are often referred to as the "Retinal Hazard Region" because these wavelengths of light can damage the retina. The amount of hazard to the retina from viewing of a laser beam in the Retinal Hazard Region increases with increased pupil size and increased duration of the laser beam. UV-A wavelengths of light are mostly absorbed in the lens of the eye and can cause photochemical damage to the lens. UV-B, UV-C, IR-B and IR-C are absorbed by the cornea of the eye. Exposure to these wavelengths can result in conjunctivitis, "milky" cornea, and inflammation.

11.5.1 Eye Exposure

Exposure to the invisible carbon dioxide laser beam (10,600 nm) can be detected by a burning pain at the site of exposure on the cornea or sclera. Exposure to a visible laser beam can be detected by a bright color flash of the emitted wavelength and an after-image of its complementary color (e.g., a green 532 nm laser light would produce a green flash followed by a red after-image). When the retina is affected, there may be difficulty in detecting blue or green colors.

Exposure to the Q-switched Nd:YAG laser beam (1064 nm) is especially hazardous and may initially go undetected because the beam is invisible and the retina lacks pain sensory nerves. Photoacoustic retinal damage may be associated with an audible "pop" at the time of exposure. Visual disorientation due to retinal damage may not be apparent to the operator until considerable thermal damage has occurred.

11.5.2   Skin Exposure

The layers of the skin are the epidermis and the dermis. The epidermis layer lies beneath the stratum corneum and is the outermost living layer of the skin. The dermis mostly consists of connective tissue and lies beneath the epidermis. To the skin, UV-A (0.315 μm - 0.400 μm) can cause hyper-pigmentation and erythema.

UV-B and UV-C often collectively referred to as "actinic UV," can cause erythema and blistering, as they are absorbed in the epidermis. UV-B is a component of sunlight that is known to have carcinogenic effects on the skin. Exposure in the UV-B range is most injurious to skin. In addition to thermal injury caused by ultraviolet energy, there is the possibility of radiation carcinogenesis from UV-B (0.280 mm - 0.315 mm) either directly on DNA or from effects on potential carcinogenic intracellular viruses.

Exposure in the shorter UV-C (0.200 μm-0.280 μm) and the longer UV-A ranges seems less harmful to human skin. The shorter wavelengths are absorbed in the outer dead layers of the epidermis (stratum corneum) and the longer wavelengths have an initial pigment-darkening effect followed by erythema if there is exposure to excessive levels. IR-A wavelengths of light are absorbed by the dermis and can cause deep heating of skin tissue (see Table 2).

11.6   NON-BEAM HAZARDS

While working with lasers one can not overlook the associated non-beam hazards. Indeed these hazards can be quite harmful, such as in the case of electrical shock.

11.6.1 Electrical Hazards

Medical lasers similar to other commercial lasers often contain high voltage electrical power supplies and circuits. Electrical safety is of paramount importance to any laser user. Currents above 6 millamps can freeze a person to an electrical device, if they become part of the current to ground path. Therefore, items like the integrity of cords, extension cords, footswitches, circuit breakers and protective housing interlocks need to be checked by a qualified person. This is extremely important after any service or maintenance has been performed on the laser equipment. Compliance with the National Electrical Code is always recommended. Remember, in medical settings accidental electrical contact with fluids is very possible, in particular IV fluids and fluids in basins.

11.6.2 Laser Generated Air Contamination

The energy supplied at the focal point of the carbon dioxide laser is so great that the tissue and fluid are vaporized. Researchers have suggested that the smoke may act as a vector for cancerous cells, which may be inhaled by the surgical team and other exposed individuals. There have been many studies on this subject. In September 1996, the National Institute for Occupational Safety and Health (NIOSH) released a Health Hazard Alert on the dangers of the smoke plume, a byproduct of the thermal destruction of tissue during sugrical procedures using a laser unit. Research has confirmed that this smoke plume can contain "toxic gases and vapors such as benzene, hydrogen cyanide, formaldehyde, bio-aerosols, dead and live cellular material (including blood fragments), and viruses". Exposure to surgical smoke has been known to cause burning, watery eyes, nausea, respiratory problems and viral contamination and re-growth. According to the Association of Operating Room Nurses, 90,000 registered nurses who work in operating rooms are potentially affected by this occupational hazard. Another study in 1987 by Camran Nezhat *et al.* [1] examined the compositions of the smoke plume produced during carbon dioxide laser surgery to determine whether the operating room team was at risk from the laser smoke. The authors were interested in calculating the probability that something the size of a whole red blood cell (7.5 μm) would be present in the smoke. Particles with an aerodynamic diameter range from 0.1-0.8 μm were found in the collected smoke plume samples but no cell-size particles, including cancer cells, were present in the plume. The findings of this study differ from some earlier studies in which intact cells or identifiable cell parts were collected from both carbon dioxide and Nd:YAG laser radiation of animal tissue. The conclusion of the Nezhat study was that although no identifiable hazard from airborne cancer cells was detected, an significant portion of the particles in the smoke were in the range of 0.5-5.0 um. These particles are too small to be effectively filtered by surgical masks. It was recommended that a mechanical smoke evacuator system with a high-efficiency, multi-stage filter be used during smoke generating laser vaporization procedures. An article by Robert Fisher [2] indicated that although mechanical smoke vacuuming systems were used in carbon dioxide laser surgery, the tube had to be held as close as 1cm from the target. At 2 cm, the evacuation ratio was down to fifty per cent. The author concluded that prudence should be exercised while the hazards presented by the laser smoke are further investigated (see Table 3). A study published in February 1988 by Garden *et al.*[3] analyzed the vapor produced by the carbon dioxide laser during vaporization of Papilloma Virus infected Verrucae. This study concluded that intact viral deoxyribonueleic acid (DNA) was liberated into the air with the plume of laser-treated verrucae.

Papillomavirus DNA has been demonstrated to be infectious. Therefore, when performing laser therapy on patients infected with viruses such as Hepatitis or the Human Immunodeficiency Virus, the smoke plume should be assumed to be infectious and appropriate precautions, such as a well maintained vacuum apparatus should be observed. These studies are only a few of a vast number published on this topic, all confirming a hazard and the need for special controls. "American National Standard for the Safe Use of Laser in Health Care Facilities," ANSI Z-136.3 provides guidance for safe use of lasers and laser systems for diagnostic and therapeutic uses in health care facilities.

Table 3. Laser plume contents, their sources and related health risks

Laser Plume Content	Source	Potential Health Problem	Control Measures
Dust	Procedures using CO_2 lasers	Lung damage	Surgical masks,Local exhaust ventilation.
Toxic chemicals: Benzene, Formaldehyde Acrolein, Aldehydes Polycyclic aromatic hydrocarbons, Cyanides Methane	Laser beam contact with human & animal tissues Plastics, polymer (Teflon) coated products	Irritation, fire mutagenic potential	Respiratory protection suitable for plume composition. Local exhaust ventilation
Biological agents	Laser beam contact, tumours, with warts, HIV bacteria, culture	Infection	Same as above plus Protective clothing and gloves
Smoke (general)	Laser beam vaporization, incision, CO_2 laser beam contact with skin	Obstruction of the field of view	Local ventilation

11.6.3 Fire

This can be caused by laser radiation interaction with a long list of materials found in medical settings (see Table 4). Gas (i.e. methane gas, bowl gas,) or other materials (paper, plastic tubing), can be electrically induced. Following are a number of laser fire accidents in medical facilities:

11.6.3.1 Fire Accidents

Event 1: After connecting the kit and laser, it was observed that the red He-Ne aiming beam was not visible at the laser kit tip. The physician elected to proceed with the procedure. When the laser control footswitch was depressed, no laser energy was emitted from the laser tip. Flames appeared on the sterile drape where the laser fiber had been resting, but were quickly extinguished. No one was injured. Analysis of the returned product pointed to a broken laser fiber probably caused by mishandling.

Event 2: During a procedure to relieve bladder outlet obstruction, the surgical Team smelled "burning rubber" and saw smoke curling up from the laser fiber catheter, close to the connection of the laser. The fiber reportedly separated completely. The lasing process was immediately halted. The reporter estimated that the laser had fired for approx. 90 seconds up to that point at a setting of 60 watts. The 3rd of a series of 30-second "swipes" of the target tissue was just being started. The case completed uneventfully with a second fiber of the same type. No injuries occurred nor was there any damage resulting from the momentary free beam release into the OR. The laser port on the device points upward at 90 degrees and there was no indication of burning on the ceiling above the unit. The fiber catheter distal and proximal portions were returned for evaluation. Analysis: the fiber was broken 1.7 cm from the nut, which secures the fiber to the connector. This is a stress point. The broken ends displayed only minor heat damage and the rubber sheath appeared torn rather than melted. It appears that the break did not occur as a result of laser energy being applied. As the fiber had delivered energy already in an apparently satisfactory manner, it is most likely that the fiber was broken due to physical stress in between periods of energy deposition. Corrective action: physician-training sessions will review this type of problem with the physician and emphasize the importance of not over bending the fibers at this critical point.

Event 3: The nurse was readjusting the laser system for the next patient. During the verification of the energy, she heard an unusual noise. The nurse put the system in "standby" and sought assistance from her supervisor. When the supervisor took the system from a "standby" mode to a "ready" mode, she heard a loud "bang" and subsequently smelled smoke. Hospital personnel extinguished a small fire which had developed and was contained within the laser system. An internal high voltage arc ignited the component's supporting plastic material resulting in an internal fire. In order to prevent this from recurring in the future, a design change increasing high voltage clearances and changes in associated materials has been made.

Event 4: An incident occurred as a result of a laser assisted TRUP procedure. Fiber was utilized with another company's laser system. The physician had initiated the procedure and had lased 3 times for approx. 60 seconds each time when the laser nurse smelled smoke and reported her clothing was in flames. Approximately, 3" x 2 " hole in the clothing was created by the burn. No injuries occurred to the patient, surgeon or nurse. The company's engineers visually examined the fiber. The failure occurred in the center of the small connector, the proximal aperture was not damaged. Since all fibers are thoroughly tested prior to shipping and the hospital reported that this fiber worked initially, the company's conclusion is that the beam output from the laser system was not compatible with the other company's fiber. This resulted in an internal hot spot causing the fiber to fracture and fail. The fiber is not intended for use with lasers producing a beam divergence from the laser system's aperture greater than 17 degrees full angle.

Table 4. List of materials found in medical settings for laser accidents.

Source	Items
Patients	Hair, gastrointestinal gases (methane, hydrogen sulfide)
Prep Agents	Degreasers (ether, acetone) tinctures
Fabric Products	Towels, surgical drapes, dressing gowns, masks shoe covers, gauze sponges caps/hoods
Plastic products	Surgical drapes, gloves, tracheal tubes, fiber optic cables
Ointments	Petroleum-based jelly
Gases	anesthetic gases (oxygen, nitrous oxide, methane, hydrogen
Ignitable solvents	Laser dye solvents, oil coolants

11.6.3.2 Preventative Measures for Laser Fire Hazards

First, train the personnel to develop an awareness about fire hazards and response procedures in case of laser fires. The following points should be kept in mind in this regard.

- Make sure the hot tip of the laser does not touch combustible items.
- Maintain precise control of laser beam.
- Eliminate surfaces, which can reflect a laser beam.
- During surgery, the laser beam should be in the stand-by position at all times except when the handpiece is in the hand of the surgeon.
- Make sure that skin preparation solutions are fully vaporized before covering the area with surgical drapes.
- Follow standard procedures in the event of fire or explosion.

11.6.4   Compressed and Toxic Gases

Some lasers carry with them the risk of toxic gases; an example of this is the Excimer laser. Excimer lasers involve the use of noble and halogen gases, such as Fluorine, or Hydrogen Chloride. The manufactures of medical Excimer devices are actively striving to improve the safety of these types of lasers with internal scrubbers and sealed systems. Procedures for dealing with compressed and toxic gases should already be part of the protocol of most medical facilities, due to the routine use of compressed gas in medical settings.

11.7   PERSONS UNDER RISK

Any person in the immediate area of a laser used in a medical application, should have laser safety and training addressed for their protection. For the patient, as with any procedure information on what to expect will ease fears. For ancillary staff, they need to be included in laser safety training, either due to their proximately to the laser, or their entering and leaving the laser use area. The physician and OR nurses are, of course, in the direct line of fire. Service personnel, due to the nature of their work, are by passing safety devices and interlocks to check or repair units. The LSO needs to be knowledgeable in laser safety in order to provide guidance at all levels.

11.8   LASER SAFETY ELEMENTS

In the field of safety, engineering controls are always preferred to administrative controls. Someone has to remember to perform the administrative controls, while well-planned engineering controls will not let an activity take place unless the engineering control is active. Much of a medical laser safety program is administrative in nature, which emphasizes the need for training, audits and attention to detail. Below are the administrative elements of a Medical laser safety program.

- A written Laser Safety Policy/Program
- Posting of warning signs
- Designation of the authority and responsibility for the evaluation and control of laser hazards to a Medical Laser Safety Officer
- Management of incidents (near accidents) and accidents including reporting, investigation, analysis and remedial action

- Training and education of personnel involved in the use and maintenance of lasers
- Formation of a Medical Laser Safety Committee.
- The establishment of a Quality Assurance Program including regular inspection of the laser equipment.
- Presence of another person (buddy system) during maintenance work to provide first aid and to call for assistance in case of an injury or accident.

11.9   DUTIES OF A LASER SAFETY OFFICER

As defined by the ANSI Z136.3 Standard for Safe Use of Lasers in Health Care Facilities section 1.3.1 the "Laser Safety Officer (LSO) is an individual with the training and experience to administer a laser safety program. The LSO is authorized and is responsible for monitoring and overseeing the control of laser hazards. The LSO shall effect the knowledgeable evaluation and control of laser hazards by utilizing, when necessary, the most appropriate clinical and technical support staff and other resources." In simple words, the LSO is responsible to see that laser safety is maintained, but not required to do everything. Some of the duties of the LSO are

- Ensure all lasers are classified correctly.
- Perform a hazard evaluation of each use area.
- Develop and see that control measures are in place.
- Review and approve standard operating procedures, along with pre and post operation checklists.
- Ensure that proper personal protective equipment is selected, i.e. protective eyewear.
- Assure proper posting is in place and accurate.
- Be involved in facility design.
- See that all personnel involved in laser procedures receive laser safety training commensurate with their possible exposure.
- Follow up on medical surveillance.

Who serves as LSO? In the majority of hospitals the role of LSO is performed by a nurse. This presents a number of unique problems. It may be difficult for some physicians when it comes to taking instructions and directions form a nurse when issues arise. In smaller medical facilities the LSO maybe the physician.

The Medical Laser Safety Officer (MLSO) might find it beneficial to establish deputy laser safety officers. These individuals will be the ones to carry out the daily laser safety assignments. They might be called Laser Safety Liaisons, Laser Safety Supervisors, and Deputy LSOs. Whatever the name, the success of the laser safety program will hinge on the work of these individuals. Their authority, training and belief in the importance of laser safety will make the difference.

11.10 LASER SAFETY COMMITTEE

Depending on the number, type and diversity of procedures performed, a medical laser safety committee maybe needed. The membership should, as a minimum, include individuals from the different disciplines using lasers at the institution. The committee should include a representative of management, the Laser Safety Officer and a representative from the laser surgical nursing staff. Membership could also include a training person, Risk Management person, biomedical engineer, and other technical safety staff. The role of the Committee is to establish and maintain adequate polices and practices for the control of laser hazards, establish training requirements, acceptable credentialing of physicians for laser use, arbitrate disagreements concerning laser safety applications, play a role in accident investigations, and set medical surveillance requirements. The committee should also review pre and postoperative laser use checklists. The Committee can be invaluable in obtaining institutional compliance for laser safety since it is composed of the peers of the general laser user community. The issue of credentials and clinical privileges can be delegated to an existing standing committee or addressed by the medical laser safety committee. This issue is of great importance and will have an effect on the medical laser safety program.

11.11 LASER SAFETY TRAINING

Any medical or industrial employer has the responsibility for the safe use of lasers operated by the employee. Along with establishing the role of the laser safety officer, training is essential to achieving that goal. The level of training can vary with the potential of laser exposure. The majority of laser's used in medicine are of the hazard classification IIIB or class 4. These represent a potential eye and skin hazard. Therefore, training must be provided to staff that have exposure to this level of laser radiation. Training needs to include:
- An understanding of warning signs
- An understanding of engineering and administrative control measures
- Emergency actions to be taken

- Bio-effects of laser radiation
- Use and care of protective equipment
- Brief non-beam description
- Meaning of reflection types and causes

Depending on audience the following are additional or optional:

1. Medical Surveillance
2. Working knowledge of laser operation (How laser work)
3. Complete Non-beam hazards
4. Laser classification
5. Laser use procedures
6. Laser types and wavelengths
7. How to do hazard calculations, MPE, OD, NHZ

11.11.1 Laser Equipment Service Staff

A group that is often forgotten in regards to laser safety, but requires training is laser service personnel. Service can be performed by, in-house technical staff or third party contractor, this group should be trained to comply with laser safety guidelines. Emphasis should be placed on the practical techniques and procedures required during high-hazard periods when portions of the medical laser protective housing are removed for various purposes, such as the highly hazardous process of optical alignment. It is essential that service personnel be knowledgeable about all potential electrical hazards of the equipment. One reason is that when service is performed on your site it usually takes place in any clear area where the service person can find to work. In addition, this population must understand the hazards related to eye and skin exposure from direct and reflected laser beams and the possibility of fire hazards with the beam.

11.12 AUTHORITY FOR LASER PROCEDURES

The issue of who has authority to perform laser procedures and how this authority is granted varies from institution to institution. No set standard exists. Below is one format, which is not universally followed. In this example the authority arises from the Medical Laser Safety Committee and follows a very regimented approach.

Only personnel approved by the Laser Safety Officer or the Laser Safety Committee shall operate the laser. In a health care facility all OR and clinical personnel who are likely to be present during laser operation or maintenance are required to attend a training seminar that will describe the principles of operating lasers, their clinical applications, attendant risks to patient and staff, safety procedures, and care of the equipment. The facility shall certify or authorize individuals to perform laser procedures, designating laser type and delivery system and procedure(s) based on at least one of the following criteria:

- Documented completion of an approved formal laser training program offered by a recognized authority (e.g. by the relevant medical college), which includes didactic training and practical experience with lasers.
- Documented completion of a manufacturer's formal training program that includes a demonstration of clinical competence under the management of a previously certified laser operator.
- On-the-job or residency training and proven proficiency while assisting an experienced, certified laser operator. In this case, the certified operator or chairman of a hospital residency-training program shall provide a formal letter.
- Stating the number of hours dedicated to such training, equipment used, procedures undertaken, and the increasing levels of responsibility assigned to the physician-in-training and monitored by the certifying physician.
- In addition to the copies of certification or approval letters that the physician should retain, copies of such documents shall be filed with the Department of Surgery and, optionally, the hospital or facility administration.
- A physician should not be allowed to use a laser to perform any procedures other than those for which he has the hospital's approval without prior notification of an approval by the LSO and Chief of the appropriate service. In emergencies, such use of the laser may be unavoidable, but the physician must then notify the Laser Safety Committee in writing after such use, noting the circumstances that necessitated emergency use and the postoperative plan for the patient.

11.13   LASER SAFETY IN DIFFERENT SETTINGS

Not all medical laser safety programs will be the same. Programs will vary with the laser use situation, size of staff, number of units, number of procedures performed, type and variety of procedures performed. Any program established will have to be one that can be maintained. Setting up an elaborate program with no hope of being followed is harmful to obtaining safety and establishing a working safety culture. Medical laser use can be found in the single physician office, clinic, hospital, teaching hospital or large university setting.

Elements of a Laser Safety Program:
* Establishment of the position and authority of the Medical Laser Safety Officer
* Establish a Medical laser safety committee (optional)
* Define roles the of laser supervisors, OR staff and Physican as it effects laser safety
* Develop Policies & Procedures
* Training Requirements
* Authorization of Users
* Standard Operating Procedures for each Activity
* Inventory tracking
* Accident reporting
* Evaluate Hazards
* Develop controls of Hazards
* Decide on Medical Surveillance
* Audit compliance

11.14 LASER SAFETY DEVICES

11.14.1 Protective Eyewear

The purpose of laser protective eyewear is to either completely prevent any laser radiation from entering the eye or reduce any laser radiation entering the eye to a level below the maximum permissible exposure level (MPE). In brief, MPE is the maximum amount of laser energy for a given wavelength that can be tolerated by the eye without causing any injury. Any exposure above the MPE will create damage to the eye, how much will depend of how far above the MPE the exposure is and the length of exposure. The need for eye protection is not limited to one category of individuals. In any laser procedure where the level of laser radiation used is above the MPE for that wavelength the patients eyes should be covered. This is to prevent any accidental exposure to the eye causing damage or even the perception of injury.

For the patient, standard patient eye covers are either made of metal or plastic. Towels and wet gauze can be used (if gauze is used it needs to be monitored and kept damp during the procedure). Even laser protective goggles can be used. The goal is to protect the patients eyes from any stray laser reflections that may cause injury. So little effort is needed to protect the patient from injury that no valid reasons exists not to protect them.

Support staff such as Anestheologists, nurses and x-ray technicians should be wearing eyewear, even if the laser radiation is being transmitted by means of a fiber optic cable. This is to provide protection in case the fiber breaks or is taken out while still in an energized state, or once removed, is accidentally engerized.

The physician performing the procedure may elect not to wear eyewear if he believes the eyewear colors the perception of the patient's condition. This rationale does not hold up when the use of an infrared laser is involved.

11.14.1.1 Factors in Choosing Laser Protective Eyewear

Proper fit and viewing ease, no matter what level of protection laser protective eyewear may provide, if the eyewear does not fit well or provide a good field of view it will not be worn. Laser protective eyewear has evolved to the point that the selection of styles/frames is wide enough that a pair can be found for any face.

Optical Density (OD) is the base 10 log of the attenuation factor, which is the ratio of the laser beam input irradiance divided by the transmitted irradiance. Generally termed OD, the higher the OD the less is transmitted through the eyewear. OD for full protection eyewear will generally be in the 4-8 OD range, while OD for diffuse viewing will be in the 1-3 OD range. When using infrared wavelength (thus an invisible beam) full protection eyewear is recommended, when using visible beam. Diffuse viewing optical density (DVO) is usually the protection range of choice, remember, OD refers to the ability of a material to reduce laser energy of a specific wavelength to a safe level below the MPE. It can be expressed by the following formula:

$$OD = \log_{10}(E_i / E_t)$$

E_i = incident beam irradiance (W/cm^2) for a "worse case exposure"

E_t = transmitted beam irradiance (MPE limit in W/cm^2)

Example: OD of 4.0 allows 1/10,000 of the laser light energy to be transmitted. The required OD for any given laser can be determined by:
      (a) Calculation,
      (b) Consulting nomograms or tables (e.g., ANSI 136.1 guidelines), or
      (c) Consulting the laser manufacturer.

The OD of the protective eyewear will decrease if the eyewear is damaged. The damage threshold refers to the maximum protection that the protective eyewear will provide for at least 5 - 10 seconds following noticeable melting or flame. Any protective eyewear, in particular laser protective eyewear, should be routinely inspected for scratches or burn marks either before each wearing at least on a regular schedule.

All the laser protective eyewears are required to have printed on them the wavelength band and the optical density they provide protection for. Eyewear that is marketed for Europe will also have a code indicating the manufacturer and whether it is DVO (sometimes called alignment eyewear) or full protection. Laser protective eyewear that provides protection across the entire spectrum of UV-Visible-IR would be useless because no one could see through it. Therefore, laser protective eyewear provides protection over limited bands.

It is the role of the LSO to make sure that the proper eyewear is available for the laser wavelength being used. For lasers that travel from one OR setting to another, the eyewear should travel with the machine. The laser user is better served to learn to look at the eyewear to see the wavelength coverage that to relay on the color of the eyewear or a color coding system. OD refers to the ability of a material to reduce laser energy of a specific wavelength to a safe level below the MPE.

11.14.2 Barriers

Barriers can be opaque in nature or have some visual transmittance. Barriers need to be considered to cover OR windows, the temporary control area around equipment being serviced, or to prevent a laser beam from exiting the OR.

11.14.3 Guard Switches

Any switch, i.e. foot pedal that controls activation of the laser beam should be guarded to prevent accidental firing of the laser beam. If multiple switches are in use, care has to be taken to ensure the wrong switch is not pressed.

11.14.4 Posting

Proper posting should serve as a warning notice to all entering a laser use area. The most important information on a laser warning sign is the indication whether or not the laser is in use, and its wavelength. Armed with these two pieces of information, one can determine if the eyewear to be worn is correct for that laser. In addition, the required optical density for the laser protective eyewear can be listed on the warning sign. If the warning sign is an illuminated one, then one might also know if the laser is in a standby mode or firing. It is rare for medical laser use rooms to be equipped with interlocks for access control. Correct posting and education on the meaning of posting becomes increasingly important.

11.14.5 Smoke Evacuators

Surgical plumes are a genuine concern. To mitigate this concern, smoke evacuators where developed. With a vacuum action they suck the generated smoke into a biohazard filter. The filter should be designed to remove odors and small particulate material. The closer the end of the tube is to the source of the smoke the more efficient it will be. This is especially true in procedures where an assist gas is used, which could spread the plume. It is preferable to have a stand-alone unit rather than a wall vacuum unit. An important issue not to overlook is changing the filters. The manufacturer instructions on frequency of filter changes need to be followed. A record should be kept on how many times the filter has been used and for how long. As suction starts to decrease, the filter effectiveness becomes less. Any tubing that relates to the smoke evacuator must be handled as if it has become contaminated. Either bagged and disposed of properly or effectively cleaned. During use the smoke evacuator tube needs to be held as close as possible to the source of the plume.

The smoke evacuator contain elements such as vacuum pump, filter, hose and an inlet nozzle. While smoke evacuators are efficient in the suction of the smoke generated by the laser procedure, the air flow speed of the smoke evacuator depends on the rate of smoke generated. Activated charcoal beds are used to remove odors and certain organic vapors. High-efficiency particulate air (HEPA) filters or ultra-low penetration air (ULPA) filters are used to remove particulate matter in the smoke. Remember, the air suction ability of filters is significantly reduced when the filter has reached its capacity.

11.14.5.1 Dedicated Exhaust Systems

Local exhaust systems remove the laser plume before it reaches people. In order to be effective, the exhaust system should include the following features:

- In-line filters to prevent clogging of the exhaust tubes
- Exhaust air outside the building to prevent re-circulation
- Located on the roof-top at the end of the line in order to maintain a negative pressure in the duct-work to prevent leakage of contaminated exhaust air.

11.14.6 Operation Room (OR) Masks

To assist in protection from any smoke exposure or unevacuated laser plumes, high filtration masks need to be worn. High filtration masks with protection levels to 0.1 μm are recommended, 0.3 μm is the minimum. These masks should be worn during any nonendoscopic procedure that generates a laser plume.

11.14.7 Respiratory Protection

Respirators can be used to provide additional protection but not as a substitute for as air exhaust system. Surgical masks tend to protect the patient from "contamination" from medical staff, but do not protect the medical staff from inhaling viruses, germs, chemical vapors, tiny dust particles, or cellular debris. If engineering controls do not offer sufficient protection, then an alternative to surgical masks is to use a properly fitted "industrial" type respirator that is suitable protection against the airborne contaminants. The practical aspects and benefits of using such respirators should be carefully evaluated.

11.14.8 Protective Clothing

Protective clothing (gown, cap, and mask), gloves, and safety eyewear may be required for working near a laser. The potential for skin damage depends on the type of laser the power of the laser beam, and the duration of exposure. The type of damage may range from localized reddening to charring and deep incision. When dealing with laser radiation in the ultra violet spectrum, protective clothing is a must due to the delay sensation effect of UV exposure. The medical laser safety officer should determine the use of gowns for other wavelengths.

11.15 REFLECTIONS

Laser beams can reflect off a wide variety of surfaces in an operating room setting. This potential hazard needs to be evaluated. Look over the room. Can tools be made non-reflective? The options include covering them with towels, sponges, or by anodizing them to make the surface matted dull to reflections.

11.15.1 Preventing Back Flash

Reflections of laser radiation (i.e. Nd:YAG and Argon) back through a fiber optic endoscope or up the optics of an ocular eyepiece can be prevented or lessened by the use of attenuating filters. These types of reflections are not only possible but have been observed. Some ophthalmic equipment contains a mechanical shutter made to block the eyepiece when the laser pulse fires.

11.16 ALIGNMENT AIDS

Since many of the wavelengths used in medical applications are invisible, a visible alignment beam is used to aid the user. The alignment beam and service beam should be focused to the same point. It is common for laser surgical equipment to be stored outside of the laser surgery room, and concern must be given to units becoming out of alignment due to movement of the unit during transportation. Some units are brought to medical facilities from outside. Here again, transportation and alignment of the units in transit is important. Prior to any procedure this alignment must be checked. A common technique is to see the alignment beam over a tongue blade and confirm that the service beam cuts at the same point where the alignment beam is reaching.

11.17 LOW POWER LASER SAFETY

In procedures where a low power class IIIA visible laser is used, laser eyewear is not required. This does not mean one can or should allow unintentional eye exposure. Such a laser might be used as an alignment aid for an invisible beam, equipment alignment or photodynamic therapy. These visible laser beams are bright enough, if they fall upon ones retina, to startle one and or produce double vision for a period of time.

11.18 LASER SAFETY POLICIES AND PROCEDURES

11.18.1 Laser Safety Check-list for Laser Control Area

The checklist should give date, lase procedure/unit used and the name of the operator. Afterwards the following points be checked.
1. Warning signs in good condition and positioned properly
2. Light blocking shades in good condition, functioning, and properly positioned
3. Safety eyewear in good condition and properly labeled

4. Reflective surfaces reviewed
5. Water supply and filter system functioning
6. Electrical cords and connections in good condition
7. Fiber optic cables in good condition
8. Laser power meter functioning
9. Footswitch/fire button functioning
10. Safety interlock(s) switches functioning
11. Disconnect switches functioning
12. Re-evaluation of direct and indirect radiation within laser control area
13. Patient protective devices in good condition
14. Explanation of any negative answers

11.18.2 Charting Procedure

1. Complete date of procedure, time arrived/left and type of laser, model of unit.
2. Indicate procedure type, and start and finish times
3. Denote preoperative diagnosis, physician name, post-op diagnosis, and assistants name
4. Physician report shall be completed and signed by the physician
5. Attendants report will vary by laser types, should include:
    a) Record exposure number, spot size (microns) exposure time (seconds), power (watts or millijuoles) and location if laser applications and or lens used
    b) Nurses/attendants notes shall include
    c) Type of laser consent
    d) History of patient health, i.e. respiratory or cardiac disorders, medication allergies
    e) Statement of patient's mental status
    f) An indication of preoperative medications given
    g) Complication or problems associated with procedure
    h) Mode of discharge, ambulation or otherwise
    i) Documentation that patient received and post operation instructions

11.18.2 Pre-operative Check-list

This list can be separate from or made part of "Laser Safety Check-list prior to patient entering laser control area".
1. Clean laser unit
2. Obtain laser on key
3. Ask physician about positioning of patient and laser
4. Place proper laser warning sign on door & maybe windows

5. Obtain required laser accessories, i.e. microscope, hand-piece, broncho-scope, etc
6. Are extra sterile drapes available
7. Bring in smoke evacuator and check filters and related equipment
8. Have safety laser protective eyewear available,
9. Check if laser protective eyewear is correct for laser procedure Have sufficient eye wear present for anesthesiologist, and rest of team staff
10. Wet eye pads or other devices to protect patients eyes
11. Position and plug in all laser(s) and related equipment
12. Go through checks on laser device to ensure it is working properly. Will need to be developed for each type of laser equipment.

11.18.4 Intra-operative Check-list

1. When surgeon requests, turn laser unit on.
2. Select mode and power requested.
3. Do not leave laser unattended when in use.
4. Place laser on standby when not in use.
5. Check system controls, such a vacuum pressure, water pressure, gas tanks periodically during procedure.
6. Maintaining communications with the surgeon is of paramount importance during procedure.

11.18.5 Post-operative Procedure Check-list

1. Put in "Off" position.
2. Move laser unit away from patient area.
3. Place articulating arm in holder, or place fiber in tray.
4. Unplug laser unit.
5. Remove laser on key & store.
6. Collect protective eyewear.
7. Clean off laser unit and replace in storage area.
8. Remove laser warning sign(s).
9. Remove window barriers/shades.
10. Complete post op notes.

11.18.6 Laser Safety Check-list

Laser Room

Warning signs.

Window and door covers (non-transparent,
non-reflecting material).
Fire extinguishers.
Storage for gas tanks.
Secure locked designated place for the laser key.
Designated place for accessories.

Personal Protection

Documented personal protection program.
Training for use and maintenance of personal protective
equipment.

Laser Equipment

Electrical outlets.
Electrical power cords.
Cooling water pressure.
Cooling water temperature.
Maintenance up-to-date.
Laser log up-to-date

Smoke Evacuator

Filter change date record.
Responsibility for filter change assigned.
Valid safety sticker.

Laser Operation.

Documented authorization procedure.
Written operating procedures.
Emergency contact telephone numbers of persons
responsible for laser safety.

11.19   LASER INCIDENTS

Despite care and safety precautions, medical laser accidents do happen. A number of laser incidents that have happened can be searched from the FDA/CDRH available on the Medical Device Reporting (MDR) database webpages as referred to in the resource material given at the end of this chapter.

REFERENCES

1. Nezhat C, Winer W, Nezhat F et. al.: Smoke from Laser Surgery: Is there a hazard? "Lasers in Surgery and Medicine" 1987; 7: 376-382.
2. Fisher RW: Laser smoke in the operating room, "Biomedical Technology Today" 1987; 191-194.

3 Garden JM, O'Banion KM, Shelnitz LS et. al.: Papillomavirus in the vapor of carbon dioxide laser-treated verrucae,"Journal of American Medical Association," 1988 ;**259**: 1199-1202.

RESOURCE MATERIAL

The resource material, including web pages, used in this chapter will be of interest to the reader and is provided below.

1. Web Pages
CDRH Home page http://www.fda.gov/cdrh/index.html
Control of Smoke from Laser/Electric Surgical Procedures
http://www.cdc.gov/niosh/hc11.html?
MAUDE Database Accidents
http://www.accessdata.fda.gov/scripts/cdrh/ctdocs/cfMAUDE/Detail.CFM?MDRFOI_ID
=17985&CRIT=Excimer%20Laser
OSHA Laser Safety http://www.osha-slc.gov/SLTC/laserhazards/index.html
Medical Device Reporting search page
http://www.accessdata.fda.gov/scripts/cdrh/cfdocs/cfmdr/search.CFM

2. Books
A.R.Henderson, A Guide to Laser Safety, Chapman & Hall1997
K.A. Ball, Lasers The perioperative Challenge, 1995 Mosby Press
LIA Guide to Medical Laser Safety, LIA Press 1997
Guidelines for Laser Safety and Hazard Assessment. OSHA Instruction PUB 8
1.7(1991 August 5), 70 pages.

3. Standards
ANSI Z87.1-1989: Practice for Occupational and
Educational Eye and Face Protection.
ANSI Z136.1-2000 American National Standard for the Safe Use of Lasers.
ANSI Z136.3-1996: American National Standard for the Safe Use of Lasers in the
Health Care Environment.
ANSI/NFPA 70-1996: The National Electrical Code.
NFPA Code #115 Laser Safety

4. Valued Miscellaneous Sources
Boswell Eye Institute, Scottsdale Az.
Laser Safety in Surgery and Medicine, Rockwell Laser Industries
Massachusetts Institute of Technology Lincoln Laboratory
Duke University Medical Center

APPENDIX

(Glossary of Terms in Lasers and Devices)*

ABSORB: To transform radiant energy into a different form, with a resultant rise in temperature.

ABSORPTION: Transformation of radiant energy to a different form of energy by the interaction of matter, depending on temperature and wavelength.

ABSORPTION COEFFICIENT: Factor describing light's ability to be absorbed per unit of path length.

ACCESSIBLE EMISSION LEVEL: The magnitude of accessible laser (or collateral) radiation of a specific wavelength or emission duration at a particular point as measured by appropriate methods and devices. Also means radiation to which human access is possible in accordance with the definitions of the laser's hazard classification.

ACTIVE MEDIUM: Collection of atoms or molecules capable of undergoing stimulated emission at a given wavelength.

AIMING BEAM: A laser (or other light source) used as a guide light. Used co-axially with infrared or other invisible light may also be a reduced level of the actual laser used for surgery or for other   applications.

AMPLIFICATION: The growth of the radiation field in the laser resonator cavity. As the light wave bounces back and forth between the cavity mirrors, it is amplified by stimulated emission on each pass through the active medium.

APERTURE: An opening through which radiation can pass.

ARGON: A gas used as a laser medium. It emits blue/green light primarily at 448 and 515 nm.

ARTICULATED : CO_2 laser beam delivery device consisting of a series of hollow tubes and mirrors interconnected in such a manner as to maintain alignment of the laser beam along the path of the   arm.

ATTENUATION: The decrease in energy (or power) as a beam passes through an absorbing or scattering medium.

AVERAGE POWER: The total energy imparted during exposure divided by the exposure duration.

AVERSION RESPONSE: Movement of the eyelid or the head to avoid an exposure to a noxious stimulant, bright light. It can occur within 0.25 seconds, and it includes the blink reflex time.

AXIS, OPTICAL AXIS: The optical centerline for a lens system; the line passing through the centers of curvature of the optical surfaces of a lens.

BEAM: A collection of rays that may be parallel, convergent, or divergent.

BEAM DIAMETER: The distance between diametrically opposed points in the cross section of a circular beam where the intensity is reduced by a factor of e^{-1} (0.368) of the level (for safety standards).   The value is normally chosen at e^{-2} (0.135) of the peak level for manufacturing specifications.

BEAM DIVERGENCE: Angle of beam spread measured in radians more milliradians (1 milliradian = 3.4 minutes-of-arc or approximately 1 mil). For small angles where the cord is approximately equal to the arc, the beam divergence can be closely approximated by the ratio of the cord length (beam diameter) divided by the distance (range) from the laser aperture.

BLINK REFLEX: See aversion response.

---

*Prepared by Ken Barat, Lawrence Berkeley National Laboratory, Berkeley, U.S.A.

BRIGHTNESS: The visual sensation of the luminous intensity of a light source. The brightness of a laser beam is most closely associated with the radio-metric concept of radiance.

CARBON DIOXIDE: Molecule used as a laser medium. Emits far energy at 10,600 nm (10.6 μm).

CO_2 LASER: A widely used laser in which the primary lasing medium is carbon dioxide gas. The output wavelength is 10.6 μm (10600 nm) in the far infrared spectrum. It can be operated in either CW or pulsed.

COHERENCE: A term describing light as waves which are in phase in both time and space. monochromaticity and low divergence are two properties of coherent light.

CONTINUOUS WAVE(CW): Constant, steady-state delivery of laser power.

CONTROLLED AREA: An locale where the activity of those within are subject to control and supervision for the purpose of laser radiation hazard protection.

CRYSTAL: A solid with a regular array of atoms. Sapphire (Ruby Laser) and YAG (Nd:YAG laser) are two crystalline materials used as laser sources.

CW: Abbreviation for continuous wave; the continuous-emission mode of a laser as opposed to pulsed operation.

DIFFRACTION: Deviation of part of a beam, determined by the wave nature of radiation and occurring when the radiation passes the edge of an opaque obstacle.

DIFFUSE REFLECTION: Takes place when different parts of a beam incident on a surface are reflected over a wide range of angles in accordance with Lambert's Law. The intensity will fall-off as the inverse of the square of the distance away from the surface and also obey a Cosine Law of reflection.

DIVERGENCE: The increase in the diameter of the laser beam with distance from the exit aperture. The value gives the full angle at the point where the laser radiant exposure or irradiance is e^{-1} or e^{-2} of the maximum value, depending upon which criteria is used.

DUTY CYCLE: Ratio of total "on" duration to total exposure duration for a repetitively pulsed laser.

ELECTROMAGNETIC RADIATION: The propagation of varying electric and magnetic fields through space at the velocity of light.

ELECTROMAGNETIC SPECTRUM: The range of frequencies and wavelengths emitted by atomic systems. The total spectrum includes radiowaves as well as short cosmic rays. Wavelengths cover a range from 1 Hz to perhaps as high as 1020 Hz.

ELECTRON: Negatively charged particle of an atom.

EMBEDDED LASER: A laser with an assigned class number higher than the inherent capability of the laser system in which it is incorporated, where the systems lower classification is appropriate to the engineering features limiting accessible emission.

EMISSION: Act of giving off radiant energy by an atom or molecule.

ENCLOSED LASER DEVICE: Any laser or laser system located within an enclosure which does not permit hazardous optical radiation emission from the enclosure. The laser inside is termed an "embedded laser."

ENERGY: The product of power (watts) and duration (seconds). One watt second = one Joule.

ENERGY (Q): The capacity for doing work. Energy is commonly used to express the output from pulsed lasers and it is generally measured in Joules (J). The product of power (watts) and duration (seconds). One watt second = one Joule.

ENERGY SOURCE: High voltage electricity, radio-waves, flashes of light, or another laser used to excite the laser medium.

EXCIMER "EXCITED DIMER": A gas mixture used as the active medium in a family of lasers emitting ultraviolet light.

EXCITATION: Energizing a material into a state of population inversion.

EXCITED STATE: Atom with an electron in a higher energy level than it normally occupies.

EXEMPTED LASER PRODUCT: In the U.S., a laser device exempted by the U.S. Food and Drug Administration from all or some of the requirements of 21 CFR 1040.

FAILSAFE INTERLOCK: An interlock where the failure of a single mechanical or electrical component of the interlock will cause the system to go into, or remain in, a safe mode.

FEMTOSECONDS: 10(-15) seconds.

FIBEROPTICS: A system of flexible quartz or glass fibers with internal reflective surfaces that pass light through thousands of glancing (total internal) reflections.

FLASHLAMP: A tube typically filled with Krypton or Xenon. Produces a high intensity white light in short duration pulses.

FLUORESCENCE: The emission of light of a particular wavelength resulting from absorption of energy typically from light of shorter wavelengths.

FOCAL POINT: That distance from the focusing lens where the laser beam has the smallest diameter.

FOCUS: As a noun, the point where rays of light meet which have been reflected by a mirror or refracted by a lens, giving rise to an image of the source. As a verb, to adjust focal length for the clearest image and smallest spot size.

FREQUENCY: The number of light waves passing a fixed point in a given unit of time, or the number of complete vibrations in that period.

GAIN: Another term for amplification.

GAS LASER: A type of laser in which the laser action takes place in a gas medium.

GROUND STATE: Lowest energy level of an atom.

HELIUM-NEON (He-Ne) LASER: A laser in which the active medium is a mixture of helium and neon. Its wavelength is usually in the visible range. Used widely for alignment, recording, printing, and measuring.

HERTZ (Hz): Unit of frequency in the International System of Units (SI), abbreviated Hz; replaces cps for cycles per second.

INCIDENT LIGHT: A ray of light that falls on the surface of a lens or any other object. The "angle of incidence" is the angle made by the ray with a perpendicular to the surface.

INFRARED RADIATION (IR): Invisible Electromagnetic radiation with wavelengths which lie within the range of 0.70 to 1000 µm. These wave-lengths are often broken up into regions: IR-A (0.7-1.4 µm), IR-B (1.4-3.0 µm) and IR-C (3.0-1000 µm).

INTENSITY: The magnitude of radiant energy.

INTRABEAM VIEWING: The viewing condition whereby the eye is exposed to all or part of a direct laser beam or a specular reflection.

ION LASER: A type of laser employing a very high discharge current, passing down a small bore to ionize a noble gas such as argon or krypton.

IONIZING RADIATION: Radiation commonly associated with X-ray or other high energy electromagnetic radiation which will cause DNA damage with no direct, immediate thermal effect. Contrasts with non-ionizing radiation of lasers.

IRRADIANCE (E): Radiant flux (radiant power) per unit area incident upon a given surface. Units: Watts per square centimeter. (Sometimes referred to as power density, although not exactly correct).

IRRADIATION: Exposure to radiant energy, such as heat, X-rays, or light.

JOULE (J): A unit of energy (1 watt-second) used to describe the rate of energy delivery. It is equal to one watt-second or 0.239 calorie.

JOULE/cm^2: A unit of radiant exposure used in measuring the amount of energy incident upon a unit area..

KTP: Potassium Titanyl Phosphate. A crystal used to change the wavelength of a Nd:YAG laser from 1060 nm (infrared) to nm (green).

LASER: An acronym for light amplification by stimulated emission of radiation. A laser is a cavity, with mirrors at the ends, filled with material such as crystal, glass, liquid, gas or dye. A device which produces an intense beam of light with the unique properties of coherency, collimation and monochromaticity.

LASER DEVICE: Either a laser or a laser system.

LASER MEDIUM (Active Medium): Material used to emit the laser light and for which the laser is named.

LASER OSCILLATION: The buildup of the coherent wave between laser cavity end mirrors producing standing waves.

LASER PRODUCT: A legal term in the U.S. See 21 CFR 1040.10, a laser or laser system or any other product that incorporates or is intended to incorporate a laser or a laser system.

LASER ROD: A solid-state, rod-shaped lasing medium in which ion excitation is caused by a source of intense light, such as a flash-lamp. Various materials are used for the rod, the earliest of which was synthetic ruby crystal.

LASER SAFETY OFFICER (LSO): One who has authority to monitor and enforce measure to the control of laser hazards and effect the knowledgeable evaluation and control of laser hazards.

LASER SYSTEM: An assembly of electrical, mechanical and optical components which includes a laser. Under the Federal Standard, a laser in combination with its power supply (energy source).

LENS: A curved piece of optically transparent material which depending on its shape is used to either converge or diverge light.

LIGHT: The range of electromagnetic radiation frequencies detected by the eye, or the wavelength range from about 400 to 780 nanometers. The term is sometimes used loosely to include radiation beyond visible limits.

MAINTENANCE: Performance of those adjustments or procedures specified in user information provided by the manufacturer with the laser or laser system, which are to be performed by the user to ensure the intended performance of the product. It does not include operation or service as defined in this glossary.

MAXIMUM PERMISSIBLE EXPOSURE (MPE): The level of laser radiation to which person may be exposed without hazardous effect or adverse biological changes in the eye or skin.

METASTABLE STATE: The state of an atom, just below a higher excited state, which an electron occupies momentarily before destabilizing and emitting light. The upper of the two lasing levels.

MICROMETER: A unit of length in the International System of Units (SI) equal to one-millionth of a meter. Often referred to as a "micron".

MICRON: An abbreviated expression for micrometer which is the unit of length equal to 1 millionth of a meter. See MICROMETER.

MODE: A term used to describe how the power of a laser beam is geometrically distributed across the cross-section of the beam. Also used to describe the operating mode of a laser such as continuous or pulsed laser.

MODE LOCKED: A method of producing laser pulses in which short pulses (approximately 10-12 second) are produced and emitted in bursts or a continuous train.

MODULATION: The ability to superimpose an external signal on the output beam of the laser as a control.

MONOCHROMATIC LIGHT: Theoretically, light consisting of just one wavelength. No light is absolutely single frequency since it will have some bandwidth. Lasers provide the narrowest of bandwidths that can be achieved.

MULTIMODE: Laser emission at several closely-spaced frequencies.

NANOMETER (nm): A unit of length in the International System of Units (SI) equal to one-billionth of a meter. Abbreviated nm - a measure of length. One nm equals 10^{-9} meter, and is the usual measure of light wavelengths. Visible light ranges from about 400 nm in the purple to about 780 nm in the deep red.

NANOSECOND: One billionth (10^{-9}) of a second. Longer than a picosecond or femtosecond, but shorter than a micro-second. Associated with Q-switched lasers.

Nd:GLASS LASER: A solid-state laser of neodymium: glass offering high power in short pulses. A Nd doped glass rod used as a laser medium to produce 1064 nm light.

Nd:YAG LASER: Neodymium:Yttrium Aluminum Garnet. A synthetic crystal used as a laser medium to produce 1064 nm light.

NEODYMIUM (Nd): The rare earth element that is the active element in Nd:YAG laser and Nd:Glass lasers.

.NOMINAL HAZARD ZONE (NHZ): The nominal hazard zone describes the space within which the level of the direct, reflected or scattered radiation during normal operation exceeds the applicable MPE. Exposure levels beyond the boundary of the NHZ are below the appropriate MPE level.

OPEN INSTALLATION: Any location where lasers are used which will be open to operating personnel during laser operation and may or may not specifically restrict entry to observers.

OPERATION: The performance of the laser or laser system over the full range of its intended functions (normal operation). It does not include maintenance or services as defined in this glossary.

OPTICAL CAVITY (Resonator): Space between the laser mirrors where lasing action occurs.

OPTICAL DENSITY: A logarithmic expression for the attenuation produced by an attenuating medium, such as an eye protection filter.

OPTICAL FIBER: A filament of quartz or other optical material capable of transmitting light along its length by multiple internal reflection and emitting it at the end.

OPTICAL PUMPING: The excitation of the lasing medium by the application of light rather than electrical discharge.

OPTICAL RADIATION: Ultraviolet, visible and infrared radiation (0.35-1.4 μm) that falls in the region of transmittance of the human eye.

OPTICAL RESONATOR: See Resonator.

OPTICALLY PUMPED LASERS: A type of laser that derives energy from another light source such as a xenon or krypton flash-lamp or other laser source.

OUTPUT COUPLER: Partially reflective mirror in laser cavity which allows emission of laser light.

OUTPUT POWER: The energy per second measured in watts emitted from the laser in the form of coherent light.

PHASE: Waves are in phase with each other when all the troughs and peaks coincide and are "locked" together. The result is a reinforced wave in increased amplitude (brightness).

PHOTO-COAGULATION: Use of the laser beam to heat tissue below vaporization temperatures with the principal objective being to stop bleeding and coagulate tissue.

PHOTON: In quantum theory, the elemental unit of light, having both wave and particle behavior. It has motion, but no mass or charge. The photon energy (E) is proportional to the EM wave frequency (v) by the relationship: $E=hv$; where h is Planck's constant $(6.63 \times 10^{-34}$ Joule-sec).

PHOTO-SENSITIZERS: Chemical substances or medications which increase the sensitivity of the skin or eye to irradiation by optical radiation, usually to UV.

PIGMENT EPITHELIUM: A layer of cells at the back of the retina containing pigment granules.

POPULATION INVERSION: A state in which a substance has been energized, or excited, so that more atoms or molecules are in a higher excited state than in a lower resting state. This is necessary prerequisite for laser action.

POWER: The rate of energy delivery expressed in watts (joules per second). Thus: 1 Watt = 1 Joule x 1 Sec.

POWER METER: An accessory used to measure laser beam power.

PRF(Pulse Repetition Frequency): The number of pulses produced per second by a laser.

PROTECTIVE HOUSING: A protective housing is a device designed to prevent access to radiant power or energy.

PULSE: A discontinuous burst of laser, light or energy, as opposed to a continuous beam. A true pulse achieves higher peak powers than that attainable in a CW output.

PULSE DURATION: The "on" time of a pulsed laser, it may be measured in terms of milliseconds, microsecond, or nanosecond as defined by half-peak-power points on the leading and trailing edges of the pulse.

PULSE MODE: Operation of a laser when the beam is intermittently on in fractions of a second.

PULSED LASER: Laser which delivers energy in the form of a single or train of pulses.

PUMP: To excite the lasing medium. See Optical Pumping or Pumping.

PUMPING: Addition of energy (thermal, electrical, or optical) into the atomic population of the laser medium, necessary to produce a state of population inversion.

Q-SWITCH: A device that has the effect of a shutter to control the laser resonator's ability to oscillate. Control allows one to spoil the resonator's "Q-factor", keeping it low to prevent lasing action. When a high level of energy is stored, the laser can emit a very high-peak-power pulse.

Q-SWITCHED LASER: A laser which stores energy in the laser media to produce extremely short, extremely high intensity bursts of energy.

RADIANCE: Brightness; the radiant power per unit solid angle and per unit area of a radiating surface.

RADIANT ENERGY (Q): Energy in the form of electromagnetic waves usually expressed in units of Joules (watt-seconds).

RADIANT EXPOSURE (H): The total energy per unit area incident upon a given surface. It is used to express exposure to pulsed laser radiation in units of J/cm^2.

RADIANT INTENSITY: The radiant power expressed per unit solid angle about the direction of the light.

RADIATION: In the context of optics, electromagnetic energy is released; the process of releasing electromagnetic energy.

REFLECTANCE OR REFLECTIVITY: The ratio of the reflected radiant power to the incident radiant power.

REFLECTION: The return of radiant energy (incident light) by a surface, with no change in wavelength.

REFRACTION: The change of direction of propagation of any wave, such as an electromagnetic wave, when it passes from one medium to another in which the wave velocity is different. The bending of incident rays as they pass from one medium to another (eg.: air to glass).

REPETITIVELY PULSED LASER: A laser with multiple pulses of radiant energy occurring in sequence with a PRF greater than or equal to 1 Hz.

RESONATOR: The mirrors (or reflectors) making up the laser cavity including the laser rod or tube. The mirrors reflect light back and forth to build up amplification.

RUBY: The first laser type; a crystal of sapphire (aluminum oxide) containing trace amounts of chromium oxide.

SCANNING LASER: A laser having a time-varying direction, origin or pattern of propagation with respect to a stationary frame of reference.

SEMICONDUCTOR LASER: A type of laser which produces its output from semiconductor materials such as GaAs.

SERVICE: Performance of adjustments, repair or procedures on a non routine basis, required to return the equipment to its intended state.

SOURCE: The term source means either laser or laser-illuminated reflecting surface, i.e., source of light.

SPECTRAL RESPONSE: The response of a device or material to monochromatic light as a function of wavelength.

SPECULAR REFLECTION: A mirror-like reflection.

SPONTANEOUS EMISSION: Decay of an excited atom to a ground or resting state by the random emission of one photon. The decay is determined by the lifetime of the excited state.

SPOT SIZE: The mathematical measurement of the diameter of the laser beam.

STABILITY: The ability of a laser system to resist changes in its operating characteristics. Temperature, electrical, dimensional and power stability are included.

STIMULATED EMISSION: When an atom, ion or molecule capable of lasing is excited to a higher energy level by an electric charge or other means, it will spontaneously emit a photon as it decays to the normal ground state. If that photon passes near another atom of the same frequency, the second atom will be stimulated to emit a photon.

SUPER-PULSE: Electronic pulsing of the laser driving circuit to produce a pulsed output (250-1000 times per second), with peak powers per pulse higher than the maximum attainable in the continuous wave mode. Average powers of super-pulse are always lower than the maximum in continuous wave. Process often used on CO_2 surgical lasers.

TEM: Abbreviation for: Transverse Electro-Magnetic modes. Used to designate the cross-sectional shape of the beam. TEM_{00} The lowest order mode possible with a bell-shaped (Gaussian) distribution of light across the laser beam.

TRANSMISSION: Passage of electromagnetic radiation through a medium.

TRANSMITTANCE: The ratio of transmitted radiant energy to incident radiant energy, or the fraction of light that passes through a medium.

TUNABLE LASER: A laser system that can be "tuned" to emit laser light over a continuous range of wavelengths or frequencies.

ULTRAVIOLET (UV) RADIATION: Electromagnetic radiation with wave-lengths between soft X-rays and visible violet light, often broken down into UV-A (315-400 nm), UV-B (280-315 nm), and UV-C (100-280 nm).

VAPORIZATION: Conversion of a solid or liquid into a vapor.

VISIBLE RADIATION (LIGHT): Electromagnetic radiation which can be detected by the human eye. It is commonly used to describe the wavelengths that fall in the range between 400 nm and 700-780 nm.

WATT: A unit of power (equivalent to one Joule per second) used to express laser power.

$WATT/cm^2$: A unit of irradiance used in measuring the amount of power per area of absorbing surface, or per area of CW laser beam.

WAVE: An sinusoidal undulation or vibration; a form of movement by which all radiant electromagnetic energy travels.

WAVELENGTH: The length of the light wave, usually measured from crest to crest, which determines its color. Common units of measurement are the micrometer (micron), the nanometer, and (earlier) the Angstrom unit.

WINDOW: A piece of glass with plane parallel sides which admits light into or through an optical system and excludes dirt and moisture.

YAG (Yttrium Aluminum Garnet): A widely used solid-state crystal which is composed of yttrium and aluminum oxides which is doped with a small amount of the rare-earth neodymium.

Fundus structures
  optimal visibility, 70

G

Gallbladder, 26
Ganglion cells, 62
Gaussian beam
  circularly symmetric, 34
  irradiance, 33
  profile, 33
Gingiva (dentistry), 304
Glaucoma surgery, 77
Glossary
  laser terms and devices, 355-61
Glucose level monitoring, 83
Gradient-index lens, 175
Guard switches, 347
Gynaecology, 309-326
  adhesions, 311
  applications of lasers in, 310
  Asherman's syndrome, 319
  electrocautery, 322
  hysteroscopic procedures, 318
  isthmic area, 315
  LEEP, 320
  laparoscopy, 311
  photodynamic therapy, 321
  photoionizing agents, 321
  pre-implantation diagnosis, 322
  resectoscope, 319
  use of lasers in, 309, 310

H

Hair
  follicles, 274
  grafts, 284
  removal by lasers, 273, 74, 75
  transplantation, 284
Hazards
  analysis surgical fibre, 331
  during use of lasers, 327
Heart surgery
  by laser catheter (figure), 101
Heat source term, 46

Helium-neon laser, 17
Helmholtz equation, 150
Hemodialysis
  by CO_2 laser, 130
Hemodynamic investigation, 116
Hemoglobin, 32
Hemolized blood, 32
Hemostasis, 196. 197
Hepatitis
  laser therapy, 337
Hexascan, 278
Hirtutism, 276
Histological
  examination, 119
  findings of
    anastomosis, 130
    laser channel, 120
Histograms of human skin images,
    187
Holmium laser fiber (figure), 244
Holmium laser lithotripsy, 217, 246-
    48
Human eye
  characteristics, 59
  ionizing effects, 68
  laser penetration depth, 69
  laser-tissue interaction, 67
  photochemical effects, 68
  photocoagulation, 68
  photovaporization, 68
  Raman spectroscopy, 83
  refractive error, 66
  thermal effets, 68
  transmittance, 70
Human sclera, 182
Human tissue
  optical properties, 52
  thermal properties, 53
Human tooth
  exposure to laser (figure), 296
  exposure to picosecond pulse laser,
    298
  exposure to femtosecond pulse laser,
    299
Humor
  aqueous, 60